Common Infectious Diseases of the Central Nervous System:

Pathologies, Diagnostics, and Therapeutics

Tabish Qidwai
Shri Ramswaroop Memorial University, India

IGI Global
Scientific Publishing
Publishing Tomorrow's Research Today

Vice President of Editorial	Melissa Wagner
Director of Acquisitions	Mikaela Felty
Director of Book Development	Jocelynn Hessler
Production Manager	Mike Brehm
Cover Design	Jose Rosado

Published in the United States of America by
IGI Global Scientific Publishing
701 East Chocolate Avenue
Hershey, PA, 17033, USA
Tel: 717-533-8845 | Fax: 717-533-7115
Website: https://www.igi-global.com E-mail: cust@igi-global.com

Library of Congress Cataloging-in-Publication Data

Names: Qidwai, Tabish editor http://id.loc.gov/rwo/agents/n2022181963
Title: Common infectious diseases of the central nervous system : pathologies, diagnostics, and therapeutics / edited by Tabish Qidwai.
Description: Hershey, PA : IGI Global, [2026] | Includes bibliographical references and index. | Summary: "This book proposal is aimed to focus on common prevalent neurological infectious diseases and their pathology, biomarkers, diagnosis, and therapy of CNS disease"-- Provided by publisher.
Identifiers: LCCN 2024047946 (print) | LCCN 2024047947 (ebook) | ISBN 9798337301051 s/c | ISBN 9798369340707 h/c | ISBN 9798337301051 eISBN
Subjects: LCSH: Central nervous system--Infections http://id.loc.gov/authorities/subjects/sh2001008632 | Central nervous system--Infections--Diagnosis | Central nervous system--Infections--Treatment
Classification: LCC RC359.5 .C66 2025 (print) | LCC RC359.5 (ebook) | DDC 616.804194--dc23/eng/20250212
LC record available at https://lccn.loc.gov/2024047946
LC ebook record available at https://lccn.loc.gov/2024047947

British Cataloguing in Publication Data
A Cataloguing in Publication record for this book is available from the British Library.

Table of Contents

Detailed Table of Contents

Bilal El-Mansoury, Faculty of Sciences, Chouaib Doukkali University, Morocco
Hanane El Fatimi, Mohammed VI University of Health Sciences, Morocco
Ayyoub Skaou, Faculty of Science Semlalia, Cadi Ayyad University, Morocco
Soraia El-Baz, Faculty of Science Semlalia, Cadi Ayyad University, Morocco
El Mehdi Dalil, Faculty of Medicine and Pharmacy, Cadi Ayyad University, Morocco
Taoufik Adoch, Faculty of Medicine and Pharmacy, Cadi Ayyad University, Morocco
Nadia Zouhairi, Faculty of Sciences and Techniques, Beni Mellal, Morocco
Abdelaati El Khiat, Higher Institute of Nursing Professions and Health Techniques, Ministry of Health, Ouarzazate, Morocco
Jawad Laadraoui, Faculty of Science Aïn Chock, Hassan II University, Morocco

Acute bacterial meningitis is an inflammation of the meninges, the protective layers of the central nervous system (CNS) and the cerebrospinal fluid (CSF), secondary to bacterial infection. Symptoms of bacterial meningitis (BM) can be manifested by stiff neck, headache, fever, confusion or altered mental status, nausea, and vomiting. The pathogens responsible for bacterial meningitis vary according to several factors, including the patient's age and geographic location. The main germs responsible for bacterial meningitis are Neisseria meningitidis (meningococcus), Streptococcus pneumoniae (pneumococcus), and Haemophilus influenzae. The neurological complications of meningitis, such as hearing loss, hydrocephalus, increased intracranial pressure and brain damage are of particular concern. Early diagnosis, preventive strategies, and appropriate treatment are of great importance to prevent serious complications. This chapter provides an overview on the BM epidemiology, pathophysiology, diagnostic, and treatment as well as preventive strategies.

Neurosyphilis is a severe complication of syphilis that appears when the bacterium Treponema pallidum invades the central nervous system (CNS). The pathogenesis of this condition is complex, due to Treponema pallidum that infiltrates the CNS at any stage of infection, which leads to diverse neurological manifestations, ranging from asymptomatic forms to severe neuropsychiatric disorders. Moreover, the diagnosis remains challenging due to the variability of symptoms and typically requires a combination of serological tests and cerebrospinal fluid analysis for accurate confirmation. Penicillin remains the most effective treatment for neurosyphilis. This chapter will explore the importance of early intervention and ongoing research in improving both treatment outcomes and diagnostic accuracy.

The cause of tuberculosis (TB) is Mycobacterium tuberculosis. It remains a global health burden in developing and developed countries. TB meningitis (TBM) can occur when M. tuberculosis spreads to other organs, such as the brain and meninges, despite its primary role as a respiratory infection. The most serious type of tuberculosis is called tuberculous meningitis (TBM). One of the most severe clinical signs of tuberculosis (TB) is the involvement of the central nervous system (CNS), which occurs in 5–10% of extrapulmonary TB patients and makes up around 1% of all TB case. TBM has a significant death rate (20–50%) even when it is identified early and treated with the right antibiotics. Traditional techniques, like the culture of cerebrospinal fluid (CSF) and acid-fast bacilli (AFB) on smears, remain the gold standard for diagnosing TBM.

Central Nervous System (CNS) infections are caused by a variety of pathogens including bacteria, virus, fungi, protozoa, and parasites. Viral CNS infections can present as meningitis, encephalitis, or localized abscesses. Such infections are challenging to diagnose and the blood brain barrier in the human body guards the entry of the pathogens into CNS. The CNS is also shielded by neuroanatomical barriers which may be blood CSF barrier or the blood brain barrier and the fibroblasts from olfactory nerve. Our immune cells enhance these barriers by activating T cells with protective function. Once invasion occurs, the viruses interact with various cell populations of CNS and can induce pro-inflammatory immune response that leads to development of pathologies like viral meningitis and encephalitis. Children have immature immune defenses and blood–brain barrier; hence, they are more vulnerable to viral CNS infections compared to adults. Viruses like enteroviruses account for more than 50% of CNS infections amongst children. Infections, either mild or severe, severely impact the quality of life in developing children and chief cause of morbidities and mortality worldwide. This chapter aims to provide an overview on viral pathogens of nervous system, their pathogenesis, diagnosis, and treatment options available in the current scenario. The authors review various viral pathogens of CNS in children and describe their casual microbiological cause, clinical features, and provide an update on the classical and latest diagnostic approaches and treatment strategies available for them. Newly developed PCR-based methods that are efficiently capable of detecting and diagnosing the neurotropic viruses in almost all sample types are discussed. The chapter finds its importance in providing an overview for management approach of viral infections of the central nervous system in children from the point of clinical presentation, diagnosis, treatment, and complications.

Central nervous system (CNS) infections involve the brain, spinal cord, optic nerves, and their protective membranes. These infections are medical emergencies with high morbidity, mortality, and potential long-term complications that significantly affect quality of life. Parasitic infections are common in regions with poor sanitation but can also occur in non-endemic areas due to international travel and immunosuppression

light on the problems caused by bacterial, fungal, and viral pathogens as it examines the complex link between neurotransmitters and CNS diseases. The authors explore the complex processes by which these diseases modify the production, release, and reception of neurotransmitters, highlighting the significant consequences for the general health of the nervous system. This chapter also looks into non-pharmacological methods as workable ways to change neurotransmitter levels in CNS diseases. The knowledge offered here serves as a basis for upcoming investigations and the treatment plans are meant to maintain brain function even in the face of infections and other challenges.

The field of medical imaging has been revolutionized by intelligent systems, especially those powered by machine learning and artificial intelligence (AI). Among various applications, brain tumor detection and classification stand out due to their critical impact on patient health outcomes. Brain tumors—whether benign or malignant—are among the most serious neurological conditions and often require prompt and accurate diagnosis. Traditionally, identifying brain tumors through imaging has been a manual and expertise-driven process, but with the integration of AI, especially deep learning, the accuracy and speed of diagnosis have improved significantly. This overview explores how machine learning contributes to brain tumor analysis, from the collection and pre-processing of MRI data to model training and classification. Key challenges such as data quality, model explainability, and tumor variability are also addressed, alongside modern advancements in deep learning models that continue to evolve in precision and clinical applicability.

Preface

Central nervous system (CNS) infections represent a critical and escalating global health challenge, characterized by their complexity, high morbidity, and significant mortality rates. These infections, caused by a diverse array of pathogens including bacteria, viruses, fungi, and parasites, pose unique diagnostic and therapeutic difficulties due to the protective barriers of the CNS and the emergence of drug-resistant strains. This book aims to provide a comprehensive exploration of CNS infections, addressing their epidemiology, pathogenesis, clinical manifestations, diagnostic advancements, and therapeutic strategies. By bringing together cutting-edge research and clinical insights, it seeks to equip researchers, healthcare professionals, and policymakers with the knowledge needed to confront this growing public health crisis.

The chapters collectively offer a multidisciplinary perspective, delving into the molecular mechanisms, diagnostic innovations, and emerging treatment modalities for CNS infections. They highlight the importance of timely diagnosis, the role of biomarkers, and the potential of novel therapeutic approaches, such as nanotechnology and non-pharmacological interventions. Additionally, the book examines specific CNS infections, including bacterial meningitis, tubercular meningitis, neurosyphilis, and viral infections in children, while exploring advanced diagnostic tools like machine learning for brain tumor segmentation and the role of neurotransmitters in infection-related neurological damage.

CHAPTER OVERVIEW

- The first chapter examines the global burden of CNS infections, emphasizing their public health implications, epidemiology, and the need for enhanced surveillance and preventive measures.
- The second chapter provides an in-depth analysis of acute bacterial meningitis, covering its epidemiology, pathophysiology, diagnostic approaches, and treatment strategies.

- The third chapter investigates neurosyphilis, discussing its complex pathogenesis, diagnostic difficulties, and the critical role of penicillin-based treatments.
- The fourth chapter explores tubercular meningitis, detailing its pathogenesis, diagnostic challenges, and therapeutic options, with a focus on its significant global impact.
- The fifth chapter focuses on viral CNS infections in children, outlining their clinical presentations, diagnostic approaches, and available treatment modalities.
- The sixth chapter addresses parasitic and fungal CNS infections, highlighting their prevalence, diagnostic methods, treatment challenges, and future research prospects.
- The seventh chapter reviews current trends in biomarkers for diagnosing neurological infectious diseases, focusing on their potential to assess disease severity and guide treatment.
- The eighth chapter explores the role of neurotransmitters in CNS infections and discusses non-pharmacological approaches to modulate their functions for improved outcomes.
- The ninth chapter introduces a novel machine learning approach for automated segmentation of brain tumor MRI images, emphasizing its potential to enhance diagnostic precision.
- The tenth chapter looks to the future, discussing innovative therapeutic approaches, such as nanotechnology and targeted drug delivery, to address the challenges posed by CNS infections.

This book serves as a vital resource for understanding the multifaceted nature of CNS infections and fostering collaborative efforts to mitigate their impact on global health.

Chapter 1
Unveiling the Burden: CNS Infections as a Growing Public Health Crisis

Bhat Ummar Nabi
https://orcid.org/0009-0007-7918-3717
Bhai Gurdas Institute of Allied Sciences, India

Swati Priyadarshi
Bhai Gurdas Institute of Engineering and Technology, India

Noopur Khare
Bhai Gurdas Institute of Engineering and Technology, India

ABSTRACT

Infections of the central nervous system (CNS) are a serious and growing public health concern that calls for immediate attention and all-encompassing approaches. This chapter explores the many facets of this emerging issue, providing insights into its epidemiology, clinical symptoms, difficulties in diagnosis, and treatment options. CNS infections are becoming more commonplace worldwide and can be caused by a variety of pathogens, including bacteria, viruses, fungi, and parasites. The advent of drug-resistant bacteria exacerbates treatment paradigms and raises rates of morbidity and mortality. A coordinated effort involving improved surveillance systems, prompt diagnosis using cutting-edge molecular tools, and the creation of innovative therapies that target resistant infections is required to address this epidemic. Additionally, public health awareness initiatives play a critical role in encouraging preventive actions and lessening the toll that CNS infections take on society and healthcare systems.

DOI: 10.4018/979-8-3693-4070-7.ch001

1. INTRODUCTION

Infections of the central nervous system (CNS) pose a serious threat to public health worldwide because of the intricate interactions between pathogens, clinical manifestations, diagnostic challenges, and treatment options. This introduction delves into the complex terrain of CNS infections, clarifying how they have become an increasingly significant issue with far-reaching consequences for global healthcare systems. CNS infection rates have significantly increased in recent years, which is indicative of both the changing epidemiological environment and our growing awareness of these illnesses. These infections are caused by a wide range of etiological agents, such as fungi, viruses, bacteria, and parasites, each of which has distinct clinical traits and therapeutic difficulties. Interestingly, CNS diseases are worldwide in nature, impacting people in a variety of geographic locations rather than being exclusive to just one (Ngarka et al., 2022). Beyond only causing personal illness and death, CNS infections have a major negative socioeconomic impact on entire communities as well as healthcare systems. The identification and treatment of central nervous system infections continue to be difficult procedures despite advancements in medical technology and treatment approaches. Delays in starting therapy and less than ideal patient outcomes are caused by difficulties in precisely identifying the causal infections, especially in environments with limited resources. Additionally, the rise in antibiotic resistance makes treatment plans even more complex, calling for a paradigm change in favour of precision medical techniques. It is critically necessary to increase efforts to combat CNS infections on a local and global level in light of these complex issues (Milburn et al., 2024). This means funding in research projects targeted at creating novel treatment approaches and diagnostic tools, encouraging multidisciplinary collaboration amongst physicians, microbiologists, and public health specialists, and improving surveillance systems to track illness patterns. Moreover, public health education programmes play a critical role in promoting preventative actions in communities and increasing public knowledge of the risk factors linked to CNS diseases. This introduction lays the groundwork for a thorough examination of this crucial healthcare issue by clarifying the subtleties of CNS infections and the diverse approaches needed to address this growing public health emergency (Budreviciute et al., 2020).

Figure 1. Diagram depicting the anatomy of the Central Nervous System (CNS). (Adapted from Gutierrez & Emmanuel, 2018).

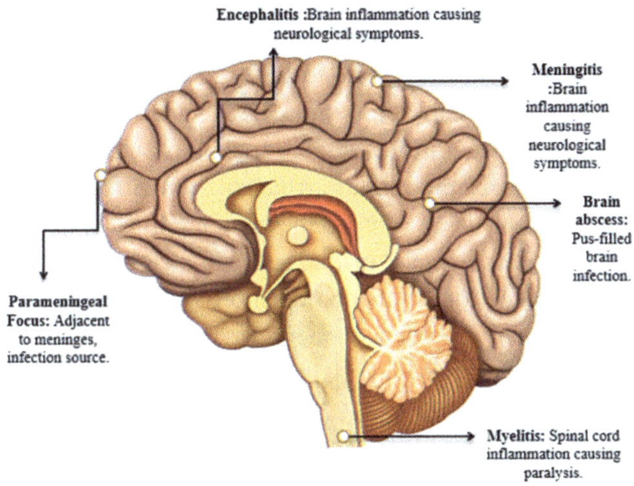

2. UNDERSTANDING CNS INFECTIONS

2.1 Etiology and Pathogenesis

The pathophysiology and etiology of CNS infections highlight the intricacy of public health emergency. Numerous pathogens, including as bacteria, viruses, fungi, and parasites, can enter the central nervous system in a number of ways, including through the cribriform plate, direct extension from nearby structures, and hematogenous spread (Rizzo et al., 2021). Once within the central nervous system, these pathogens set off inflammatory reactions that destroy neurons and compromise the blood-brain barrier. While bacteria like Neisseria meningitidis can cause meningitis by colonising the nasopharynx and then invading the meninges, viruses like the West Nile virus and herpes simplex virus can directly infect neurons and cause encephalitis. Toxins or immune-mediated harm are additional ways that some infections might exacerbate neurological dysfunction. Comprehending the complex interactions between infections and the host immune response is essential for creating diagnostic and therapeutic strategies that effectively address this rapidly growing public health emergency (Singh et al., 2024).

2.1.1 Infectious Agents (Viruses, Bacteria, Fungi, Parasites)

Comprising a wide range of infectious organisms, such as bacteria, fungi, viruses, and parasites, CNS illnesses provide distinct obstacles to public health. A large percentage of CNS infections are caused by viruses; prominent culprits include the varicella-zoster virus, the herpes simplex virus, and enteroviruses, which can cause encephalitis and meningitis (Le Govic et al., 2022). Bacterial infections such as Neisseria meningitidis, Haemophilus influenzae, and Streptococcus pneumoniae continue to pose a serious threat, especially when it comes to bacterial meningitis, which can quickly worsen and result in fatal consequences. Even though they are less frequent, fungal CNS infections are becoming more well acknowledged. Species like Aspergillus fumigatus and Cryptococcus neoformans can cause meningitis and brain abscesses, particularly in those with impaired immune systems (Nathan et al., 2021).

2.1.2 Routes of Transmission

There are many different ways that CNS diseases can spread, and they frequently rely on the particular infectious agent at play. Viral infections, such enteroviruses and herpes simplex virus, are typically spread by direct contact with saliva, respiratory secretions, or contaminated surfaces. Similar to this, close contact with infected individuals or respiratory droplets can spread bacterial diseases like Streptococcus pneumoniae and Neisseria meningitides (Sivapathasundharam, et al., 2020). Certain pathogens can be breathed from environmental sources including dirt or bird droppings, such as Cryptococcus neoformans. Furthermore, consuming tainted food or drink or coming into contact with contaminated cat excrement can spread some parasites, such as Toxoplasma gondii. Implementing effective preventative measures, such as immunisation, hygiene habits, and vector control, is essential to reducing the development of CNS illnesses and the corresponding public health burden. This involves understanding and disrupting the many channels of transmission (Srivastava et al., 2022).

Figure 2. Transmission routes of CNS disease.

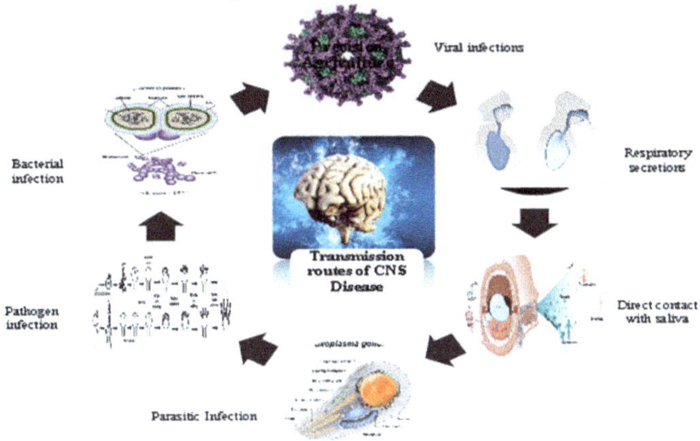

2.1.3 Host Factors

The susceptibility, severity, and outcome of CNS infections are significantly influenced by host variables, which further complicate this public health issue. One important factor is immune status. People who are immunocompromised due to HIV/AIDS, chemotherapy, or immunosuppressive treatments are more vulnerable to opportunistic infections like progressive multifocal leukoencephalopathy or cryptococcal meningitis (Littera et al., 2020). Age is another important determinant. Because of their underdeveloped or diminishing immune systems, babies and the elderly are frequently more susceptible to serious CNS infections. Chronic respiratory disorders or diabetes, for example, might weaken the host's defence mechanisms, making a person more vulnerable to certain infections. Additionally, vulnerability to particular infections or the intensity of the host immune response may be influenced by genetic variables (Tsafaras et al., 2020).

2.2 Clinical Manifestations

CNS infections can present with a wide range of clinical signs, from mild neurological disorders to potentially fatal consequences. Patients frequently arrive with fever, headaches, changed mental status, and stiff necks, which are indicators of meningeal irritation (Guadarrama-Ortiz et al., 2020). Additional neurological signs and symptoms, including as seizures, focal impairments, altered consciousness, and behavioural disturbances, may appear depending on the particular infectious agent implicated. While disorientation, hallucinations, and focal neurological impairments are common symptoms of viral encephalitis, severe headache, photophobia, and altered sensorium are frequently the first signs of bacterial meningitis. Fungal infections can cause subacute or progressive neurological deterioration in addition to chronic, indolent manifestations. Serious cases of CNS infections may cause paralysis, seizures, coma, or even death (Kozyolkin et al., 2023).

2.2.1 Common Symptoms

Depending on the precise infectious agent and the part of the central nervous system that is impacted, common symptoms of CNS infections can range across a spectrum of neurological and systemic manifestations. A common trademark symptom that can range from little discomfort to severe and incapacitating is fever, which is frequently accompanied by headaches. Indicators of meningeal irritation, such as photophobia, nausea, and vomiting, can also be experienced by patients (Li et al., 2020). It is common to witness altered mental status, which can lead to coma in extreme circumstances and includes confusion, disorientation, and impaired consciousness. The location and severity of the infection can also lead to focal neurological problems, such as weakness, abnormalities of the cranial nerve, or difficulties in sensory perception. Particularly in cases of viral encephalitis, seizures, both localised and generalised, can be a prominent symptom. It is essential to identify these typical symptoms in order to initiate appropriate therapy promptly, avoid complications, and enhance patient outcomes (Chaudhuri et al., 2022).

2.2.2 Variability in Presentation

It is remarkable how different CNS diseases can appear, as this is a reflection of the wide range of microorganisms that can cause them, the particular anatomical structures that they can damage, and the immune system of the host. The wide range of symptoms might make diagnosis difficult because they can be mild and vague or severe and progress quickly. Certain infections can primarily exhibit as neurological abnormalities, such as altered mental state, seizures, or localised neurological findings suggestive of encephalitis or brain abscess (Taha et al., 2020). While certain infections can show conventional symptoms like fever, headache, and stiff neck indicative of meningitis, others may not. Furthermore, the clinical course can differ greatly; some infections have an abrupt beginning and rapidly worsen, while others may progress more slowly or chronically, resembling other systemic or neurological disorders. Additionally, variables like age, immunological status, underlying medical disorders, and previous use of antibiotics or antivirals may have an impact on the presentation. Clinicians must be aware of the wide range of presentation types and keep an eye out for unusual characteristics in order to guarantee prompt diagnosis and effective treatment of CNS infections (Muschol et al., 2022).

2.3 Diagnosis and Laboratory Techniques

A combination of laboratory tests, neuro-imaging studies, and clinical assessment is crucial in the diagnosis of CNS infections. In order to identify specific signs and symptoms suggestive of CNS infection, an extensive neurological examination and a full medical history are usually part of the initial evaluation process (Surianarayanan et al., 2023). Serological testing, viral cultures, and molecular assays on blood, urine, or other body fluids may also be used in addition to CSF analysis to help in the diagnosing process. The use of neuroimaging investigations, such as magnetic resonance imaging (MRI) and computed tomography (CT), is crucial for determining the degree of central nervous system involvement, identifying consequences such hydrocephalus or abscess formation, and directing treatment approaches. In general, a multidisciplinary strategy that incorporates data from radiographic, laboratory, and clinical settings is essential for precise diagnosis of CNS infections and prompt commencement of suitable treatment (Li, et al., 2020).

2.3.1 Imaging Modalities

The diagnosis and treatment of CNS infections are greatly aided by advanced imaging modalities, which provide precise anatomical and pathological data essential for prognosis and therapy planning. The mainstay of neuroimaging is magnetic resonance imaging (MRI), which offers excellent soft tissue contrast and multiplanar imaging capabilities (Shahzad et al., 2020). MRI sequences such as T1-weighted, T2-weighted, fluid-attenuated inversion recovery (FLAIR), and diffusion-weighted imaging (DWI) can show characteristic findings such as inflammation-indicating leptomeningeal enhancement, meningeal enhancement, parenchymal abnormalities, and abscess formation in cases of suspected CNS infection. Furthermore, sophisticated MRI methods like perfusion-weighted imaging (PWI) and magnetic resonance spectroscopy (MRS) provide information about alterations in brain perfusion and metabolism, which helps distinguish viral lesions from inflammatory or malignant processes (Rahman et al., 2023).

2.3.2 Laboratory Tests

Laboratory testing is essential for the diagnosis and treatment of CNS infections because they provide important information about the underlying pathogen and help determine the best course of treatment. A crucial component of the diagnostic workup is the study of cerebrospinal fluid (CSF), which yields vital information about factors like cell count, protein, glucose levels, and microbiological studies (Czarniak,et al., 2023). Microbiological methods such as polymerase chain reaction

(PCR) assays, Gramme staining, and culture allow the identification of bacteria, viruses, fungi, and parasites in CSF samples. Diagnosis may also be aided by molecular assays, viral cultures, and serological testing on bodily fluids such as blood or urine. Furthermore, imaging methods like computed tomography (CT) and magnetic resonance imaging (MRI) provide further data regarding the degree of central nervous system involvement, the existence of problems, and direct targeted(Martín-Noguerol et al.,2019).

2.3.3 Challenges in Diagnosis

Due to the intricate nature of the central nervous system, the wide range of possible pathogens, and the variation in clinical manifestations, diagnosing CNS infections is fraught with difficulties. The ability to differentiate between infectious and non-infectious causes of neurological symptoms is a major challenge because symptoms like fever, headaches, and altered mental state can coexist with other neurological or systemic diseases (Zinserling et al., 2022). Further complicating diagnostic attempts is the fact that lumbar puncture, which is the method used to obtain cerebrospinal fluid (CSF) for investigation, contains inherent hazards and may not be appropriate in some clinical settings. Furthermore, because CNS infections can develop and spread quickly, it may be necessary to begin empiric treatment right away before final diagnostic results are obtained. This could cause delays in the proper course of care or needless exposure to antimicrobial drugs. Another major issue is the emergence of antimicrobial resistance, since certain infections have unusual susceptibility patterns or contain resistance mechanisms that require customised antibiotic regimens based on microbiological results (Abushaheen et al., 2020).

3. EPIDEMIOLOGY OF CNS INFECTIONS

The wide range of pathogens and risk factors that contribute to the occurrence and spread of CNS diseases is encompassed by the epidemiology of these infections. Neurological infections are a major global public health concern that impact people of all ages and socioeconomic backgrounds. Among the most common CNS infections are bacterial meningitis, viral encephalitis, and fungal meningitis; these infections vary in prevalence and distribution across different regions of the world (Ding et al., 2022). The epidemiology of CNS infections is influenced by variables like geography, socioeconomic position, vaccination coverage, and the existence of underlying medical disorders. Furthermore, efforts to monitor and control disease are continuously hampered by newly emerging infections, antibiotic resistance, and shifting travel and migration patterns. To mitigate the burden of CNS infections on global health, optimize healthcare resources, and implement focused preventative initiatives, it is imperative to comprehend the epidemiological trends and drivers of these illnesses (Owolabi, et al., 2023).

Table 1. Pathogens that commonly cause meningitis Adapted from (Riddell IV & Shuman, 2012).

Pathogen that can cause meningitis	Risk Factor	Incidence
Parasites		
Strongyloides stercoralis	Regional exposure, immune compromise	Rare
Naegleria fowleri	Warm fresh water	Very rare
Bacterial/mycobacterial pathogens		
Streptococcus pneumoniae	Day care, HIV infection	Most common
Listeria monocytogenes	Immune compromise, elderly	Less common
Viral pathogens		
Enteroviruses	Warm weather	Most common
Herpes simplex virus	Presence of latent virus	common
Fungal organisms		
Cryptococcus neoformans	Immune compromise, older age	Most Common
Candida spp	Systemic infection	Rare

3.1 Global Burden

The prevalence of CNS infections around the world is a complex public health issue that has a big impact on global morbidity, mortality, and the use of healthcare resources. Brain infections comprise a range of illnesses brought on by different pathogens, such as bacteria, viruses, fungi, and parasites, and they can impact people of different ages and backgrounds (Salam et al., 2023). CNS infections continue to be a major cause of neurological impairment and mortality despite advances in medical research, especially in areas with limited resources where access to treatment and preventive measures is restricted. In addition, the dynamic character of the worldwide burden of CNS infections is influenced by new pathogens, antibiotic resistance, and shifting migration and travel patterns. Comprehending the extent and dispersion of CNS infections globally is crucial for shaping public health policies, distributing resources efficiently, and executing focused interventions aimed at diminishing the impact of these illnesses and enhancing global health outcomes (Yadav et al., 2023).

3.1.1 Incidence and Prevalence

The incidence and prevalence of CNS diseases exhibit considerable regional and population-level variation, which can be attributed to the intricate interaction of various factors including geographic location, socioeconomic position, immunisation coverage, and healthcare accessibility. For example, bacterial meningitis is more common in low- and middle-income nations, especially in children under five, while viral encephalitis can be more common in temperate regions with seasonal outbreaks. The frequency of fungal meningitis, which is frequently linked to immunocompromised people, varies according to the presence of risk factors such organ transplantation or HIV/AIDS (Kanungo et al., 2023). New pathogens, patterns of antibiotic resistance, and shifting demographic trends all have an impact on the frequency of CNS infections. Precise surveillance data are necessary to guide preventive initiatives to lessen the worldwide burden of these diseases, to understand the epidemiology of CNS infections, and to improve public health policies (Feigin et al., 2020).

3.1.2 Geographical Distribution

There is significant heterogeneity in the geographical distribution of CNS infections, which can be attributed to various factors like climate, environmental circumstances, and healthcare infrastructure. For example, bacterial meningitis has a greater frequency in the "meningitis belt" of sub-Saharan Africa, which is recognised for being hyperendemic because of pathogen transmission-promoting climate conditions, overcrowding, and poor access to healthcare (Weaver, et al., 2022). It's possible that viral encephalitis is more widely distributed than thought. For example, the Japanese encephalitis virus is more common in Asia, while the West Nile virus is present in areas ranging from Africa to North America. Certain regions of Southeast Asia and sub-Saharan Africa may have higher incidence rates of fungal meningitis, which is frequently linked to environmental exposure to organisms such as Cryptococcus neoformans. Comprehending the spatial arrangement of CNS illnesses is pivotal in the allocation of resources, execution of focused therapies, and resolution of inequalities in healthcare accessibility and consequences among diverse areas (Almubaslat et al., 2023).

3.2 Risk Factors

Immunocompromised states (HIV/AIDS, organ transplantation), extremes of age (infants, elderly), close contact with sick people, low vaccination rates, and environmental variables (overcrowding, inadequate sanitation) are risk factors for

CNS infections. Differentiating susceptibility and outcomes are also influenced by new infections, healthcare availability, and geographic location. Prevention requires early identification and mitigation of these dangers (Kaslow et al., 2022).

3.2.1 Age

The susceptibility and clinical manifestation of CNS infections are strongly influenced by age. Due to their developing immune systems, infants and young children are more vulnerable and typically exhibit vague symptoms like fever and irritability (Littera, et al., 2020). On the other hand, deteriorating immune function and underlying medical conditions make older people more vulnerable to more severe symptoms, such as focal neurological impairments and disturbed mental status. Teens and young adults may be more vulnerable to specific diseases as a result of high-risk lifestyle choices like travelling. Comprehending age-related vulnerabilities is essential for developing customised preventative measures and enhancing therapeutic management to lessen the effects of CNS illnesses in people of all ages (Kesidou et al., 2023).

3.2.2 Immune Status

The ability to fight against infections is crucial for both the likelihood and severity of CNS illnesses. People with impaired immune systems, such as those suffering from HIV/AIDS, chemotherapy, or immunosuppressive treatments, are more vulnerable to opportunistic infections such progressive multifocal leukoencephalopathy or cryptococcal meningitis (Balaji et al., 2024). CNS infections may advance quickly or present atypically in these populations, resulting in severe morbidity and mortality. On the other hand, those with healthy immune systems could react strongly to infections, reducing the intensity and length of the illness. Even yet, in immunocompetent people, some viral infections, such the herpes simplex virus, can result in grave central nervous system consequences. Comprehending the subtleties of immune state is crucial for risk assessment, timely identification, and suitable handling of central nervous system infections, especially in susceptible groups where immunological dysregulation could lead to more severe disease consequences (Kakooza-Mwesige et al., 2019).

3.2.3 Socioeconomic Factors

The prevalence and consequences of CNS infections are significantly influenced by socioeconomic conditions. Marginalised people are disproportionately affected by limited access to healthcare services, including diagnostic facilities and treatment alternatives, which can result in delayed diagnosis and subpar management. Increased transmission rates are a result of inadequate sanitation, congested housing, and a lack of hygiene education, especially in underdeveloped rural areas or densely populated urban areas. Socioeconomic differences have an effect on vaccination rates as well. Those with lower incomes frequently encounter obstacles to vaccination, which makes them more vulnerable to avoidable CNS illnesses (Barach et al., 2020). Moreover, socioeconomic position has an impact on general health and nutrition, which can then have an impact on immune system performance and susceptibility to infectious pathogens. It is imperative to tackle socioeconomic disparities by means of enhanced healthcare accessibility, public health initiatives, and social welfare schemes to mitigate the incidence of central nervous system infections and foster health parity among heterogeneous communities (Gotlieb et al., 2023).

3.3 Emerging Trends

Emerging trends in CNS infections, which are influenced by things like globalisation, antibiotic resistance, and technological advancements in medicine, signify dynamic changes in the epidemiology, diagnosis, and treatment of these illnesses. Novel infections have surfaced recently, posing a challenge to established paradigms for diagnosis and treatment. The geographic distribution and seasonality of CNS infections may also shift due to changing environmental factors as urbanisation and climate change (Yadav et al., 2023). Additionally, new developments in diagnostic methods like next-generation sequencing and molecular tests provide never-before-seen insights into the genetic diversity and evolution of infectious pathogens. The growing issue of antibiotic resistance calls for creative strategies to effectively combat resistant bacteria. Furthermore, there is a new frontier in our understanding of disease etiology as the role of the microbiome in modifying host susceptibility to CNS diseases becomes increasingly apparent. In order to successfully address the changing problems of CNS infections, future research agendas and public health policies must take into account these rising tendencies (Fisher, et al., 2022).

3.3.1 Changes in Incidence Rates

Variations in the incidence rates of CNS infections are indicative of changing epidemiological dynamics that are impacted by antimicrobial resistance, vaccination campaigns, and demographic changes in the population. The incidence of bacterial meningitis has significantly decreased as a result of vaccination programmes against prevalent infections such as Streptococcus pneumoniae and Haemophilus influenzae type B, especially in youngsters (Straif-Bourgeois et al., 2023). Globalisation, changing climatic conditions, and newly developing infections, however, can possibly offset these advantages by bringing along new infectious dangers. Antimicrobial resistance is a serious problem that makes managing diseases more difficult and affects the effectiveness of treatments. The distribution and burden of CNS infections may also shift due to changes in population demography, such as ageing populations and increased travel. For early detection, prompt intervention, and efficient public health measures to lessen the impact of shifting CNS infection incidence rates on global health, surveillance systems keeping an eye on these patterns are crucial (Robertson et al., 2018).

3.3.2 Impact of Climate Change

The distribution, seasonality, and dynamics of infectious agent transmission are all altered by changing environmental circumstances, making the effects of climate change on CNS diseases complex and challenging. Changes in precipitation patterns and rising temperatures have an impact on vector ecology, which may lead to an expansion in the geographic range of vector-borne illnesses including Lyme neuroborreliosis and West Nile virus encephalitis (Yadav et al., 2023). In addition, severe weather events such as hurricanes and floods have the potential to cause damage to the healthcare system, hinder the availability of medical care, and promote the spread of waterborne diseases linked to encephalitis and meningitis. Furthermore, changes in wildlife populations may result from habitat loss and environmental degradation, raising the possibility of zoonotic illnesses like rabies or hantavirus pulmonary syndrome. In order to reduce the increasing risks that environmental disturbances offer to the security of global health, addressing the effect of climate change on CNS diseases necessitates a comprehensive strategy combining environmental stewardship, public health initiatives, and adaptive healthcare techniques (Tazerjiet al., 2022).

3.3.3 Antimicrobial Resistance

The therapy of CNS infections is significantly hampered by antimicrobial resistance (AMR), which also affects patient outcomes and treatment efficacy. Conventional treatment techniques become unproductive due to the growth and spread of resistant bacteria caused by the misuse and overuse of antimicrobial drugs. Because bacteria like Neisseria meningitidis and Streptococcus pneumoniae have become resistant to several antibiotics, including beta-lactams and fluoroquinolones, there are fewer treatment options available and a higher chance of treatment failure when CNS infections occur (Salam et al., 2023). The issue is further compounded by resistance mechanisms in fungal pathogens such as Candida species and antiviral drugs against herpesviruses. A multimodal strategy is needed to address antimicrobial resistance (AMR) in CNS infections. This strategy should include prudent antibiotic use, improved surveillance systems, the development of innovative therapies, and public health initiatives to encourage antimicrobial stewardship. The effectiveness of current treatments could be jeopardised if AMR is not addressed, which emphasises the urgent need for concerted measures to counter this danger to world health (Azak et al., 2023).

4. IMPACT ON VULNERABLE POPULATIONS

The way that CNS infections affect communities who are already at risk highlights the ways in which socioeconomic injustices, systemic barriers to accessing healthcare, and health disparities interact. Immunocompromised people, the elderly, children, and people living in resource-poor environments are among the vulnerable groups that are more vulnerable to CNS infections because of things like weakening or immature immune systems, underlying medical conditions, and limited access to vaccinations and other preventive measures (Parenteau et al., 2022). Furthermore, the burden of CNS infections is increased by socioeconomic factors such poverty, congested living conditions, and a lack of access to quality healthcare, which can result in delayed diagnosis, inadequate treatment, and unfavourable health outcomes. A comprehensive strategy that includes targeted public health interventions, equal access to healthcare services, and measures to address social determinants of health is required to address the burden of CNS infections on vulnerable groups. In the care of CNS infections, we might endeavour to reduce health disparities and promote health equity by giving priority to the needs of disadvantaged populations (Ha et al., 2023).

4.1 Pediatrics

CNS infections have a significant and diverse effect on vulnerable groups, including children. As a result of their immature immune systems and restricted capacity for symptom communication, children—especially infants—are more vulnerable to severe CNS illness symptoms (Singh et al., 2022). For example, if bacterial meningitis is not identified and treated right once, it can advance quickly in infants and cause permanent neurological damage or even death. Furthermore, socioeconomic variables that impair timely access to medical care and preventive measures like immunisations, such as poverty and limited access to healthcare increase the vulnerability of paediatric populations. In order to lessen the effects of these illnesses and guarantee the best possible health outcomes for children everywhere, there is an urgent need for focused public health initiatives, better access to healthcare, and raised awareness. This is highlighted by the burden of CNS infections on susceptible paediatric populations (Mannebach et al., 2022).

4.1.1 Neonatal Infections

A significant subclass of CNS infections, neonatal infections present unique clinical difficulties and consequences. Due to certain prenatal risk factors and their undeveloped immune systems, newborns are especially susceptible to CNS infections. In this population, meningitis is frequently caused by bacterial pathogens including Escherichia coli and Group B Streptococcus, which are frequently acquired vertically after childbirth or through maternal-fetal transmission (Mohebalizadeh et al., 2023). Neonates with CNS infections might present in subtle, nonspecific ways that make diagnosis difficult and require a high index of suspicion. Timely identification and intervention are essential to avoid severe consequences like sepsis, neurodevelopmental damage, or even death. In addition, the prevalence of neonatal CNS infections has decreased significantly as a result of preventative measures including intrapartum antibiotic prophylaxis and mother screening, underscoring the need of comprehensive perinatal care in preserving the health of newborns (Gaur, et al., 2020).

4.1.2 Childhood Infections (e.g., Meningitis)

Meningitis is one of the most common childhood illnesses and accounts for a large portion of CNS infections, which has serious consequences for children's health. Because of their developing immune systems and the close social interactions they have in school and nursery settings, children are particularly vulnerable to meningitis, regardless of its bacterial, viral, or fungal aetiology (du Preez et al., 2022). If bacterial meningitis is not identified quickly and treated with the right medications, it can result in potentially fatal consequences like sepsis and neurological aftereffects. Bacterial meningitis is frequently caused by pathogens such as Neisseria meningitidis and Streptococcus pneumoniae. Even while viral meningitis is typically less severe, it still needs to be treated carefully because it might have serious side effects (Mahmoudinezhad et al., 2021).

4.2 Elderly Population

The effects of CNS infections on susceptible groups, such the elderly, highlight the particular difficulties brought on by aging-related changes in immunological function, comorbidities, and access to treatment. The ageing population's weakened immune system makes them more vulnerable to central nervous system infections

(CNS) infections because of age-related immunosenescence (Palacios-Pedrero et al., 2021). Furthermore, underlying illnesses including diabetes, heart disease, and neurological diseases make patients more vulnerable to CNS infections and make therapeutic management more difficult. The aged population is particularly vulnerable due to social isolation, institutionalisation, and limited access to healthcare services, which makes it more difficult to diagnose and treat CNS infections in a timely manner. Targeted preventive interventions, such as vaccination programmes and increased healthcare resources, are essential to lessen the impact of these diseases and improve outcomes in this vulnerable cohort, given the considerable morbidity and mortality associated with CNS infections in the elderly (Gold et al., 2020).

4.2.1 Increased Susceptibility

The ageing population is more vulnerable to CNS infections because of immunosenescence, a term used to describe changes in immune function brought on by ageing. Due to the body's diminished capacity to fight off diseases, infections like fungal meningitis, viral encephalitis, and bacterial meningitis are more common in older persons (Xu, et al., 2020). Furthermore, the immune system is further weakened by underlying chronic illnesses like diabetes, cardiovascular disease, and neurological disorders, which increases susceptibility. Moreover, alterations in the blood-brain barrier brought on by ageing and a reduction in cerebral blood flow may make it easier for infections to enter the central nervous system. The elderly population is more susceptible to CNS infections than other populations due to social isolation, institutionalization, and limited access to healthcare. This highlights the significance of early detection, prompt treatment, and targeted preventive measures in reducing the impact of infections on health outcomes in this vulnerable population (Noe et al., 2020).

4.2.2 Challenges in Diagnosis and Management

Given the potentially serious implications connected with CNS infections, the aged population is particularly vulnerable to these illnesses, which is a major worry in the healthcare industry. Due to changes in immune function brought on by ageing, diseases such fungal meningitis, viral encephalitis, and bacterial meningitis are more common in older persons. Furthermore, the immune system's capacity to successfully fight infections is further undermined by the existence of underlying chronic illnesses, such as diabetes, cardiovascular disease, and neurodegenerative disorders (Chee, et al., 2021). In addition to reduced cerebral blood flow and age-related alterations in the blood-brain barrier, older adults are more vulnerable to CNS infections. The danger is further increased by elements like institutionalization, social isolation, and restricted access to healthcare. To minimize the impact of CNS diseases on the health and well-being of the senior population, targeted preventative efforts, such as health education programmes and vaccination campaigns, increased healthcare resources, and early detection methods, are essential (World Health Organization., 2020).

4.3 Immunocompromised Individuals

Those with damaged immune systems—a result of underlying illnesses or medical interventions—represent a particularly susceptible segment of the population. These people are more vulnerable to CNS infections as a result of their weakened immune systems, which can have serious consequences. Conditions including HIV/AIDS, cancer, organ transplantation, autoimmune illnesses, or immunosuppressive medications can all lead to immunocompromised states. Immunocompromised people are more vulnerable to CNS infections due to a variety of factors, including weakened immune systems, a heightened vulnerability to opportunistic microorganisms, and difficulties with prompt diagnosis and treatment (Henao-Martínez et al., 2018).

4.3.1 HIV/AIDS

Due to the severe immune suppression brought on by the disease, people living with HIV/AIDS represent a particularly susceptible subset among immunocompromised people and are at heightened risk of CNS infections. HIV/AIDS patients are more vulnerable to opportunistic infections such progressive multifocal leukoencephalopathy (PML), toxoplasmosis, and cryptococcal meningitis because they are less able to develop a strong immune response against pathogens (Agnihotri, et al., 2019). HIV/AIDS-related CNS involvement can result in severe neurological side effects, such as motor dysfunction, cognitive decline, and even death if treatment is not received. Furthermore, the burden of CNS infections is increased among populations with low resources due to the high prevalence of HIV/AIDS in these settings, where access to antiretroviral medication and comprehensive healthcare services may be restricted. In order to maximise outcomes and quality of life for impacted individuals, treating CNS infections in HIV/AIDS patients necessitates a multidisciplinary strategy that includes early diagnosis, timely antiretroviral therapy initiation, adjunctive treatments for opportunistic infections, and continuous monitoring (Bremer, et al., 2021).

4.3.2 Organ Transplant Recipients

Organ transplant patients are a distinct subgroup of immunocompromised people who are more vulnerable to central nervous system infections because they must take immunosuppressive medication for the rest of their lives in order to prevent organ rejection. These people experience severe immunological suppression, which makes them more susceptible to opportunistic infections, such as those that damage the central nervous system (Kennedy et al., 2021). Organ transplant recipients may develop new infections after receiving an organ transplant, or CNS infections may arise from the reactivation of latent diseases like Epstein-Barr virus (EBV) or cytomegalovirus (CMV). Furthermore, immunosuppressive medications, such corticosteroids and calcineurin inhibitors, impair immune function even more, making transplant recipients more vulnerable to infections like toxoplasmosis, progressive multifocal leukoencephalopathy, and cryptococcal meningitis (PML). In order to balance the need for immunosuppression with the control of infection and preservation of graft function, timely diagnosis and management of CNS infections in organ transplant recipients is critical. This frequently necessitates a multidisciplinary approach involving infectious disease specialists, neurologists, and transplant physicians (Pruitt et al., 2021).

4.3.3 Cancer Patients

Because chemotherapy and radiation therapy depress the immune system, people with cancer who are receiving these therapies are more susceptible to CNS infections. Myelosuppression brought on by chemotherapy impairs the bone marrow's capacity to generate immune cells, resulting in neutropenia and weakened immunity, both of which raise the risk of infection (Pruitt et al., 2021). Radiation therapy can also result in tissue damage and mucositis, which open up pathways for infections to enter the central nervous system. Patients with cancer may experience opportunistic infections such as viral encephalitis, bacterial brain abscesses, or fungal meningitis as a result of CNS illnesses. Furthermore, leukemic cells or lymphomatous masses can infiltrate the central nervous system as a direct result of hematologic malignancies including lymphoma and leukaemia. In order to maximise results and reduce treatment-related problems, oncologists, infectious disease specialists, and neurologists must frequently work together to diagnose and treat CNS infections in cancer patients promptly and aggressively (Pruitt et al., 2018).

5. PUBLIC HEALTH STRATEGIES AND INTERVENTIONS

In order to address the issues raised by CNS infections, public health policies and interventions—which include a range of preventative measures, surveillance systems, and healthcare interventions aimed at lessening the impact of these diseases on global health—are essential. Among these tactics are immunisation campaigns that focus on common infections such as Neisseria meningitidis and Streptococcus pneumoniae, which have been shown to be successful in lowering the prevalence of bacterial meningitis (Coordination et al., 2022). In order to avoid outbreaks in healthcare settings, public health initiatives also prioritise raising knowledge of risk factors and symptoms, enabling prompt diagnosis and treatment initiation, and putting infection control measures into place. Monitoring illness patterns, identifying new pathogens, and directing focused actions to lessen the effects of CNS infections are all made possible by surveillance systems. Furthermore, improving public health responses to CNS illnesses and developing new diagnostic tools, vaccinations, and antimicrobial medicines require study into these areas. Public health initiatives aim to prevent and control CNS infections while also promoting health equity, protecting vulnerable groups, and lowering morbidity and mortality rates through the integration of various multimodal approaches (Straif-Bourgeois et al., 2022).

5.1 Prevention Measures

A variety of tactics are used in CNS infection prevention techniques with the goal of lowering the risk of infection and transmission, with a focus on vulnerable populations. The mainstay of preventative efforts is vaccination, which lowers the risk of bacterial meningitis by targeting common pathogens like Haemophilus influenzae type b, Neisseria meningitidis, and Streptococcus pneumoniae. Furthermore, maintaining proper hygiene habits reduces the transmission of respiratory viruses and bacteria linked to central nervous system diseases (Deghmane et al., 2021). These behaviours include frequent handwashing and respiratory etiquette. Prophylactic antibiotic medication or immunisation against particular pathogens may be advised for immunocompromised persons in order to prevent opportunistic infections. Campaigns for public health are essential in bringing attention to the value of immunisation, the signs of CNS diseases, and the need for quick medical care. Preventing infections related to healthcare is further enhanced by implementing infection control measures in healthcare settings, such as tight adherence to aseptic procedures and isolation precautions. Public health programmes seek to reduce the burden of CNS infections and protect population health by using these preventive approaches (World Health Organization., 2021).

5.1.1 Vaccination Programs

Because vaccinations provide immunity against common pathogens that cause disorders like viral encephalitis and bacterial meningitis, they are essential in preventing CNS infections. These initiatives usually aim to lower the prevalence of illnesses and the problems they cause by focusing on immunocompromised people, children, and newborns (Ngarka et al., 2022). Immunisations against Streptococcus pneumoniae and Neisseria meningitidis, respectively, have significantly decreased the incidence of bacterial meningitis. Examples of these vaccinations are the meningococcal conjugate vaccine and the pneumococcal conjugate vaccine. Vaccines against viruses like rubella, measles, mumps, and varicella-zoster virus also aid in preventing neurological consequences such viral encephalitis. Through regular immunisation schedules, catch-up campaigns, and focused vaccination efforts in response to outbreaks or endemic transmission, public health initiatives aim to ensure high vaccine coverage rates. Vaccination programmes play a major role in shielding people from the devastation caused by CNS illnesses by advocating vaccination as the cornerstone of disease prevention (Dudley et al., 2018).

5.1.2 Hygiene Practices

By reducing the spread of the bacteria that cause CNS infections, good hygiene habits are essential for preventing these infections. In crowded environments like schools, nursery schools and healthcare facilities, basic yet efficient precautions like routine hand washing with soap and water can drastically prevent the spread of respiratory viruses and germs linked to CNS diseases (Cristina et al., 2021). The spread of respiratory droplets carrying infectious pathogens can be avoided by practicing proper respiratory etiquette, which includes covering coughs and sneezes with a tissue or elbow. Furthermore, preserving sanitary and uncontaminated living spaces, which includes routinely cleaning high-touch surfaces and appropriately disposing of garbage, lowers the chance of pathogen contamination and spread. Campaigns for public health that encourage proper hygiene habits help to create healthier communities by increasing awareness of the role that personal hygiene has in reducing CNS diseases. People can actively prevent the spread of infectious diseases to others and themselves by incorporating good hygiene practices into daily activities (Rios, et al., 2020).

5.1.3 Vector Control

In order to prevent CNS illnesses spread by vectors like ticks and mosquitoes, vector management is an essential tactic. Insecticide spraying, larval habitat reduction and mosquito surveillance programmes are examples of vector management techniques that can help reduce the spread of mosquito-borne illnesses such West Nile virus encephalitis and Japanese encephalitis (Socha et al., 2022).

5.2 Surveillance Systems

In order to prevent and control CNS infections, surveillance systems are essential because they provide vital information on disease patterns, spot new pathogens, and direct public health initiatives. These systems consist of a network of public health organisations, labs, and healthcare institutions that methodically gather, process, and distribute data about CNS illnesses (Hawker et al., 2019). Aspects of CNS infections such as incidence rates, regional distribution, demographic trends, and profiles of antibiotic resistance are all captured by surveillance activities. Surveillance systems are able to identify outbreaks, evaluate the efficacy of preventative interventions, and provide information for policy decisions that aim to lower the incidence of CNS infections by tracking illness trends over time (Ludden et al., 2019).

5.2.1 Importance of Surveillance

For the purpose of early identification, monitoring, and response to infectious disease concerns, CNS infection surveillance is an essential tool in public health endeavours. Surveillance systems gather and analyse data on disease incidence, prevalence, and trends in a systematic manner, which offers valuable insights into the epidemiology of CNS diseases. Public health officials can use this data to pinpoint outbreaks, monitor the transmission of infectious pathogens, and evaluate the efficacy of preventative measures (Akinyemi et al., 2021).

5.2.2 Role of Technology

Technology is essential to improving CNS infection surveillance, diagnosis, and treatment, and it has completely changed how medical professionals treat infectious disorders. Next-generation sequencing (NGS) and polymerase chain reaction (PCR) assays are two examples of advanced molecular diagnostic tools that enable quick and precise identification of pathogens from clinical samples, facilitating early diagnosis and focused therapy. In remote or underserved locations, telemedicine platforms and electronic health records facilitate prompt consultations and collaborations among healthcare practitioners for the management of CNS infections (Shrestha et al., 2024).

5.3 Treatment Guidelines

Guidelines for the treatment of CNS infections give medical personnel the fundamental foundations they need to manage patients and improve their results. These guidelines cover expert consensus and evidence-based advice for the diagnosis, management, and prophylaxis of a variety of central nervous system diseases, such as fungal meningitis, viral encephalitis, and bacterial meningitis. Treatment recommendations serve to standardize care procedures, encourage consistency in treatment approaches, and guarantee the provision of high-quality healthcare services by synthesizing the most recent scientific data and clinical experience (Sharma et al., 2021).

5.3.1 Antimicrobial Therapy

An essential component of treating CNS infections is antimicrobial therapy, which attempts to destroy the causing microorganisms and avoid sequelae. The hypothesised or confirmed etiological agent determines which antimicrobial drugs are used; broad-spectrum antibiotics are usually started empirically before receiving microbiological confirmation (Sutharet al., 2019). Examples of such medicines are vancomycin and third-generation cephalosporin's. Certain antiviral medications, such as ganciclovir for the cytomegalovirus or acyclovir for the herpes simplex virus, may be necessary for treating viral encephalitis. Antifungal medications, such as fluconazole or amphotericin B, must be used to treat fungal meningitis, frequently for extended periods of time (Molloy et al., 2018).

5.3.2 Supportive Care

In order to reduce symptoms, stabilise patients, and improve their general health, supportive care is essential in the treatment of CNS infections. In order to identify and treat problems as soon as possible, supportive measures may include careful monitoring of vital signs, neurological function, and fluid balance. Furthermore, improving patient comfort can be achieved by providing symptomatic relief via the use of antipyretics for fever, analgesics for headaches, and antiemetics for nausea and vomiting. To prevent further deterioration in cases of altered mental state or seizures, supportive treatment may include neurological monitoring, airway management, and seizure control (Strein et al., 2019).

5.3.3 Rehabilitation Services

In cases where patients develop neurological deficits or functional impairment as a result of the infection or its treatment, rehabilitation services are especially important to the entire care of CNS diseases. Physical therapy can help with motor impairments; occupational therapy can help with daily living tasks; speech therapy can help with language and swallowing issues; and cognitive rehabilitation can help with memory and executive function issues. Patients may also receive counselling and psychological support to help them deal with the psychological and emotional fallout from CNS illnesses (Khan et al., 2020).

6. SOCIOECONOMIC AND CULTURAL CONSIDERATIONS

A thorough understanding and treatment of CNS illnesses must take socioeconomic and cultural factors into account. In addition to their medical effects, these illnesses also have an impact on broader social, economic, and cultural aspects that affect treatment outcomes, healthcare access, and the spread of disease. In underprivileged populations in particular, socioeconomic disadvantages such as poverty, poor access to healthcare, and low health literacy might increase the incidence of CNS infections. People's reactions to CNS infections and adherence to treatment regimens may also be influenced by cultural traditions, attitudes, and beliefs about sickness, treatment-seeking behaviour, and healthcare decision-making (Towfighi et al., 2023).

6.1 Access to Healthcare

One of the most important factors in the therapy, diagnosis, and prevention of CNS infections is access to healthcare. The ability of individuals to obtain timely and adequate healthcare treatments is substantially influenced by socioeconomic characteristics, including income level, education, and geographic location. For those with CNS infections, inadequate access to healthcare facilities can result in delayed diagnosis, fewer treatment options, and worse results. This is especially true in rural or underserved locations. Furthermore, obstacles including a lack of health insurance, problems with transportation, and language hurdles make it harder for people to get the care they need, especially those who are marginalised. Multifaceted strategies are needed to address healthcare disparities (McMaughan et al., 2020).

6.1.1 Disparities in Healthcare Access

The problems associated with CNS infections are made worse by disparities in healthcare access, which disproportionately impact underprivileged and marginalised groups. The intersection of socioeconomic factors such as education level, work status, and income inequality results in impediments to healthcare access that sustain inequalities in the diagnosis, treatment, and prevention of CNS infections. Minority groups, people living in remote areas, and those with low socioeconomic level sometimes have trouble accessing healthcare facilities, which can lead to delayed diagnosis, inadequate care, and worse health outcomes (Towfighi et al., 2023).

6.1.2 Impact on Diagnosis and Treatment Outcomes

The diagnosis and course of treatment for CNS infections are greatly influenced by socioeconomic and cultural factors. Individuals from poor origins may experience delayed diagnosis and suboptimal treatment initiation due to limited access to healthcare facilities, financial constraints, and low health literacy. The inequalities in diagnostic and treatment accessibility lead to severe consequences, such as higher rates of morbidity and death among marginalised communities afflicted with CNS illnesses (Amezcua et al., 2021).

6.2 Stigma and Discrimination

The difficulties that impacted people and communities must overcome might be made worse by the stigma and discrimination associated with CNS illnesses. People who are diagnosed with or suspected of having a CNS infection may face social stigma, isolation, and discrimination as a result of misconceptions and fear surrounding these infections. This stigma can take many different forms, such as obstacles to receiving healthcare services, discrimination in the workplace, and social rejection. Furthermore, members of marginalised groups—such as members of racial or ethnic minorities, LGBTQ+ people, and people living with HIV/AIDS—may encounter many forms of discrimination and stigma, which makes them even more vulnerable (Dahalan et al., 2022).

6.2.1 Perceptions of Infectious Diseases

Cultural, societal, and historical variables impact people's perceptions of infectious diseases, particularly CNS infections, which in turn affect their understanding, attitudes, and behaviours about these disorders. Cultural values, customs, and life events frequently influence how people view the causes of illnesses, the ways in which they spread, and the best ways to cure them. Furthermore, societal reactions to infectious diseases can be shaped by historical events, such as previous epidemics or pandemics, which can alter perceptions of risk, dread, and shame. In order to address how contagious diseases are seen, culturally sensitive methods must be used, such as community involvement, education, and communication techniques that take into account different viewpoints and beliefs (Bayeh et al., 2021).

6.2.2 Psychological Impact on Patients and Families

Beyond the disease's outward symptoms, CNS infections can have a significant psychological impact on patients and their relatives. Concerns regarding their diagnosis, prognosis, and course of therapy can cause dread, anxiety, and uncertainty among patients. Additional factors that may exacerbate emotional discomfort, emotions of loss, or frustration include neurological deficiencies or cognitive impairments brought on by the infection. Families may experience worry, remorse, and helplessness when they see a loved one suffer and deal with the unpredictability of the condition. In addition, family dynamics and relationships may be strained by the interruption of daily routines, financial difficulties, and the requirement for care giving (Testa et al., 2019).

6.3 Community Engagement

In order to address the complex issues surrounding CNS infections, community participation is essential for promoting cooperation between local communities, public health officials, and healthcare practitioners. Community engagement projects provide individuals with the opportunity to actively participate in promoting health and reducing the spread of infectious diseases by incorporating members of the community in the development, execution, and assessment of interventions. Community engagement initiatives, which include education campaigns, support groups, and outreach programmes, seek to decrease stigma and discrimination related to CNS infections, promote preventive measures like vaccinations and good hygiene, and increase public knowledge of the warning signs and symptoms of these illnesses (Calnan, et al., 2019).

6.3.1 Education Campaigns

In order to lessen the impact of CNS illnesses on communities, education programmes play a crucial role in promoting preventive measures and increasing public awareness. These campaigns spread correct information about the symptoms, signs, and pathways of CNS diseases through a variety of communication platforms, such as social media, mainstream media, and community outreach initiatives. Education campaigns seek to raise awareness of the dangers of CNS infections and the significance of early detection and timely treatment by focusing on a variety of audiences, including individuals, families, medical professionals, and community leaders. Furthermore, education initiatives are essential for busting stereotypes, lowering stigma, and creating a supportive atmosphere for those with CNS diseases (Fancourt et al., 2019).

6.3.2 Empowerment of Local Communities

Investing in local communities is crucial to the holistic strategy for treating CNS illnesses. Local communities take an active role in promoting health and halting the spread of infectious illnesses by including community members in decision-making procedures, resource distribution, and intervention execution. Through empowerment programmes, community people are given the information, tools, and resources needed to take charge of their own health and wellbeing. This could entail putting community health workers through training, founding neighbourhood associations, and supporting neighborhood-led campaigns aimed at advocacy, education, and prevention (Platt et al., 2018).

Figure 3. Socio-Cultural CNS Considerations.

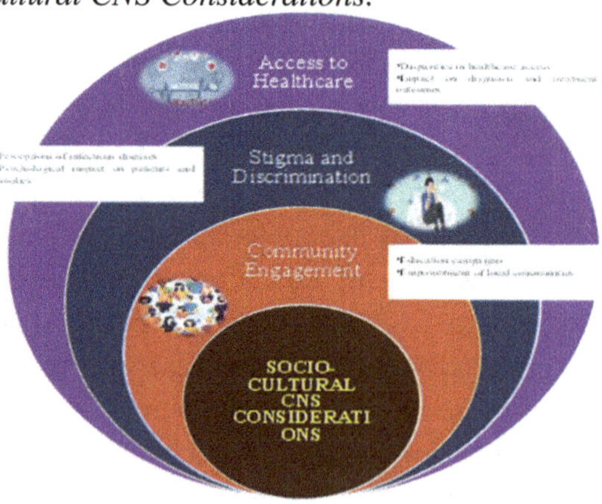

7. CHALLENGES AND FUTURE DIRECTIONS

It is essential to address the issues and map out future strategies in the field of CNS infections in order to advance public health initiatives and enhance patient outcomes. There are many difficulties, such as the differences in access to healthcare due to socioeconomic status and the complexity of diagnosis and treatment. Furthermore, there are constant risks from newly developing infectious agents and antibiotic resistance, which calls for creativity and attentiveness in the monitoring and treatment of illnesses. Furthermore, successful preventative and control initiatives are still hampered by stigma, discrimination, and cultural hurdles. But amid these difficulties, there are chances for creativity, cooperation, and advancement. The field's future prospects could involve the creation of innovative medicines, improvements in diagnostic tools, and focused initiatives to close the gaps in healthcare access (Dash et al., 2019).

7.1 Diagnostic Challenges

Effective patient care and public health initiatives are severely hampered by the difficulties in diagnosing CNS infections. It is necessary to navigate a vast terrain of pathogens, each with a distinct clinical presentation and diagnostic nuances, in order to determine the causative agent of a CNS infection. Furthermore, CNS infection symptoms might be vague and mimic those of other neurological disorders, delaying diagnosis and treatment commencement. Diagnostic procedures like lumbar punctures are intrusive, which increases complexity, especially for vulnerable populations. Furthermore, particularly in low-resource environments, resource constraints, such as lack of access to cutting-edge diagnostic technologies and knowledge, can impede prompt and accurate diagnosis (Karvouniaris et al., 2022).

7.1.1 Lack of Specific Diagnostic Tests

One major obstacle to accurately detecting CNS infections is the lack of specialised diagnostic assays. Diagnosing CNS infections frequently involves a combination of clinical assessment, imaging studies, and laboratory tests, unlike other infectious disorders where diagnostic techniques may provide clear and definite answers. Many of these tests, meanwhile, lack the specificity required to correctly identify the infection's causal agent. This is especially true when there is a possibility that more than one pathogen is causing similar clinical presentations, which can cause ambiguity in the diagnosis process and postpone the start of appropriate therapy. Moreover, extra dangers and difficulties arise from the intrusive nature of certain diagnostic procedures, such as lumbar punctures for the examination of cerebrospinal fluid, particularly in vulnerable populations (Hahn et al., 2020).

7.1.2 Delayed Diagnosis

Prompt detection of central nervous system infections presents notable obstacles to patient care and results. Uncertain diagnosis arises because the vague symptoms, such fever, headache, and altered mental status, that are frequently linked to these diseases might also be caused by other neurological disorders. Additionally, patient pain or resistance combined with the invasive nature of diagnostic procedures like lumbar punctures may cause delays in the diagnostic evaluation process. As a result, a delayed diagnosis may lead to a delayed start of the necessary therapy, allowing the infection to spread unchecked and perhaps resulting in fatal consequences or serious neurological side effects (Bransfield et al., 2019).

7.2 Therapeutic Challenges

Therapeutic problems related to CNS infections provide complex obstacles to the efficient care and treatment of afflicted patients. The blood-brain barrier, which restricts the amount of antibiotics that may enter the central nervous system, makes CNS infections different from many other illnesses in that they present special difficulties. Treatment plans are further complicated by the variety of bacteria that can cause CNS infections and the possibility of antibiotic resistance. Individualised approaches to therapy are also necessary due to the heterogeneity of clinical presentations and the variability in patient responses to treatment. A multidisciplinary strategy that incorporates developments in antimicrobial treatments, neurocritical care, and supportive interventions is necessary to address therapeutic obstacles (Edelmann et al., 2020).

7.2.1 Antimicrobial Resistance

Treatment options for CNS infections are severely limited by antimicrobial resistance, which complicates therapeutic approaches. The effectiveness of frequently used antimicrobial drugs, such as antibiotics, is diminished by the rise of resistance strains, especially among bacterial pathogens. Many things can lead to this resistance, such as selective pressure in hospital settings, improper or excessive use of antibiotics, and unfinished treatment regimens. Furthermore, the blood-brain barrier limits the ability of several antibiotics to enter the central nervous system, which further reduces the number of CNS infection treatments available. A multimodal approach is needed to combat antimicrobial resistance, involving the creation of new antimicrobial agents, infection control strategies, and antimicrobial stewardship programmes (Haddad et al., 2022).

7.2.2 Neurological Sequelae

Commonly, CNS infections result in neurological sequelae, which frequently cause long-term issues and disabilities in those who are impacted. The consequences of these events might take many different forms, such as defects in perception, motor skills, seizures, and cognitive decline. Among the CNS infections linked to a significant risk of neurological consequences are bacterial meningitis, viral encephalitis, and fungal meningitis; this risk increases if diagnosis and treatment are postponed. The degree and gravity of neurological aftereffects can differ based on the underlying cause, when therapy is started, and the patient's general condition (Wang et al., 2020).

7.3 Research Needs

In order to improve patient outcomes, advance our understanding, and develop more effective diagnostic and treatment approaches, there is an urgent need for research on CNS infections. Many obstacles still remain in the face of tremendous advancements, including confusion about the diagnosis, restrictions on treatment options, and long-term neurological effects. A concentrated research effort focused on creating novel strategies for prevention, diagnosis, and therapy is necessary to address these issues. Enhancing the quality of life for those impacted by CNS diseases also requires study into the long-term neurological effects of the infections and the creation of efficient rehabilitation plans (Li et al., 2021).

7.3.1 Development of Novel Therapeutics

To overcome the difficulties brought on by antibiotic resistance and the constraints of current treatment choices, innovative treatments for CNS infections must be developed. The blood-brain barrier presents challenges for conventional antibacterial drugs, which reduces their efficacy in treating CNS illnesses. As a result, research efforts are concentrated on finding and creating cutting-edge therapy strategies that can successfully target infections inside the central nervous system. This include looking into novel antimicrobial substances with improved CNS penetration, repurposing already-approved medications to treat CNS infections, and researching alternate forms of therapy such immunomodulatory medicines and phage therapy (Terreni et al., 2021).

7.3.2 Advancements in Diagnostics

For CNS infections, improvements in early detection, precise diagnosis, and prompt treatment initiation are essential. Traditional diagnostic techniques have drawbacks with regard to invasiveness, specificity, and sensitivity. Examples include imaging studies and cerebrospinal fluid analysis. As a result, research efforts are concentrated on creating innovative diagnostic techniques that provide enhanced precision, speed, and usability. This involves the creation of point-of-care diagnostics for quick pathogen identification, sophisticated imaging methods for better disease visualisation in the central nervous system, and the application of genomic and molecular technology for accurate causative agent identification. Furthermore, developments in machine learning and artificial intelligence show promise for supporting the interpretation of diagnostic data and forecasting the course of disease (Schwartz, et al., 2018).

7.3.3 Long-Term Outcomes Studies

Comprehensive therapeutic techniques and a complete understanding of the full impact of CNS illnesses on afflicted persons depend on long-term outcomes research. These investigations offer important new understandings of the neurological, cognitive, and functional effects of the virus that might last after its acute stage. Researchers can evaluate the frequency and severity of long-term consequences such cognitive impairment, motor impairments, epilepsy, and psychiatric illnesses by following patients for longer periods of time. Furthermore, long-term outcome studies clarify the variables affecting prognosis, such as the underlying cause, promptness of therapy, and existence of comorbidities (Azzollini et al., 2021).

8. CONCLUSION AND CALL TO ACTION

In summary, tackling the complex issues brought about by CNS infections necessitates an all-encompassing, multidisciplinary strategy that incorporates developments in long-term outcomes research, diagnostics, and treatments. The intricate nature of these illnesses necessitates creative approaches and cooperative efforts from a range of sectors, including public health, industry, academia, and healthcare. There is still much to be done, despite the fact that understanding the pathogenesis and developing diagnostic and therapy techniques have advanced significantly. The creation of novel treatments with improved CNS penetration, cutting-edge diagnostic instruments for quick and precise pathogen identification, and long-term outcome studies to clarify the whole picture of CNS infections on afflicted people should be the top priorities for future research.

Moreover, coordinated actions are required to alleviate inequalities in healthcare access, enhance health literacy, and lessen the stigma associated with CNS illnesses. Initiatives aimed at empowering and involving the community are essential for spreading knowledge, encouraging preventative measures, and building resilience in impacted communities. Furthermore, financing and support for research projects that attempt to improve our knowledge of CNS infections and integrate scientific findings into clinical practice must be given top priority by legislators.

We must act together in unity to address the persistent problems caused by CNS illnesses. Through the integration of resources and knowledge from all stakeholders throughout the healthcare continuum, evidence-based solutions to reduce the incidence of CNS infections, enhance patient outcomes, and protect public health can be developed. In order to successfully prevent, diagnose, and treat CNS infections in the future for the benefit of all, let's commit to advancing research, improving healthcare infrastructure, and fostering equity in access to care.

REFERENCES

Abushaheen, M. A., Fatani, A. J., Alosaimi, M., Mansy, W., George, M., Acharya, S., & Jhugroo, P. (2020). Antimicrobial resistance, mechanisms and its clinical significance. *Disease-a-Month, 66*(6), 100971. DOI: 10.1016/j.disamonth.2020.100971 PMID: 32201008

Agnihotri, S. P. (2019, June). Central nervous system opportunistic infections. *Seminars in Neurology, 39*(03), 383–390. DOI: 10.1055/s-0039-1687842 PMID: 31378873

Akinyemi, R. O., Ovbiagele, B., Adeniji, O. A., Sarfo, F. S., Abd-Allah, F., Adoukonou, T., Ogah, O. S., Naidoo, P., Damasceno, A., Walker, R. W., Ogunniyi, A., Kalaria, R. N., & Owolabi, M. O. (2021). Stroke in Africa: Profile, progress, prospects and priorities. *Nature Reviews. Neurology, 17*(10), 634–656. DOI: 10.1038/s41582-021-00542-4 PMID: 34526674

Almubaslat, F., Sanchez-Boluarte, S. S., & Diaz, M. M. (2023). A review of neurological health disparities in Peru. *Frontiers in Public Health, 11*, 1210238. DOI: 10.3389/fpubh.2023.1210238 PMID: 37744515

Amezcua, L., Rivera, V. M., Vazquez, T. C., Baezconde-Garbanati, L., & Langer-Gould, A. (2021). Health disparities, inequities, and social determinants of health in multiple sclerosis and related disorders in the US: A review. *JAMA Neurology, 78*(12), 1515–1524. DOI: 10.1001/jamaneurol.2021.3416 PMID: 34605866

Azak, E., Sertcelik, A., Ersoz, G., Celebi, G., Eser, F., Batirel, A., & Alp, E. (2023). Evaluation of the implementation of WHO infection prevention and control core components in Turkish health care facilities: Results from a WHO infection prevention and control assessment framework (IPCAF)—based survey. *Antimicrobial Resistance and Infection Control, 12*(1), 11. DOI: 10.1186/s13756-023-01208-0 PMID: 36782267

Azzollini, V., Dalise, S., & Chisari, C. (2021). How does stroke affect skeletal muscle? State of the art and rehabilitation perspective. *Frontiers in Neurology, 12*, 797559. DOI: 10.3389/fneur.2021.797559 PMID: 35002937

Balaji, S., Chakraborty, R., & Aggarwal, S. (2024). Neurological complications caused by human immunodeficiency virus (HIV) and associated opportunistic co-infections: a review on their diagnosis and therapeutic insights. *CNS & Neurological Disorders-Drug Targets (Formerly Current Drug Targets-CNS & Neurological Disorders), 23*(3), 284-305.

Barach, P., Fisher, S. D., Adams, M. J., Burstein, G. R., Brophy, P. D., Kuo, D. Z., & Lipshultz, S. E. (2020). Disruption of healthcare: Will the COVID pandemic worsen non-COVID outcomes and disease outbreaks? *Progress in Pediatric Cardiology, 59*, 101254. DOI: 10.1016/j.ppedcard.2020.101254 PMID: 32837144

Bayeh, R., Yampolsky, M. A., & Ryder, A. G. (2021). The social lives of infectious diseases: Why culture matters to COVID-19. *Frontiers in Psychology, 12*, 648086. DOI: 10.3389/fpsyg.2021.648086 PMID: 34630195

Bransfield, R. C., & Friedman, K. J. (2019, October). Differentiating psychosomatic, somatopsychic, multisystem illnesses and medical uncertainty. *Health Care, 7*(4), 114. PMID: 31597359

Bremer, M., Kadernani, Y. E., Wasserman, S., Wilkinson, R. J., & Davis, A. G. (2021). Strategies for the diagnosis and management of meningitis in HIV-infected adults in resource limited settings. *Expert Opinion on Pharmacotherapy, 22*(15), 2053–2070. DOI: 10.1080/14656566.2021.1940954 PMID: 34154509

Budreviciute, A., Damiati, S., Sabir, D. K., & Kodzius, R. (2020). Management and prevention strategies for non-communicable diseases (NCDs) and their risk factors. *Frontiers in Public Health, 8*, 574111. DOI: 10.3389/fpubh.2020.574111 PMID: 33324597

Calnan, M., Gadsby, E. W., Kondé, M. K., Diallo, A., & Rossman, J. S. (2018). The response to and impact of the Ebola epidemic: Towards an agenda for interdisciplinary research. *International Journal of Health Policy and Management, 7*(5), 402–411. DOI: 10.15171/ijhpm.2017.104 PMID: 29764104

Chaudhuri, A., & Kennedy, P. G. (2002). Diagnosis and treatment of viral encephalitis. *Postgraduate Medical Journal, 78*(924), 575–583. DOI: 10.1136/pmj.78.924.575 PMID: 12415078

Chee, S. E. J., & Solito, E. (2021). The impact of ageing on the CNS immune response in Alzheimer's disease. *Frontiers in Immunology, 12*, 738511. DOI: 10.3389/fimmu.2021.738511 PMID: 34603320

Coordination, G., Alastruey-Izquierdo, A., World Health Organization, & World Health Organization. (2022). *WHO fungal priority pathogens list to guide research, development and public health action*. Organización Mundial de la Salud (OMS).

Cristina, M. L., Spagnolo, A. M., Giribone, L., Demartini, A., & Sartini, M. (2021). Epidemiology and prevention of healthcare-associated infections in geriatric patients: A narrative review. *International Journal of Environmental Research and Public Health, 18*(10), 5333. DOI: 10.3390/ijerph18105333 PMID: 34067797

Czarniak, N., Kamińska, J., Matowicka-Karna, J., & Koper-Lenkiewicz, O. M. (2023). Cerebrospinal fluid–basic concepts review. *Biomedicines, 11*(5), 1461. DOI: 10.3390/biomedicines11051461 PMID: 37239132

Dash, S., Shakyawar, S. K., Sharma, M., & Kaushik, S. (2019). Big data in healthcare: Management, analysis and future prospects. *Journal of Big Data*, *6*(1), 1–25. DOI: 10.1186/s40537-019-0217-0

Deghmane, A. E., & Taha, M. K. (2021). Invasive bacterial infections in subjects with genetic and acquired susceptibility and impacts on recommendations for vaccination: A narrative review. *Microorganisms*, *9*(3), 467. DOI: 10.3390/microorganisms9030467 PMID: 33668334

Ding, C., Wu, Y., Chen, X., Chen, Y., Wu, Z., Lin, Z., Kang, D., Fang, W., & Chen, F. (2022). Global, regional, and national burden and attributable risk factors of neurological disorders: The Global Burden of Disease study 1990–2019. *Frontiers in Public Health*, *10*, 952161. DOI: 10.3389/fpubh.2022.952161 PMID: 36523572

du Preez, K., Jenkins, H. E., Donald, P. R., Solomons, R. S., Graham, S. M., Schaaf, H. S., Starke, J. R., Hesseling, A. C., & Seddon, J. A. (2022). Tuberculous meningitis in children: A forgotten public health emergency. *Frontiers in Neurology*, *13*, 751133. DOI: 10.3389/fneur.2022.751133 PMID: 35370901

Dudley, M. Z., Salmon, D. A., Halsey, N. A., Orenstein, W. A., Limaye, R. J., O'Leary, S. T., ... & Omer, S. B. (2018). Do Vaccines Cause Meningitis or Encephalitis/Encephalopathy?. *The Clinician's Vaccine Safety Resource Guide: Optimizing Prevention of Vaccine-Preventable Diseases Across the Lifespan*, 281-289.

Edelmann, M. J., & Maegawa, G. H. (2020). CNS-targeting therapies for lysosomal storage diseases: Current advances and challenges. *Frontiers in Molecular Biosciences*, *7*, 559804. DOI: 10.3389/fmolb.2020.559804 PMID: 33304924

Fancourt, D., & Finn, S. (2019). *What is the evidence on the role of the arts in improving health and well-being? A scoping review*. World Health Organization. Regional Office for Europe.

Feigin, V. L., Vos, T., Nichols, E., Owolabi, M. O., Carroll, W. M., Dichgans, M., Deuschl, G., Parmar, P., Brainin, M., & Murray, C. (2020). The global burden of neurological disorders: Translating evidence into policy. *Lancet Neurology*, *19*(3), 255–265. DOI: 10.1016/S1474-4422(19)30411-9 PMID: 31813850

Fisher, M. C., Alastruey-Izquierdo, A., Berman, J., Bicanic, T., Bignell, E. M., Bowyer, P., Bromley, M., Brüggemann, R., Garber, G., Cornely, O. A., Gurr, S. J., Harrison, T. S., Kuijper, E., Rhodes, J., Sheppard, D. C., Warris, A., White, P. L., Xu, J., Zwaan, B., & Verweij, P. E. (2022). Tackling the emerging threat of antifungal resistance to human health. *Nature Reviews. Microbiology*, *20*(9), 557–571. DOI: 10.1038/s41579-022-00720-1 PMID: 35352028

Gaur, P., Kachramanoglou, C., Lyall, H., & Jan, W. (2020). Is it not time for international guidelines to combat congenital cytomegalovirus infection? A review of central nervous system manifestations. *Clinical Radiology*, *75*(8), 644–e7. DOI: 10.1016/j.crad.2020.02.009 PMID: 32216960

Gold, S. M., Köhler-Forsberg, O., Moss-Morris, R., Mehnert, A., Miranda, J. J., Bullinger, M., Steptoe, A., Whooley, M. A., & Otte, C. (2020). Comorbid depression in medical diseases. *Nature Reviews. Disease Primers*, *6*(1), 69. DOI: 10.1038/s41572-020-0200-2 PMID: 32820163

Gotlieb, E. G., Blank, L., Willis, A. W., Agarwal, P., & Jette, N. (2023). Health equity integrated epilepsy care and research: A narrative review. *Epilepsia*, *64*(11), 2878–2890. DOI: 10.1111/epi.17728 PMID: 37725065

Guadarrama-Ortiz, P., Choreno-Parra, J. A., Sanchez-Martinez, C. M., Pacheco-Sanchez, F. J., Rodriguez-Nava, A. I., & Garcia-Quintero, G. (2020). Neurological aspects of SARS-CoV-2 infection: Mechanisms and manifestations. *Frontiers in Neurology*, *11*, 1039. DOI: 10.3389/fneur.2020.01039 PMID: 33013675

Gutierrez, M., & Emmanuel, P. J. (2018). Expanding molecular diagnostics for central nervous system infections. *Advances in Pediatrics*, *65*(1), 209–227. DOI: 10.1016/j.yapd.2018.04.005 PMID: 30053925

Ha, S., Ho, S. H., Bae, Y. H., Lee, M., Kim, J. H., Kim, J. H., & Lee, J. (2023). Digital Health Equity and Tailored Health Care Service for People With Disability: User-Centered Design and Usability Study. *Journal of Medical Internet Research*, *25*, e50029. DOI: 10.2196/50029 PMID: 38015589

Haddad, N., Carr, M., Balian, S., Lannin, J., Kim, Y., Toth, C., & Jarvis, J. (2022). The blood–brain barrier and pharmacokinetic/pharmacodynamic optimization of antibiotics for the treatment of central nervous system infections in adults. *Antibiotics (Basel, Switzerland)*, *11*(12), 1843. DOI: 10.3390/antibiotics11121843 PMID: 36551500

Hahn, A., Podbielski, A., Meyer, T., Zautner, A. E., Loderstädt, U., Schwarz, N. G., Krüger, A., Cadar, D., & Frickmann, H. (2020). On detection thresholds–a review on diagnostic approaches in the infectious disease laboratory and the interpretation of their results. *Acta Tropica, 205*, 105377. DOI: 10.1016/j.actatropica.2020.105377 PMID: 32007448

Hawker, J., Begg, N., Reintjes, R., Ekdahl, K., Edeghere, O., & Van Steenbergen, J. E. (2019). *Communicable disease control and health protection handbook*. John Wiley & Sons. DOI: 10.1002/9781119328070

Henao-Martínez, A. F., & Vela-Duarte, D. (2018). Cryptococcal meningitis and other opportunistic fungal infections of the central nervous system: epidemiology, pathogenesis, diagnosis, and treatment. In *The Microbiology of Central Nervous System Infections* (pp. 261–278). Academic Press. DOI: 10.1016/B978-0-12-813806-9.00013-5

Kakooza-Mwesige, A., Tshala-Katumbay, D., & Juliano, S. L. (2019). Viral infections of the central nervous system in Africa. *Brain Research Bulletin, 145*, 2–17. DOI: 10.1016/j.brainresbull.2018.12.019 PMID: 30658129

Kanungo, R., & Anupurba, S. (2023). Association of Viral and Fungal Infections of the CNS During Immunosuppression. In *Viral and Fungal Infections of the Central Nervous System: A Microbiological Perspective* (pp. 465–482). Springer Nature Singapore. DOI: 10.1007/978-981-99-6445-1_20

Karvouniaris, M., Brotis, A., Tsiakos, K., Palli, E., & Koulenti, D. (2022). Current perspectives on the diagnosis and management of healthcare-associated ventriculitis and meningitis. *Infection and Drug Resistance, 15*, 697–721. DOI: 10.2147/IDR.S326456 PMID: 35250284

Kaslow, R. A., & Bell, D. M. (2022). Epidemiology and Control: From Principles to Pandemics. In *Viral Infections of Humans: Epidemiology and Control* (pp. 1–80). Springer US. DOI: 10.1007/978-1-4939-9544-8_1-1

Kennedy, P. G. (2021). An overview of viral infections of the nervous system in the immunosuppressed. *Journal of Neurology, 268*(8), 3026–3030. DOI: 10.1007/s00415-020-10265-z PMID: 33048220

Kesidou, E., Theotokis, P., Damianidou, O., Boziki, M., Konstantinidou, N., Taloumtzis, C., Sintila, S.-A., Grigoriadis, P., Evangelopoulos, M. E., Bakirtzis, C., & Simeonidou, C. (2023). CNS Ageing in health and neurodegenerative disorders. *Journal of Clinical Medicine, 12*(6), 2255. DOI: 10.3390/jcm12062255 PMID: 36983254

Khan, F., & Amatya, B. (2020). Medical rehabilitation in pandemics: Towards a new perspective. *Journal of Rehabilitation Medicine*, *52*(4), 1–4. DOI: 10.2340/16501977-2676 PMID: 32271393

Kozyolkin, O. A., Vizir, I. V., & Sikorskay, M. V. (2023). Infectious and parasitic disease of the nervous system: Textbook for students-foreign citizen IV course of medical faculties of the speciality. *Medicine*.

Le Govic, Y., Demey, B., Cassereau, J., Bahn, Y. S., & Papon, N. (2022). Pathogens infecting the central nervous system. *PLoS Pathogens*, *18*(2), e1010234. DOI: 10.1371/journal.ppat.1010234 PMID: 35202445

Li, P., Lee, G. H., Kim, S. Y., Kwon, S. Y., Kim, H. R., & Park, S. (2021). From diagnosis to treatment: Recent advances in patient-friendly biosensors and implantable devices. *ACS Nano*, *15*(2), 1960–2004. DOI: 10.1021/acsnano.0c06688 PMID: 33534541

Li, S., Nguyen, I. P., & Urbanczyk, K. (2020). Common infectious diseases of the central nervous system—Clinical features and imaging characteristics. *Quantitative Imaging in Medicine and Surgery*, *10*(12), 2227–2259. DOI: 10.21037/qims-20-886 PMID: 33269224

Li, S., Nguyen, I. P., & Urbanczyk, K. (2020). Common infectious diseases of the central nervous system—Clinical features and imaging characteristics. *Quantitative Imaging in Medicine and Surgery*, *10*(12), 2227–2259. DOI: 10.21037/qims-20-886 PMID: 33269224

Littera, R., Campagna, M., Deidda, S., Angioni, G., Cipri, S., Melis, M., Firinu, D., Santus, S., Lai, A., Porcella, R., Lai, S., Rassu, S., Scioscia, R., Meloni, F., Schirru, D., Cordeddu, W., Kowalik, M. A., Serra, M., Ragatzu, P., & Chessa, L. (2020). Human leukocyte antigen complex and other immunogenetic and clinical factors influence susceptibility or protection to SARS-CoV-2 infection and severity of the disease course. The Sardinian experience. *Frontiers in Immunology*, *11*, 605688. DOI: 10.3389/fimmu.2020.605688 PMID: 33343579

Littera, R., Campagna, M., Deidda, S., Angioni, G., Cipri, S., Melis, M., Firinu, D., Santus, S., Lai, A., Porcella, R., Lai, S., Rassu, S., Scioscia, R., Meloni, F., Schirru, D., Cordeddu, W., Kowalik, M. A., Serra, M., Ragatzu, P., & Chessa, L. (2020). Human leukocyte antigen complex and other immunogenetic and clinical factors influence susceptibility or protection to SARS-CoV-2 infection and severity of the disease course. The Sardinian experience. *Frontiers in Immunology*, *11*, 605688. DOI: 10.3389/fimmu.2020.605688 PMID: 33343579

Ludden, C., Raven, K. E., Jamrozy, D., Gouliouris, T., Blane, B., Coll, F., de Goffau, M., Naydenova, P., Horner, C., Hernandez-Garcia, J., Wood, P., Hadjirin, N., Radakovic, M., Brown, N. M., Holmes, M., Parkhill, J., & Peacock, S. J. (2019). One health genomic surveillance of Escherichia coli demonstrates distinct lineages and mobile genetic elements in isolates from humans versus livestock. *mBio*, *10*(1), 10–1128. DOI: 10.1128/mBio.02693-18 PMID: 30670621

Mahmoudinezhad Dezfouli, S. M., & Khosravi, S. (2021). Impact of Meningitis on Cognitive Skills and Development in Children. *Indian Journal of Forensic Medicine Toxicology*, *15*(1).

Mannebach, K., Dressel, A., & Eason, L. (2022). Pediatric tuberculosis in India: Justice and human rights. *Public Health Nursing (Boston, Mass.)*, *39*(5), 1058–1064. DOI: 10.1111/phn.13061 PMID: 35152480

Martín-Noguerol, T., Paulano-Godino, F., Riascos, R. F., Calabia-del-Campo, J., Márquez-Rivas, J., & Luna, A. (2019). Hybrid computed tomography and magnetic resonance imaging 3D printed models for neurosurgery planning. *Annals of Translational Medicine*, *7*(22), 684. DOI: 10.21037/atm.2019.10.109 PMID: 31930085

McMaughan, D. J., Oloruntoba, O., & Smith, M. L. (2020). Socioeconomic status and access to healthcare: Interrelated drivers for healthy aging. *Frontiers in Public Health*, *8*, 512143. DOI: 10.3389/fpubh.2020.00231 PMID: 32626678

Milburn, J., Suresh, R., Doyle, R., & Jarvis, J. N. (2024). The diagnosis of central nervous system infections in resource-limited settings and the use of novel and molecular diagnostic platforms to improve diagnosis. *Expert Review of Molecular Diagnostics*, *24*(3), 1–12. DOI: 10.1080/14737159.2024.2317414 PMID: 38369939

Mohebalizadeh, M., Babapour, G., Maleki Aghdam, M., Mohammadi, T., Jafari, R., & Shafiei-Irannejad, V. (2023). Role of Maternal Immune Factors in Neuroimmunology of Brain Development. *Molecular Neurobiology*, 1–13. PMID: 38057641

Molloy, S. F., Kanyama, C., Heyderman, R. S., Loyse, A., Kouanfack, C., Chanda, D., Mfinanga, S., Temfack, E., Lakhi, S., Lesikari, S., Chan, A. K., Stone, N., Kalata, N., Karunaharan, N., Gaskell, K., Peirse, M., Ellis, J., Chawinga, C., Lontsi, S., & Harrison, T. S. (2018). Antifungal combinations for treatment of cryptococcal meningitis in Africa. *The New England Journal of Medicine*, *378*(11), 1004–1017. DOI: 10.1056/NEJMoa1710922 PMID: 29539274

Muschol, N., Giugliani, R., Jones, S. A., Muenzer, J., Smith, N. J., Whitley, C. B., Donnell, M., Drake, E., Elvidge, K., Melton, L., & O'Neill, C.MPS III Guideline Development Group. (2022). Sanfilippo syndrome: Consensus guidelines for clinical care. *Orphanet Journal of Rare Diseases*, *17*(1), 391. DOI: 10.1186/s13023-022-02484-6 PMID: 36303195

Nathan, C. L., Emmert, B. E., Nelson, E., & Berger, J. R. (2021). CNS fungal infections: A review. *Journal of the Neurological Sciences*, *422*, 117325. DOI: 10.1016/j.jns.2021.117325 PMID: 33516057

Ngarka, L., Siewe Fodjo, J. N., Aly, E., Masocha, W., & Njamnshi, A. K. (2022). The interplay between neuroinfections, the immune system and neurological disorders: A focus on Africa. *Frontiers in Immunology*, *12*, 803475. DOI: 10.3389/fimmu.2021.803475 PMID: 35095888

Noe, C. R., Noe-Letschnig, M., Handschuh, P., Noe, C. A., & Lanzenberger, R. (2020). Dysfunction of the blood-brain barrier—A key step in neurodegeneration and dementia. *Frontiers in Aging Neuroscience*, *12*, 185. DOI: 10.3389/fnagi.2020.00185 PMID: 32848697

Owolabi, M. O., Leonardi, M., Bassetti, C., Jaarsma, J., Hawrot, T., Makanjuola, A. I., Dhamija, R. K., Feng, W., Straub, V., Camaradou, J., Dodick, D. W., Sunna, R., Menon, B., Wright, C., Lynch, C., Chadha, A. S., Ferretti, M. T., Dé, A., Catsman-Berrevoets, C. E., & Servadei, F. (2023). Global synergistic actions to improve brain health for human development. *Nature Reviews. Neurology*, *19*(6), 371–383. DOI: 10.1038/s41582-023-00808-z PMID: 37208496

Palacios-Pedrero, M. Á., Osterhaus, A. D., Becker, T., Elbahesh, H., Rimmelzwaan, G. F., & Saletti, G. (2021). Aging and options to halt declining immunity to virus infections. *Frontiers in Immunology*, *12*, 681449. DOI: 10.3389/fimmu.2021.681449 PMID: 34054872

Parenteau, A. M., Boyer, C. J., Campos, L. J., Carranza, A. F., Deer, L. K., Hartman, D. T., & Hostinar, C. E. (2022). A review of mental health disparities during COVID-19: Evidence, mechanisms, and policy recommendations for promoting societal resilience. *Development and Psychopathology*, 1–22. PMID: 36097815

Platt, F. M. (2018). Emptying the stores: Lysosomal diseases and therapeutic strategies. *Nature Reviews. Drug Discovery*, *17*(2), 133–150. DOI: 10.1038/nrd.2017.214 PMID: 29147032

Pruitt, A. A. (2018). Central Nervous System Infections in Patients Receiving Cancer Therapies. *Cancer Neurology in Clinical Practice: Neurological Complications of Cancer and its Treatment*, 377-396.

Pruitt, A. A. (2021). Central nervous system infections in immunocompromised patients. *Current Neurology and Neuroscience Reports*, *21*(7), 37. DOI: 10.1007/s11910-021-01119-w PMID: 34037866

Pruitt, A. A. (2021). Central nervous system infections in immunocompromised patients. *Current Neurology and Neuroscience Reports*, *21*(7), 37. DOI: 10.1007/s11910-021-01119-w PMID: 34037866

Rahman, M. (2023). Magnetic resonance imaging in personalized medicine. In *Metabolomics* (pp. 199–238). Academic Press. DOI: 10.1016/B978-0-323-99924-3.00001-7

Riddell, I. V. J.IV, & Shuman, E. K. (2012). Epidemiology of central nervous system infection. *Neuroimaging Clinics of North America*, *22*(4), 543–556. DOI: 10.1016/j.nic.2012.05.003 PMID: 23122256

Rios, P., Radhakrishnan, A., Thomas, S. M., Darvesh, N., Straus, S. E., & Tricco, A. C. (2020). Guidelines for preventing respiratory illness in older adults aged 60 years and above living in long-term care: A rapid review of clinical practice guidelines. medRxiv, 2020-03.

Rizzo, M. R., & Paolisso, G. (2021). SARS-CoV-2 emergency and long-term cognitive impairment in older people. *Aging and Disease*, *12*(2), 345. DOI: 10.14336/AD.2021.0109 PMID: 33815868

Robertson, F. C., Lepard, J. R., Mekary, R. A., Davis, M. C., Yunusa, I., Gormley, W. B., Baticulon, R. E., Mahmud, M. R., Misra, B. K., Rattani, A., Dewan, M. C., & Park, K. B. (2018). Epidemiology of central nervous system infectious diseases: A meta-analysis and systematic review with implications for neurosurgeons worldwide. *Journal of Neurosurgery*, *130*(4), 1107–1126. DOI: 10.3171/2017.10.JNS17359 PMID: 29905514

Salam, M. A., Al-Amin, M. Y., Salam, M. T., Pawar, J. S., Akhter, N., Rabaan, A. A., & Alqumber, M. A. (2023, July). Antimicrobial resistance: A growing serious threat for global public health. *Health Care*, *11*(13), 1946. PMID: 37444780

Schwartz, S., Kontoyiannis, D. P., Harrison, T., & Ruhnke, M. (2018). Advances in the diagnosis and treatment of fungal infections of the CNS. *Lancet Neurology*, *17*(4), 362–372. DOI: 10.1016/S1474-4422(18)30030-9 PMID: 29477506

Shahzad, K., & Mati, W. (2020). Advances in magnetic resonance imaging (MRI). In *Advances in Medical and Surgical Engineering* (pp. 121-142). Academic Press.

Sharma, S., & Sethi, G. R. (2021). *Standard Treatment Guidelines—A Manual for Medical Therapeutics, 6e*. Wolters Kluwer India Pvt. Ltd.

Shrestha, G. S., Nepal, G., & Prust, M. L. (2024, March). Developing Systems of Emergency and Inpatient Neurologic Care in Resource-Limited Settings. In *Seminars in neurology*. Thieme Medical Publishers, Inc. DOI: 10.1055/s-0043-1778638

Singh, G., Tucker, E. W., & Rohlwink, U. K. (2022). Infection in the developing brain: The role of unique systemic Immune Vulnerabilities. *Frontiers in Neurology*, *12*, 805643. DOI: 10.3389/fneur.2021.805643 PMID: 35140675

Singh, P., Gupta, K., Sharma, M., & Kumar, S. (2024). Molecular and Cellular Mechanism of Pathogen Invasion into the Central Nervous System: Meningitis. In *Mechanism and Genetic Susceptibility of Neurological Disorders* (pp. 317–340). Springer Nature Singapore. DOI: 10.1007/978-981-99-9404-5_14

Sivapathasundharam, B., Gururaj, N., & Ranganathan, K. (2020). Viral infections. *Shafer's Textbook of Oral Pathology E-book*, 327.

Socha, W., Kwasnik, M., Larska, M., Rola, J., & Rozek, W. (2022). Vector-borne viral diseases as a current threat for human and animal health—One Health perspective. *Journal of Clinical Medicine*, *11*(11), 3026. DOI: 10.3390/jcm11113026 PMID: 35683413

Srivastava, N., Deval, H., Mittal, M., Kant, R., & Bondre, V. P. (2022). The outbreaks of acute encephalitis syndrome in Uttar Pradesh, India (1978–2020) and its effective management: A remarkable public health success story. *Frontiers in Public Health*, *9*, 793268. DOI: 10.3389/fpubh.2021.793268 PMID: 35223759

Straif-Bourgeois, S., Tonzel, J. L., Kretzschmar, M., & Ratard, R. (2023). Infectious disease epidemiology. In *Handbook of epidemiology* (pp. 1–79). Springer New York. DOI: 10.1007/978-1-4614-6625-3_34-1

Strein, M., Holton-Burke, J. P., Smith, L. R., & Brophy, G. M. (2019). Prevention, treatment, and monitoring of seizures in the intensive care unit. *Journal of Clinical Medicine*, *8*(8), 1177. DOI: 10.3390/jcm8081177 PMID: 31394791

Surianarayanan, C., Lawrence, J. J., Chelliah, P. R., Prakash, E., & Hewage, C. (2023). Convergence of Artificial Intelligence and Neuroscience towards the Diagnosis of Neurological Disorders—A Scoping Review. *Sensors (Basel)*, *23*(6), 3062. DOI: 10.3390/s23063062 PMID: 36991773

Suthar, R., & Sankhyan, N. (2019). Bacterial infections of the central nervous system. *Indian Journal of Pediatrics*, *86*(1), 60–69. DOI: 10.1007/s12098-017-2477-z PMID: 29297142

Taha, A. R. (2020). Central Nervous System Infection. *Highly Infectious Diseases in Critical Care: A Comprehensive Clinical Guide*, 147-174.

Tazerji, S. S., Nardini, R., Safdar, M., Shehata, A. A., & Duarte, P. M. (2022). An overview of anthropogenic actions as drivers for emerging and re-emerging zoonotic diseases. *Pathogens (Basel, Switzerland), 11*(11), 1376. DOI: 10.3390/pathogens11111376 PMID: 36422627

Terreni, M., Taccani, M., & Pregnolato, M. (2021). New antibiotics for multidrug-resistant bacterial strains: Latest research developments and future perspectives. *Molecules (Basel, Switzerland), 26*(9), 2671. DOI: 10.3390/molecules26092671 PMID: 34063264

Testa, C. M., & Jankovic, J. (2019). Huntington disease: A quarter century of progress since the gene discovery. *Journal of the Neurological Sciences, 396*, 52–68. DOI: 10.1016/j.jns.2018.09.022 PMID: 30419368

Towfighi, A., Berger, R. P., Corley, A. M., Glymour, M. M., Manly, J. J., & Skolarus, L. E. (2023). Recommendations on social determinants of health in neurologic disease. *Neurology, 101*(7, Supplement_1), S17–S26. DOI: 10.1212/WNL.0000000000207562 PMID: 37580147

Tsafaras, G. P., Ntontsi, P., & Xanthou, G. (2020). Advantages and limitations of the neonatal immune system. *Frontiers in Pediatrics, 8*, 5. DOI: 10.3389/fped.2020.00005 PMID: 32047730

Wang, F., Kream, R. M., & Stefano, G. B. (2020). Long-term respiratory and neurological sequelae of COVID-19. *Medical Science Monitor, 26*, e928996–e1. DOI: 10.12659/MSM.928996 PMID: 33177481

Weaver, A. K., Head, J. R., Gould, C. F., Carlton, E. J., & Remais, J. V. (2022). Environmental factors influencing COVID-19 incidence and severity. *Annual Review of Public Health, 43*(1), 271–291. DOI: 10.1146/annurev-publhealth-052120-101420 PMID: 34982587

World Health Organization. 2. (2020). *Guidance on COVID-19 for the care of older people and people living in long-term care facilities, other non-acute care facilities and home care* (No. WPR/DSE/2020/015). WHO Regional Office for the Western Pacific.

World Health Organization. (2021). *Consolidated guidelines on HIV prevention, testing, treatment, service delivery and monitoring: recommendations for a public health approach*. World Health Organization.

Xu, W., Wong, G., Hwang, Y. Y., & Larbi, A. (2020, October). The untwining of immunosenescence and aging. *Seminars in Immunopathology, 42*(5), 559–572. DOI: 10.1007/s00281-020-00824-x PMID: 33165716

Yadav, N., & Upadhyay, R. K. (2023). Global effect of climate change on seasonal cycles, vector population and rising challenges of communicable diseases: A review. *Journal of Atmospheric Science Research*, *6*(1), 21–59. DOI: 10.30564/jasr.v6i1.5165

Zinserling, V. (2022). *Infectious Lesions of the Central Nervous System*. Springer Nature. DOI: 10.1007/978-3-030-96260-9

Chapter 2
Acute Bacterial Meningitis:
Current Perspectives on Epidemiology, Pathophysiology, Diagnosis, and Treatment

Bilal El-Mansoury
https://orcid.org/0000-0002-2583-7515
Faculty of Sciences, Chouaib Doukkali University, Morocco

Hanane El Fatimi
Mohammed VI University of Health Sciences, Morocco

Ayyoub Skaou
https://orcid.org/0009-0003-7981-2473
Faculty of Science Semlalia, Cadi Ayyad University, Morocco

Soraia El-Baz
Faculty of Science Semlalia, Cadi Ayyad University, Morocco

El Mehdi Dalil
Faculty of Medicine and Pharmacy, Cadi Ayyad University, Morocco

Taoufik Adoch
Faculty of Medicine and Pharmacy, Cadi Ayyad University, Morocco

Nadia Zouhairi
Faculty of Sciences and Techniques, Beni Mellal, Morocco

Abdelaati El Khiat
Higher Institute of Nursing Professions and Health Techniques, Ministry of Health, Ouarzazate, Morocco

Jawad Laadraoui
https://orcid.org/0000-0002-9784-1265
Faculty of Science Aïn Chock, Hassan II University, Morocco

DOI: 10.4018/979-8-3693-4070-7.ch002

ABSTRACT

Acute bacterial meningitis is an inflammation of the meninges, the protective layers of the central nervous system (CNS) and the cerebrospinal fluid (CSF), secondary to bacterial infection. Symptoms of bacterial meningitis (BM) can be manifested by stiff neck, headache, fever, confusion or altered mental status, nausea, and vomiting. The pathogens responsible for bacterial meningitis vary according to several factors, including the patient's age and geographic location. The main germs responsible for bacterial meningitis are Neisseria meningitidis (meningococcus), Streptococcus pneumoniae (pneumococcus), and Haemophilus influenzae. The neurological complications of meningitis, such as hearing loss, hydrocephalus, increased intracranial pressure and brain damage are of particular concern. Early diagnosis, preventive strategies, and appropriate treatment are of great importance to prevent serious complications. This chapter provides an overview on the BM epidemiology, pathophysiology, diagnostic, and treatment as well as preventive strategies.

INTRODUCTION

Acute bacterial meningitis (acute BM) is a life-threatening infection characterized by a rapid onset of inflammation in the meninges, the protective membranes surrounding the brain and spinal cord. It typically results from bacterial invasion of the central nervous system (CNS), often following bloodstream infection, direct extension from nearby structures, or trauma. The most common causative pathogens include *Streptococcus pneumoniae*, *Neisseria meningitidis*, and *Haemophilus influenzae*. The establishment of an infection in an anatomical region with compromised host resistance necessitates a comprehensive understanding of its pathogenesis and pathophysiology. This is crucial for deciphering the mechanisms driving disease progression and for developing effective therapeutic interventions. The study of infectious diseases has historically centered on non-indigenous microorganisms, often termed "pathogens," as primary contributors to disease etiopathogenesis. Their role in triggering and sustaining infections has been a cornerstone of research, guiding the development of diagnostic, preventive, and therapeutic strategies (El-Mansoury et al., 2023).

BM remains a major public health issue worldwide. The development of the *Haemophilus influenzae* type b vaccine relied on well-designed animal models of MB. These simulations, as well as those using tissue culture, have helped to advance our understanding of BM. Despite adequate antimicrobial therapy, the disease is fatal in 5% to 40% of patients and results in neurological consequences in up to 30% of survivors. The neurological consequences are primarily of three types: deafness or hearing loss caused by extension of inflammation from the subarachnoid space (SAS) to the inner ear; obstructed hydrocephalus; and damage to the brain parenchyma, resulting in seizures, mental retardation, focal sensory/motor deficits, or a combination of these symptoms (Leib & Tauber, 1999).

MB is prevalent worldwide and evolves in two modes: the first is the endemic-sporadic or ubiquitous mode with variable pathogens. This form occurs globally, although predominant in tropical areas. The second mode is epidemic due mainly to meningococci and which is prevalent especially in the African meningitis belt. Several germs are responsible for these MBs, among which the most frequent are: *N. meningitidis* (the meningococcus) and *S. pneumoniae* (the pneumococcus).

To improve treatment results, research on the pathogenesis and pathophysiology of MB has focused on bacterial and host factors that are responsible for some notable pathophysiological alterations, such as CSF pleocytosis, an increase in intracranial pressure, cerebral edema, and neuronal injury. In addition, immediate diagnosis is necessary to treat the disease and avoid its complications. This chapter provides a recent literature review on acute BM focusing on several aspects including epidemiology, and pathogenesis as well as treatment and prevention.

EPIDEMIOLOGY

Acute BM causes substantial illness and death globally, with the greatest burden in developing countries where healthcare resources are limited. This is largely due to the high incidence of certain pathogenic bacteria such as Streptococcus pneumoniae (pneumococcus), *Neisseria meningitidis* (meningococcus), and *Haemophilus influenzae* type b (HIB), which are the main causes of BM accounting for more than 80% of cases (Nudelman & Tunkel, 2009). The occurrence of acute bacterial meningitis differs from one region of the world to another and is affected by factors such as access to healthcare, vaccination, socio-economic and environmental conditions, as well as epidemiological surveillance. The epidemiology of BM has significantly changed. In the UK and Western Europe, the incidence is 1-2 cases per 100,000 people per year, while it can reach 1,000 cases per 100,000 people per year in the African meningitis belt (Lamridi, 2017). The frequency of BM significantly decreased in a surveillance study carried out in 1995 in laboratories servicing all acute care hospitals in four states with populations more than 10 million (Schuchat et al., 1997). A study conducted in Brazil has shown a mortality rate of 33% among infected patients (Zender et al, 2009). In the United States, *Streptococcus pneumoniae* has been previously reported as the most commonly observed bacterium, accounting for nearly half of acute BM cases (Schuchat et al., 1997). Thus, BM in the United States shifted from being a condition mostly affecting children and adults (Nudelman & Tunkel, 2009).

The introduction of the pneumococcal conjugate vaccine in 2000 resulted in a further drop in incidence, according to a different surveillance study that collected data from 1998 to 2003 (Thigpen et al., 2011). The largest review of about 4100 cases of BM in Salvador, Brazil, between 1973 and 1982 found that the overall attack rate was 45.8 cases per 100,000 people, with *H. influenzae*, *N. meningitidis*, and *S. pneumoniae* accounting for 62% of cases (Bryan et al., 1990). In a UK study, these same micorganisms were responsible for 74% of cases (Noah, 1987). In a another single-center analysis of 103 cases of bacterial meningitis from Canada between 1985 and 1996, *S. pneumoniae* was the most common pathogen (~53% of cases) (Hussein & Shafran, 2000), and *L. monocytogenes* was the second most common isolate (~13% of cases). In certain impoverished parts of the world, BM is an even more serious issue. Meningeal pathogens are responsible for one of the highest illness burdens in the world, which is found in Sub-Saharan Africa (Nudelman & Tunkel, 2009). Additionally, in 2000, *S. pneumoniae* and *H. influenzae* type B caused 500 000 deaths in the region (Peltola, 2000). Over the previous ten years, *N. meningitidis* caused recurring epidemics of meningitis that resulted in about 700 000 cases (Nudelman & Tunkel, 2009). Vaccination programs against these pathogens have played a crucial role in reducing the incidence of bacterial meningitis in many countries where they are widely applied. As a result, vaccination has helped to reduce the prevalence of these devastating diseases and saved many lives.

PATHOPHYSIOLOGY

The most common bacteria causing acute BM (*S. pneumoniae*, *N. meningitidis*, and *H. influenzae*) have neurotrophic potential, which allows them to invade the host mucosal epithelium multiply in the bloodstream, and pass through the blood-brain barrier (BBB) into the CSF (Roos et al., 2014). The bacteria adhere to the respiratory tract's epithelial lining in order to colonize the nasopharyngeal epithelium, and the mechanisms involved vary by species (Roos et al., 2014). Hence, Gram-negative bacteria such as *N. meningitidis* cling to surfaces through pili, whereas *S. pneumoniae* attaches itself to surfaces through pneumococcal surface-associated proteins like choline-binding protein A (CbpA) or pneumococcal surface adhesion A (PsaA) (Koedel et al., 2002). There are multiple ways that bacteria can penetrate the BBB: (1) by breaking down tight junctions; (2) by transcytosing across cells; and (3) by living inside phagocytes through a "Trojan horse" mechanism (*Fig. 1*). Additionally, certain interactions between bacteria and hosts can occur, such as those involving cell signal transduction pathways that impact actin cytoskeleton configurations (Kim, 2003).

To survive in the bloodstream, the bacteria must evade the host's defense, especially complement-dependent death. Both *N. meningitidis* and *S. pneumoniae* enlist complement factor H, which is the primary regulator of the alternative complement pathway that governs the early activation of the complement cascade. The proteins CbpA and PspC, which are produced by *S. pneumoniae*, bind complement factor H, while *N. meningitidis* generates factor H binding protein (Roos et al., 2014). Despite epithelial invasion, most immunocompetent individuals have mucosal immunity that eliminates *S. pneumoniae* and *N. meningitidis* colonization of the nasopharynx (Weight et al., 2019). Pneumococcal and meningococcal invasion are linked to co-infection with S. pneumoniae and respiratory viruses, such as influenza (Aguilera & Lenz, 2020; Jochems et al., 2018; Loh et al., 2013). In addition, influenza infection preceding the influenza season has been linked to seasonal acute BM (Salomon et al., 2020). Typically, bacteremia occurs prior to translocation into the CNS through the CSF or the BBB (Wall et al., 2021).

INFECTION MODE

Most cases of meningeal infection occur via the bloodstream, from a distant source of infection, notably the naso-oropharyngeal sphere, or in infants, from a maternal infection. In this way, meningitis is preceded or followed by a bacterial infection. Much more rarely, meningitis is caused by bacterial invasion through continuity, following otitis or sinus disease, dermal sinus, myelomeningocele, direct communication between the mucosa and meninges caused by various bone malformations, or fracture of the skull base, particularly the cribriform lamina (Leib & Tauber, 1999). When bacteria enter the body, they migrate to the oropharynx, where they form “commensal bacteria”. With the help of certain factors, the body's immunity is lowered, allowing the infection to spread through the bloodstream and into the brain. This marks the start of a new episode of meningitis, which can lead to multiple complications and neurosensory sequelae. The seriousness of these conditions lies in the inflammatory phenomena they can generate.

Penetration of Germs Into the CSF

BM develops when bacteria enter the CSF, multiply and produce inflammation. The first step is colonization of the oropharyngeal mucosa by surface pili (meningococcus, Haemophilus), proteases destroying secretory IgA and capsule polysaccharides (pneumococcus, Haemophilus). Under certain, as yet unidentified conditions, bacteria become invasive and access the CSF through multiple mechanisms:

- ✓ Bacteremia increases thanks to capsulation, which enables bacteria to escape phagocytosis and complement. The meninges are hematogenously seeded and the CSF is invaded, followed by crossing of the BBB at the ECM and choroid plexus levels. During this reaction, the presence of circulating post-vaccination serum antibodies can help prevent infection;
- ✓ Invasion by contiguity, favored by a neighboring infection or anatomical breach;
- ✓ Direct contamination may result from a cranio-vertebral wound, paraclinical investigations, spinal anesthesia or neurosurgery;
- ✓ In around 20% of cases, the origin of CNS infection remains unknown.

Inflammatory Response

An inflammatory reaction is triggered by bacterial multiplication and autolysis. Damage to the brain parenchyma is caused by the host's inflammatory response, rather than by the pathogen itself, overcoming its purpose (Deckert, 2018). As a result of the inflammation, the BBB is altered and vasculitis occurs. When bacteria enter the CSF, they multiply easily, given the immune defense mechanisms deficiency (complement is almost absent in CSF, with very low levels of immunoglobulin) (Elmakrini, 2014).

Thanks to bacterial virulence factors (lipopolysaccharides, peptidoglycan, techoic acids), meningeal macrophages synthesize cytokines: interleukin 1 (IL-1) and tumor necrosis factor alpha (TNFα), as well as IL-6 and IL-8. These cytokines are responsible for the expression of several adhesins on the surface of neutrophils and endothelial cells in meningeal venules, enabling the adhesion of neutrophils to endothelial cells and their subsequent influx into the CSF.

The BBB is altered by several mechanisms:

- Decreased sealing (mediated mainly by IL-1 in synergy with TNFα), through the opening of tight junctions in cerebral capillaries,
- Release by cytokine-activated polynuclear cells of various mediators, especially free radicals. Increased permeability of the BBB, which causes hyperproteinorachia due to albumin infiltration, and also favors the influx of inflammatory cells that will help to excite the inflammatory reaction (with risk of cerebral edema), also favoring the diffusion of antibiotics into the CSF.

Brain Consequences of These Events

The neurological consequences of BM can be classified into three categories: firstly, hearing loss, mainly due to direct invasion of the inner ear by inflammation of the subarachnoid space; secondly, obstructive hydrocephalus; and thirdly, damage to the brain parenchyma, leading to neurological consequences such as focal sensorimotor deficits, mental retardation and seizure disorders. It has become clear over the last three decades that bacterial proliferation in the CNS compartment provokes a host response accompanied by an excessive increase in inflammation. In recent years, some of the inflammatory and neurotoxic factors that contribute to neuronal damage in meningitis have been discovered (Tunkel & Scheld, 1993). Consequently, treatment strategies for bacterial meningitis have expanded beyond eradication of the causative pathogen with antibiotics to include approaches aimed at mitigating the harmful effects of the host immune response. The use of corticosteroids is one example of therapies aimed at regulating and reducing inflammation in BM. Current concepts in the pathophysiology of the disease are reviewed in this article, with an emphasis on the various therapeutic strategies available to prevent brain damage.

Figure 1. Pathogenesis of bacterial meningitis. Neisseria meningitidis entry into the CNS, initiate by the adherence and colonization of mucosal epithelium then invasion into systemic circulation and they multiplied. After that, they penetrate the BBB by living inside phagocytes through a "Trojan horse'' pathway. Infiltration of CSF by white cells elicits the release of pro-inflammatory cytokines. Additionally, the bacterial products that stimulate the inflammatory cascade, all these result inflammations of the meninges. Consequently, bacterial invasion and the host response to infection lead to neuronal injury, edema and increased intracranial pressure.

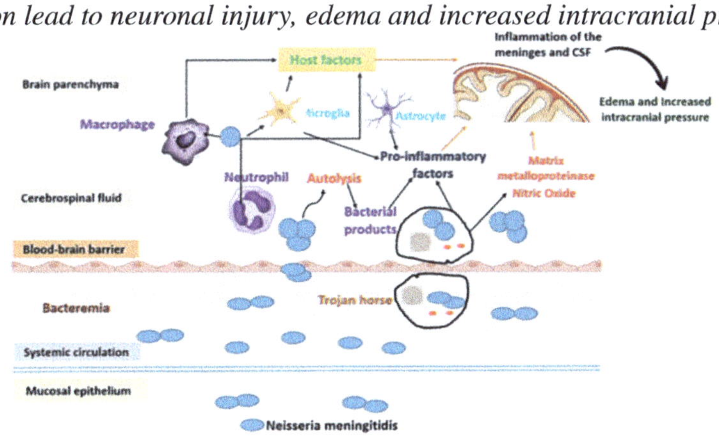

ETIOLOGY

The etiology of BM varies with age and geography. The three most common germs are Haemophilus, pneumococcus and meningococcus.

Bacteriological Characteristics of Causative Germs

Neisseria Meningitidis

The morphology of *N. meningitidis* is asymmetrical, coffee-bean shaped. They are Gram-negative, measuring 0.8 to 1 micron in diameter, and there are several serogroups: A, B, C, X, Y, Z, 29-E, and W-135 (WHO, 1995). *N. meningitidis* is a strictly human germ that colonizes asymptomatic nasopharyngeal carriage (Organization, 1995). It is a Gram-negative, immobile coccis, organized as diplococci with a flattened face, or as aerobically strict tetrads (but requiring CO2 enrichment). Bacteria are vulnerable to temperature changes, requiring rich culture media such as cooked blood or chocolate agar (Arsalane et al., 2023), whether supplemented or not (Polyvitex®, Supplement G).

Haemophilus Influenza

The *Haemophilus influenzae* bacillus is small (0.3 to 0.4 µm in diameter and 1.5 µm long), highly diverse, often Cocco bacillus-shaped, immobile, sporeless and sometimes enveloped. They are gram-negative. The rod usually forms in small clusters, similar to schools of fish moving along the water's edge. This grouping is rather typical. It can adopt a longer, filamentous form, and some strains possess pili or fimbriae that give the bacterium characteristics of adherence to epithelial cells and agglutination of red blood cells. Electron microscopy shows that its wall is made up of three layers, with the characteristic structure of Gram-negative bacilli (Lemkhoudem, 2022).

Streptococcus Pneumonia

S. pneumoniae is a bacterial species in the Streptococcaceae family, which includes over 80 species. It includes gram-positive cocci, which have neither catalases nor cytochrome oxidases, and ferment glucose to produce lactic acid. Humans are colonized by a commensal bacterium called *S. pneumoniae*. It lives mainly in the nasopharynx. The proportion of people colonized depends mainly on age, childcare, siblings, socio-economic conditions, season, concomitant viral infection, vaccination status and recent antibiotic therapy. Microscopically, a gram-positive cocci can be observed, usually encapsulated (with a clear halo around the bacterium), with a lanceolate shape (like a candle flame), usually grouped together in diplococci or sometimes isolated in chains (Arsalane et al., 2023).

DIAGNOSTIC

Clinical Diagnosis

The Meningeal Syndrome

It is distinguished by key symptoms such as headache, vomiting and constipation, all of which are referred to as the "meningeal tripod". When vomiting and constipation persist, headaches become more intense. Physical examination is complicated by hyperesthesia of the skin, leading to stiffness of the neck and KERNIG and BURDZINSKI signs. Separate paralysis of the external eye musculature and photophobia may also be present (Keita, 2011).

Infectious Syndrome

The infectious syndrome is characterized by fever, rapid heartbeat and skin vulnerability. Certain clues suggest a meningococcal infection. For example, in addition to herpes labialis, cutaneous purpura, joint pain and a palpable spleen would be observed, confirming the septicemic spread confirmed by blood cultures (Keita, 2011).

Biological Diagnosis

BM is quite common, can develop rapidly and cause death or permanent loss of strength. The presence of this infection legitimately provokes intense emotional reactions and, hopefully, prompt medical intervention. For clinical microbiology laboratory professionals, it is essential to be familiar with the methods used to detect bacteria and bacterial antigens present in CSF, and to always be aware that the results of these tests must always be communicated immediately. The academic and practical aspects of laboratory diagnosis of BM, such as: Meningeal anatomy, pathogenesis, change in CSF composition, etiological agents, treating CSF, CSF microscopy, CSF culture, approaches to detecting bacterial antigens and bacterial components in CSF (counterimmunoelectrophoresis, coagglutination, latex agglutination, enzyme-linked immunosorbent assay, Limulus amebocyte lysate test and gas-liquid chromatography), the use of polymerase chain reaction, and practical considerations for evaluating bacterial antigens in vitro (Gray & Fedorko, 1992).

On the other hand, the most important investigation is lumbar puncture (LP), which allows for quick confirmation of the type of infecting organism and meningitis. Diagnostic yield of LP can be reduced, especially for mycobacterium, by collecting small volumes of CSF. Since many patients with acute BM present with altered consciousness, clinicians often request cranial imaging before performing a diagnostic lumbar puncture. Early LP is strongly associated with higher diagnostic yield from the CSF; delays in LP for cranial imaging lead to significant reductions in yield from either CSF bacterial culture or PCR (McGill et al., 2018). Postponement of LP is linked to worsen clinical outcomes (Hasbun et al., 2001; McGill et al., 2018; Michael et al., 2010). Therefore, for the majority of patients with suspected acute BM, cranial imaging (either CT or MRI) is not advised in those with obvious clinical signs and symptoms of meningitis without focal neurology (Glimåker et al., 2018; Salazar & Hasbun, 2017). When predicting the probability of cerebral herniation in acute BM, CT exhibits low inter-reporting reliability (Costerus et al., 2018).

The examination of CSF is necessary for the diagnosis of acute BM. The leukocyte count continues to be the most reliable indicator of acute BM. Clinical judgement alone is the primary source of advantage when using diagnostic models that incorporate blood, CSF, and clinical data (Azad et al., 2014). Since giving antibiotics before LP frequently makes the CSF sterile, doctors are depending more and more on diagnostic PCR. In cases where there is a high index of clinical suspicion of ABM but no positive PCR test, metagenomics of CSF and direct next generation sequencing (NGS) have been suggested as contemporary methods to identify pathogens (Wilson et al., 2019). According to all guidelines, individuals who have been diagnosed with ABM should start parenteral antibiotics within one hour. Delays in the emergency department, however, restricted the number of patients who met this goal in a clinical research study to just 46% (Costerus et al., 2016). The patient's risk category, allergies, and local recommendations based on epidemiology which takes antimicrobial resistance into account should all be taken into consideration when choosing an antibiotic. In certain situations, penicillin resistance in *S. pneumoniae* can reach 15–20%, while it stays below 5% in *N. meningitidis* (Cornick et al., 2011; Nhantumbo et al., 2016). Nonetheless, *N. meningitidis* quinolone resistance exceeds 70% in Southeast Asia (Wen et al., 2020). Long-term dual antibiotic and antiviral therapy frequently result from diagnostic ambiguity in culture-negative meningitis, which can have unfavorable nosocomial consequences (McGill et al., 2018; Tenforde et al., 2019).

Treatment

Antibiotic Therapy

The most important aspect is initiating treatment as soon as bacterial meningitis is suspected, with prompt administration of empirical antibiotics being crucial to improving survival rates and minimizing complications (Van De Beek et al., 2012), taking into account local epidemiological patterns, the patient's age, and any underlying conditions or risk factors (Brouwer et al., 2010; Tunkel et al., 2004). Hospitalization is mandatory in case of severe symptoms such as loss of consciousness, signs of localization, respiratory failure, coughing, prolonged purpura or frail terrain (Nagafuchi et al., 2006).

In regions where cephalosporin-resistant *Streptococcus pneumoniae* is uncommon (with resistance rates below 1%), third-generation cephalosporins such as cefotaxime or ceftriaxone are generally adequate for empirical treatment. Additionally, vancomycin is costly and often inaccessible in low-income nations (Scarborough & Thwaites, 2008). In such settings, alternative options include antipneumococcal fluoroquinolones (like moxifloxacin) and rifampicin, though there is limited clinical evidence supporting their use (Van De Beek et al., 2012).

Addressing challenges like antibiotic resistance and limited access to healthcare in resource-poor settings requires coordinated global efforts. Antibiotic resistance is driven by overuse and misuse of antibiotics, particularly in regions lacking proper diagnostic tools and regulation, making it a growing public health threat (WHO, 2020). Additionally, many low-income areas face shortages of healthcare providers, medications, and infrastructure, hindering effective treatment. Combating these issues demands strengthening healthcare systems, investing in education, and promoting stewardship programs to manage antibiotic use (Laxminarayan et al., 2016). International support and funding are also crucial for improving access to affordable healthcare services. Without intervention, these challenges may worsen, undermining global health progress.

Treatment According to Isolated Germs

Antibiotic selection should be made carefully based on available data, but treatment should proceed while awaiting lab test results (Brouwer et al., 2012). The length of antibiotic therapy depends on the identified pathogen and typically lasts 21 days or more (Van de Beek et al., 2012). Once the causative microorganism is identified through in vitro testing, the treatment plan can be adjusted accordingly (Mehrdadi, 2019). Additionally, the BBB characteristics and the physicochemical properties of the antibiotics significantly impact their ability to penetrate the CSF (Van de Beek et al., 2012).

In case of positive progression, the attitude depends on the analysis of MICs to amoxicillin and cephalosporins. In the event of positive progression, the attitude depends on the analysis of MICs to amoxicillin and cephalosporins.

- MIC less than or equal to 0.5 mg/L to amoxicillin: return to amoxicillin.
- MIC greater than 0.5 mg/L with amoxicillin but greater than 0.5 mg/L with third-generation cephalosporins: cefotaxime or ceftriaxone.
- MIC greater than 0.5 mg/L to third-generation cephalosporins: cefotaxime or high-dose ceftriaxone + vancomycin; alternatively: vancomycin + rifampin.

Corticosteroid Therapy

Most clinical studies evaluating the efficacy of corticosteroids as adjunctive therapy for community-acquired purulent meningitis have been carried out in children, particularly in cases of *Haemophilus influenzae* meningitis. The frequency of pneumococcal disease explains the mortality and neurological sequelae in adults, underscoring the importance of this issue. Streptococcus pneumoniae wall elements play a similar role to H. influenzae endotoxin in experimental meningitis models, triggering a local inflammatory cascade with adverse consequences. Early administration of dexamethasone also reduces the effects of experimental meningitis, particularly on cerebral edema. Previously published research on subgroups of pneumococcal meningitis in pediatric or mixed series also appears to have a positive impact on reducing hearing sequelae and on most of a group of patients hospitalized in Cairo. A randomized, double-blind trial was conducted to evaluate dexamethasone therapy (40 mg/day for 3 days) in primary bacterial meningitis in adults treated with amoxicillin. Of the 60 patients included, 83% were admitted to intensive care and 43% required intubation. There were 31 cases of S. pneumoniae, five of which had reduced penicillin sensitivity, and 18 cases of Neisseria meningitidis. The primary endpoint of the study, the rate of recovery without neurological sequelae at D30, was 52% for the placebo group and 74% for the treatment group (NS). Corticosteroid treatment did not produce any significant adverse effects, as the 2 gastroduodenal ulceration hemorrhages were observed in the placebo group. No definitive proof of the efficacy of adjunctive corticosteroid treatment of purulent meningitis in adults is therefore currently available. This is mainly due to the absence of trials of the required quality or power. The increasing resistance of pneumococcus to betalactam antibiotics may maintain the answer to this question, as this treatment considerably reduces the intrathecal passage of usable antibiotics, which risks diminishing the therapeutic efficacy of betalactam antibiotics, and even more so of glycopeptides (Thomas et al., 1996).

Use of Non-Bacteriolytic Antibiotics

Practically, combined treatments of ampicillin/an aminoglycoside or ampicillin/cefotaxime are recommended in neonates (Principi & Esposito, 2020). In children and adults over 50, ampicillin plus cefotaxime or ceftriaxone is preferred when S. pneumoniae resistance is low; vancomycin is added to these drugs if there are high risks of the inefficacy of third-generation cephalosporins (Principi & Esposito, 2020). However, this proposed BM therapy approach ignores the evidence that strongly bacteriolytic agents, such as third-generation cephalosporins, can exacerbate the host inflammatory response triggered by pathogen penetration in the central nervous system (Principi & Esposito, 2020). Large volumes of microbial components are abruptly released during bacteriolysis, which causes a greater degree of inflammation than what is seen during natural bacterial autolysis (Principi & Esposito, 2020).

The use of bactericidal but nonbacteriolytic antibiotics has been proposed as a solution to this issue (Principi & Esposito, 2020). Among these agents are lipopeptides, quinolones, ketolides, rifamycin, and clindamycin (Wehrli & Staehelin, 1971). The most researched cyclic lipopeptide in this context is daptomycin (DAP). DAP disrupts multiple aspects of cell membrane function and inhibits protein, DNA and RNA synthesis. Through this complex mode of action, pathogens are promptly destroyed, but no bacteriolysis occurs (Heidary et al., 2018; Principi et al., 2015).

DAP is effective against Gram-positive bacteria, including multi-drug-resistant *S. pneumoniae* and *S. aureus*. DAP is considered a potential alternative to vancomycin, the drug currently used to treat beta-lactam-resistant Gram-positive rods. This activity has been evidenced in several experimental studies in which DAP was found to be as effective as vancomycin for the treatment of S. pneumoniae meningitis (Gerber et al., 2006; Mook-Kanamori et al., 2009) and superior to vancomycin (Cottagnoud et al., 2004) or various antibiotic combinations in the case of *S. aureus meningitis* and multidrug-resistant *S. pneumoniae meningitis* (Cottagnoud et al., 2004; Gerber et al., 2006), respectively. Moreover, the efficacy of DAP against Gram-positive bacteria, including multidrug-resistant *S. pneumoniae* and *S. aureus*, has been demonstrated in a number of experimental studies, where DAP was found to be superior to vancomycin (Cottagnoud et al., 2004) or various antibiotic combinations in the case of *S. aureus* meningitis and multidrug-resistant *S. pneumoniae* meningitis (Gerber et al., 2006; Mook-Kanamori et al., 2009) and as effective as vancomycin for the treatment of *S. pneumoniae* meningitis and *S. pneumoniae* meningitis in general.

Modulation of Neutrophil Activity

The hallmarks of BM include the massive recruitment of neutrophils with the goal of phagocytosing invasive bacteria and lowering the generation of reactive oxygen species; the degranulation of antimicrobial substances; and the secretion of decondensed nuclear DNA coated with antimicrobial proteins derived from granules known as neutrophil extracellular traps (NETs) (Brinkmann, 2018; Nauseef & Borregaard, 2014). Additionally, the evidence showing that giving mice granulocyte-colony-stimulating factor (G-CSF) prior to infection decreased mortality and brain damage supported the role of neutrophils in host defences (Brinkmann, 2018). Furthermore, the administration of medications, like fucoidan, prevents leukocyte formation in infected locations, raising mortality even if it had no effect on CSF bacterial load or brain injury (Brandt et al., 2005). But too much neutrophilic activity during BM can be harmful to the brain's tissue. Disruption of NETs findings suggests a second possible strategy for BM therapy through the control of neutrophil activity. According to certain recent studies. NETs have been found in the CSF, inner ear, and blood of animals as well as humans who have S. pneumoniae meningitis. This finding is linked to the survival of the infecting pathogens and the spread of the infection outside of the central nervous system (de Buhr et al., 2017; Erni et al., 2019; Mohanty et al., 2019). NETs may have antibacterial properties (Principi & Esposito, 2020). Pathogens can, avoid being killed by NETs and continue to have a harmful function (Principi & Esposito, 2020). The bacterial burden in the brain, lungs, spleen homogenates, and blood plasma was successfully decreased in a rat model by intravenous and intrathecal DNase treatment (Principi & Esposito, 2020). As IL-1β concentration dropped, NETs decreased as well, indicating a beneficial influence on inflammation. Nevertheless, little effort has been made to investigate human neutrophil activity suppression (Principi & Esposito, 2020).

Administration of Metalloproteinases Modulators (MPM)

MPs, including the disintegrin and metalloproteinase (ADAM) family and matrix metalloproteinases (MMPs), are crucial for controlling the processes that occur during brain injury in BM (Principi & Esposito, 2020). The BBB's disintegration, bacterial invasion, neutrophil infiltration, and inflammatory cytokine production are all regulated by MPs. A high level of MP activity damages the brain (Principi & Esposito, 2020). These findings suggest that the use of MP inhibitors may protect the integrity of the BBB, decrease neuroinflammation, and, in some cases, prevent brain injury (Muri et al., 2019). Studies on rodent BM have generally shown that administration of MMP and ADAM inhibitors, either alone as part of a pre-treatment regimen or in combination with antibiotics for therapy, can enhance acute and neurofunctional results (Leib et al., 2000, 2001; Liechti et al., 2014; Majeed et al., 2016; Meli et al., 2004; Muri et al., 2018). When mice infected with *N. meningitidis* that had received the broad-spectrum MP inhibitor batimastat (BM-94) either before or 24 hours after infection, the number of MMP-9 levels, intracerebral haemorrhage, and BBB disintegration was considerably lower than that of untreated controls (Ricci et al., 2014).

Rats infected with *S. pneumoniae* and treated at the time of infection with GM6001, a broad-spectrum inhibitor of the hydroxamic acid type, had significantly lower amounts of TNF-α and MMP-9 in the CSF. Additionally, after about 24 hours of infection, the amount of cortical necrosis indicated the degree of neuronal impairment, which was much lower (Meli et al., 2004). In order to assess TNF484's impact on disease parameters and brain damage, the water-soluble hydroxamate-based inhibitor of several MMPs and ADAM 17 (TACE) was investigated in a neonatal rat model of pneumococcal meningitis. There was a decrease in soluble TNF-α and the collagen degradation product hydroxyproline in the CSF, which was linked to a decreased incidence of seizures and cortical necrosis (Meli et al., 2004). Unfortunately, no study on the usage of MP inhibitors in BM patients has been done. However, as the MP expression patterns in BM-affected humans are comparable to those in experimental animals (Green et al., 2009, 2011; Shapiro et al., 2003; Thwaites et al., 2004; Tsai et al., 2011; Yushchenko et al., 2000), using one or more of these substances either alone or in conjunction with antibiotic treatment may help lessen the inflammatory damage to BM. This hypothesis is supported by the observation that corticosteroids can effectively lower mortality in patients with tuberculous meningitis (Thwaites et al., 2004), and that this beneficial impact is linked to a decrease in MMP-9 (Green et al., 2009). Any medication that restricts MP expression may be useful in lessening the brain damage caused by BM (Principi & Esposito, 2020).

PREVENTION

Preventing pneumococcal meningitis through vaccination remains controversial. People at risk (the immunocompromised, pregnant women, the elderly and very young children) should not consume soft cheeses or foods made from unpasteurized milk as far as Listeria is concerned. The main topic of this chapter is therefore the prevention of meningococcal meningitis. The presence of meningococcus in the nasopharynx is temporary, intermittent and affects 18% of people. This results in immunity to meningococcus, which means that most young adults are protected. Unlike the main meningococcal serogroups A, B, C, Y and W-135 (Goldschneider et al., 1969). The main serogroups in Switzerland are A, B and C. Given this high level of colonization, it is surprising that there are not more cases of meningococcal meningitis. Invasive meningococcal infection generally manifests itself ten days after colonization. This short period offers an opportunity for placement. Antibiotic chemoprophylaxis is in progress. Infection favors nasopharyngeal colonization. Meningitis occurs when immunity is absent, asplenia, lack of supplements (C3 and C5 to C9) and travel to regions where it is particularly prevalent (mainly sub-Saharan Africa and Saudi Arabia).

Vaccination

The main meningococcal serogroups are vaccinated, with the exception of serogroup B, which unfortunately accounts for almost 50% of meningitis cases in Switzerland. It is important to note that a protective antibody level is only reached after seven to ten days after vaccination. Vaccines in Switzerland are either exclusively against serogroup C, or against serogroups A, C, Y and W-135. It is recommended to take the latter vaccine for patients who travel to a highly endemic area (for example on a pilgrimage to Mecca). It provides protection in approximately 95% of vaccinated individuals within four weeks after a single dose and this protection persists for three to five years in children and two years in adults. It is recommended to vaccinate children and young adults housed in a dormitory (boarding school, etc.), microbiologists handling strains of Meningococcus, the population affected by an epidemic, travelers to hyperendemic areas and military personnel, particularly recruits (Zender et al, 2009). In low- and middle-income countries, the Global Alliance for Vaccines and Immunization (Gavi) has supported the rollout of PCVs, with varying coverage levels and challenges in sustained vaccine access (O'Brien et al., 2019). In sub-Saharan Africa, where the burden of pneumococcal meningitis remains high, the deployment of PCVs has shown promising results, though gaps in cold chain infrastructure and healthcare access persist (Kwambana-Adams et al., 2020).

Chemoprophylaxis

It is essential to take antibiotics as chemoprophylaxis to treat close contacts of the source patient in order to prevent any possible colonization. A "close contact" is defined as anyone who has spent eight hours or more near the source patient or who has been in contact with his or her nasopharyngeal secretions within a week before the meningitis. This therefore mainly includes people in the same household and close classmates or workmates. Mass antibiotic treatment is not recommended for those who do not meet these criteria. Those who have received a recent vaccination should also receive antibiotic chemoprophylaxis because protection is not 100%. It is recommended to start antibiotic chemoprophylaxis within 24 hours of identification of meningococcus in the source patient. Thereafter, the effectiveness of this prophylaxis decreases day by day and remains useless after two weeks(Woodard & Berman, 2006). Table 1 presents three recommended antibiotics.

Table 1. Antibiotic chemoprophylaxis in meningococcal meningitis (Zender et al, 2009).

Antibiotiques	Posologie adulte	Posologie pédiatrique
▪ **Ciprofloxacine***	500 mg p.o. en dose unique	Proscrit
▪ **Rifampicine****	2×600 mg/j p.o. pendant 2jours	2×10 mg/kg/j p.o. pendant 2jours
▪ **Ceftriaxone**	250 mg i.m. en dose unique	125 mg i.m. en dose unique

*proscrit chez la femme enceinte

** attention aux interactions médicamenteuses, colore toutes les sécrétions en orange

CONCLUSION

Despite recent successes, bacterial meningitis remains a major public health problem worldwide. The mortality rate remains high and almost unchanged since the introduction of antibiotics. Research into the pathophysiology of bacterial meningitis continues, with the aim of improving diagnostic methods and developing additional treatments to reduce mortality and improve survivor outcomes. A deep understanding of the pathophysiologic mechanisms underlying acute bacterial meningitis is essential to provide accurate treatments. Additionally, preventive measures include vaccination, maintaining good hygiene, and chemoprophylaxis are also quite important.

REFERENCES

Aguilera, E. R., & Lenz, L. L. (2020). Inflammation as a modulator of host susceptibility to pulmonary influenza, pneumococcal, and co-infections. *Frontiers in Immunology*, *11*, 105. DOI: 10.3389/fimmu.2020.00105 PMID: 32117259

Arsalane, L., De Microbiologie-virologie, P., Zouhair, S., De Microbiologie-virologie, P., Bourrous, M., Zahlane, K., & De Microbiologie-virologie, P. (2023). *Les méningites de l ' enfant dans la région d ' Agadir.*

Azad, A. K., Chakrabarti, S., Xu, Z., Davidge, S. T., & Fu, Y. (2014). Coiled-coil domain containing 3 (CCDC3) represses tumor necrosis factor-α/nuclear factor κB-induced endothelial inflammation. *Cellular Signalling*, *26*(12), 2793–2800. DOI: 10.1016/j.cellsig.2014.08.025 PMID: 25193116

Brandt, C. T., Lundgren, J. D., Frimodt-Møller, N., Christensen, T., Benfield, T., Espersen, F., Hougaard, D. M., & Østergaard, C. (2005). Blocking of leukocyte accumulation in the cerebrospinal fluid augments bacteremia and increases lethality in experimental pneumococcal meningitis. *Journal of Neuroimmunology*, *166*(1–2), 126–131. DOI: 10.1016/j.jneuroim.2005.05.014 PMID: 15982752

Brinkmann, V. (2018). Neutrophil extracellular traps in the second decade. *Journal of Innate Immunity*, *10*(5–6), 414–421. DOI: 10.1159/000489829 PMID: 29909412

Brouwer, M. C., Thwaites, G. E., Tunkel, A. R., & van de Beek, D. (2012). Dilemmas in the diagnosis of acute community-acquired bacterial meningitis. *Lancet*, *380*(9854), 1684–1692. DOI: 10.1016/S0140-6736(12)61185-4 PMID: 23141617

Brouwer, M. C., Tunkel, A. R., & van de Beek, D. (2010). Epidemiology, diagnosis, and antimicrobial treatment of acute bacterial meningitis. *Clinical Microbiology Reviews*, *23*(3), 467–492. DOI: 10.1128/CMR.00070-09 PMID: 20610819

Bryan, J. P., de Silva, H. R., Tavares, A., Rocha, H., & Scheld, W. M. (1990). Etiology and mortality of bacterial meningitis in northeastern Brazil. *Reviews of Infectious Diseases*, *12*(1), 128–135. DOI: 10.1093/clinids/12.1.128 PMID: 2300734

Cornick, J. E., Everett, D. B., Broughton, C., Denis, B. B., Banda, D. L., Carrol, E. D., & Parry, C. M. (2011). Invasive Streptococcus pneumoniae in children, Malawi, 2004–2006. *Emerging Infectious Diseases*, *17*(6), 1107–1109. DOI: 10.3201/eid1706.101404 PMID: 21749782

Costerus, J. M., Brouwer, M. C., Bijlsma, M. W., Tanck, M. W., van der Ende, A., & van de Beek, D. (2016). Impact of an evidence-based guideline on the management of community-acquired bacterial meningitis: A prospective cohort study. *Clinical Microbiology and Infection*, *22*(11), 928–933. DOI: 10.1016/j.cmi.2016.07.026 PMID: 27484018

Costerus, J. M., Brouwer, M. C., Sprengers, M. E. S., Roosendaal, S. D., van der Ende, A., & van de Beek, D. (2018). Cranial computed tomography, lumbar puncture, and clinical deterioration in bacterial meningitis: A nationwide cohort study. *Clinical Infectious Diseases*, *67*(6), 920–926. DOI: 10.1093/cid/ciy200 PMID: 29522090

Cottagnoud, P., Pfister, M., Acosta, F., Cottagnoud, M., Flatz, L., Kühn, F., Müller, H.-P., & Stucki, A. (2004). Daptomycin is highly efficacious against penicillin-resistant and penicillin-and quinolone-resistant pneumococci in experimental meningitis. *Antimicrobial Agents and Chemotherapy*, *48*(10), 3928–3933. DOI: 10.1128/AAC.48.10.3928-3933.2004 PMID: 15388454

de Buhr, N., Reuner, F., Neumann, A., Stump-Guthier, C., Tenenbaum, T., Schroten, H., Ishikawa, H., Müller, K., Beineke, A., Hennig-Pauka, I., Gutsmann, T., Valentin-Weigand, P., Baums, C. G., & von Köckritz-Blickwede, M. (2017). Neutrophil extracellular trap formation in the Streptococcus suis-infected cerebrospinal fluid compartment. *Cellular Microbiology*, *19*(2), e12649. DOI: 10.1111/cmi.12649 PMID: 27450700

El-Mansoury, B., Smimih, K., Hamdan, Y. A., El Khiat, A., Elouali, S., El Fatimi, H., Draoui, A., El Hiba, O., & Jayakumar, A. R. (2023). The Interplay Between Environmental Pollutants, Gut Microbiota, and Infections: Current Concepts and Therapies. *Ecological and Evolutionary Perspectives on Infections and Morbidity*, 173–207.

Elmakrini, N. (2014). *Méningites Infectieuses Communautaires: Profil Microbiologique et Épidémiologique à l'Hôpital Militaire Moulay Ismaïl de Meknès (De 2011 à 2013).*

Erni, S. T., Fernandes, G., Buri, M., Perny, M., Rutten, R. J., Van Noort, J. M., Senn, P., Grandgirard, D., Roccio, M., & Leib, S. L. (2019). Anti-inflammatory and oto-protective effect of the small heat shock protein alpha B-crystallin (HspB5) in experimental pneumococcal meningitis. *Frontiers in Neurology*, *10*, 570. DOI: 10.3389/fneur.2019.00570 PMID: 31244750

Gerber, P., Stucki, A., Acosta, F., Cottagnoud, M., & Cottagnoud, P. (2006). Daptomycin is more efficacious than vancomycin against a methicillin-susceptible Staphylococcus aureus in experimental meningitis. *The Journal of Antimicrobial Chemotherapy*, *57*(4), 720–723. DOI: 10.1093/jac/dkl007 PMID: 16459345

Glimåker, M., Sjölin, J., Åkesson, S., & Naucler, P. (2018). Lumbar puncture performed promptly or after neuroimaging in acute bacterial meningitis in adults: A prospective national cohort study evaluating different guidelines. *Clinical Infectious Diseases*, *66*(3), 321–328. DOI: 10.1093/cid/cix806 PMID: 29020334

Goldschneider, B. Y. I., Gotschlich, E. C., & Artenstein, M. S. (1969). Immunity in the Adult : The Carrier State as an Immunizing Process. *Serum, 2191*.

Gray, L. D., & Fedorko, D. P. (1992). Laboratory diagnosis of bacterial meningitis. *Clinical Microbiology Reviews*, *5*(2), 130–145. DOI: 10.1128/CMR.5.2.130 PMID: 1576585

Green, J. A., Thi Hong Chau, T., Farrar, J. J., Friedland, J. S., & Thwaites, G. E. (2011). CNS infection, CSF matrix metalloproteinase concentrations, and clinical/laboratory features. *Neurology*, *76*(6), 577–579. DOI: 10.1212/WNL.0b013e31820b7600 PMID: 21300974

Green, J. A., Tran, C. T. H., Farrar, J. J., Nguyen, M. T. H., Nguyen, P. H., Dinh, S. X., Ho, N. D. T., Ly, C. V., Tran, H. T., Friedland, J. S., & Thwaites, G. E. (2009). Dexamethasone, cerebrospinal fluid matrix metalloproteinase concentrations and clinical outcomes in tuberculous meningitis. *PLoS One*, *4*(9), e7277. DOI: 10.1371/journal.pone.0007277 PMID: 19789647

Hasbun, R., Abrahams, J., Jekel, J., & Quagliarello, V. J. (2001). Computed tomography of the head before lumbar puncture in adults with suspected meningitis. *The New England Journal of Medicine*, *345*(24), 1727–1733. DOI: 10.1056/NEJMoa010399 PMID: 11742046

Heidary, M., Khosravi, A. D., Khoshnood, S., Nasiri, M. J., Soleimani, S., & Goudarzi, M. (2018). Daptomycin. *The Journal of Antimicrobial Chemotherapy*, *73*(1), 1–11. DOI: 10.1093/jac/dkx349 PMID: 29059358

Hussein, A. S., & Shafran, S. D. (2000). Acute bacterial meningitis in adults: A 12-year review. *Medicine*, *79*(6), 360–368. DOI: 10.1097/00005792-200011000-00002 PMID: 11144034

Jochems, S. P., Marcon, F., Carniel, B. F., Holloway, M., Mitsi, E., Smith, E., Gritzfeld, J. F., Solórzano, C., Reiné, J., Pojar, S., Nikolaou, E., German, E. L., Hyder-Wright, A., Hill, H., Hales, C., de Steenhuijsen Piters, W. A. A., Bogaert, D., Adler, H., Zaidi, S., & Ferreira, D. M. (2018). Inflammation induced by influenza virus impairs human innate immune control of pneumococcus. *Nature Immunology*, *19*(12), 1299–1308. DOI: 10.1038/s41590-018-0231-y PMID: 30374129

Kim, K. S. (2003). Pathogenesis of bacterial meningitis: From bacteraemia to neuronal injury. *Nature Reviews. Neuroscience*, *4*(5), 376–385. DOI: 10.1038/nrn1103 PMID: 12728265

Koedel, U., Scheld, W. M., & Pfister, H.-W. (2002). Pathogenesis and pathophysiology of pneumococcal meningitis. *The Lancet. Infectious Diseases*, *2*(12), 721–736. DOI: 10.1016/S1473-3099(02)00450-4 PMID: 12467688

Lamridi, O. (2017). *Les facteurs pronostiques des méningites bactériennes communautaires de l'adulte.*

Leib, S. L., Clements, J. M., Lindberg, R. L. P., Heimgartner, C., Loeffler, J. M., Pfister, L.-A., Täuber, M. G., & Leppert, D. (2001). Inhibition of matrix metalloproteinases and tumour necrosis factor α converting enzyme as adjuvant therapy in pneumococcal meningitis. *Brain*, *124*(9), 1734–1742. DOI: 10.1093/brain/124.9.1734 PMID: 11522576

Leib, S. L., Leppert, D., Clements, J., & Täuber, M. G. (2000). Matrix metalloproteinases contribute to brain damage in experimental pneumococcal meningitis. *Infection and Immunity*, *68*(2), 615–620. DOI: 10.1128/IAI.68.2.615-620.2000 PMID: 10639424

Leib, S. L., & Tauber, M. G. (1999). Pathogenesis of Bacterial meningitis. *Infectious Disease Clinics of North America*, *13*(3), 527–548. DOI: 10.1016/S0891-5520(05)70093-3 PMID: 10470554

Lemkhoudem, M. A. (2022). *évolutif et préventif des méningites à Haemophilus à Marrakech.*

Liechti, F. D., Grandgirard, D., Leppert, D., & Leib, S. L. (2014). Matrix metalloproteinase inhibition lowers mortality and brain injury in experimental pneumococcal meningitis. *Infection and Immunity*, *82*(4), 1710–1718. DOI: 10.1128/IAI.00073-14 PMID: 24491581

Loh, E., Kugelberg, E., Tracy, A., Zhang, Q., Gollan, B., Ewles, H., Chalmers, R., Pelicic, V., & Tang, C. M. (2013). Temperature triggers immune evasion by Neisseria meningitidis. *Nature*, *502*(7470), 237–240. DOI: 10.1038/nature12616 PMID: 24067614

Majeed, S., Radotra, B. D., & Sharma, S. (2016). Adjunctive role of MMP-9 inhibition along with conventional anti-tubercular drugs against experimental tuberculous meningitis. *International Journal of Experimental Pathology*, *97*(3), 230–237. DOI: 10.1111/iep.12191 PMID: 27385155

McGill, F., Griffiths, M. J., Bonnett, L. J., Geretti, A. M., Michael, B. D., Beeching, N. J., McKee, D., Scarlett, P., Hart, I. J., Mutton, K. J., Jung, A., Adan, G., Gummery, A., Sulaiman, W. A. W., Ennis, K., Martin, A. P., Haycox, A., Miller, A., Solomon, T., & Martin, W. (2018). Incidence, aetiology, and sequelae of viral meningitis in UK adults: A multicentre prospective observational cohort study. *The Lancet. Infectious Diseases*, *18*(9), 992–1003. DOI: 10.1016/S1473-3099(18)30245-7 PMID: 30153934

Mehrdadi, S. (2019). Acute Bacterial Meningitis: Diagnosis, Treatment and Prevention. *Journal of Archives in Military Medicine*. Advance online publication. DOI: 10.5812/jamm.84749

Meli, D. N., Loeffler, J. M., Baumann, P., Neumann, U., Buhl, T., Leppert, D., & Leib, S. L. (2004). In pneumococcal meningitis a novel water-soluble inhibitor of matrix metalloproteinases and TNF-α converting enzyme attenuates seizures and injury of the cerebral cortex. *Journal of Neuroimmunology*, *151*(1–2), 6–11. DOI: 10.1016/j.jneuroim.2004.01.026 PMID: 15145598

Michael, B., Menezes, B. F., Cunniffe, J., Miller, A., Kneen, R., Francis, G., Beeching, N. J., & Solomon, T. (2010). Effect of delayed lumbar punctures on the diagnosis of acute bacterial meningitis in adults. *Emergency Medicine Journal : EMJ*, *27*(6), 433–438. DOI: 10.1136/emj.2009.075598 PMID: 20360497

Mohanty, T., Fisher, J., Bakochi, A., Neumann, A., Cardoso, J. F. P., Karlsson, C. A. Q., Pavan, C., Lundgaard, I., Nilson, B., Reinstrup, P., Bonnevier, J., Cederberg, D., Malmström, J., Bentzer, P., & Linder, A. (2019). Neutrophil extracellular traps in the central nervous system hinder bacterial clearance during pneumococcal meningitis. *Nature Communications*, *10*(1), 1667. DOI: 10.1038/s41467-019-09040-0 PMID: 30971685

Mook-Kanamori, B. B., Rouse, M. S., Kang, C.-I., van de Beek, D., Steckelberg, J. M., & Patel, R. (2009). Daptomycin in experimental murine pneumococcal meningitis. *BMC Infectious Diseases*, *9*(1), 1–9. DOI: 10.1186/1471-2334-9-50 PMID: 19405978

Muri, L., Grandgirard, D., Buri, M., Perny, M., & Leib, S. L. (2018). Combined effect of non-bacteriolytic antibiotic and inhibition of matrix metalloproteinases prevents brain injury and preserves learning, memory and hearing function in experimental paediatric pneumococcal meningitis. *Journal of Neuroinflammation*, *15*(1), 1–14. DOI: 10.1186/s12974-018-1272-8 PMID: 30131074

Muri, L., Leppert, D., Grandgirard, D., & Leib, S. L. (2019). MMPs and ADAMs in neurological infectious diseases and multiple sclerosis. *Cellular and Molecular Life Sciences : CMLS*, *76*(16), 3097–3116. DOI: 10.1007/s00018-019-03174-6 PMID: 31172218

Nagafuchi, M., Nagafuchi, Y., Sato, R., Imaizumi, T., Ayabe, M., Shoji, H., & Ichiyama, T. (2006). Adult meningism and viral meningitis, 1997-2004: Clinical data and cerebrospinal fluid cytokines. *Internal Medicine (Tokyo, Japan)*, *45*(21), 1209–1212. DOI: 10.2169/internalmedicine.45.1769 PMID: 17139119

Nauseef, W. M., & Borregaard, N. (2014). Neutrophils at work. *Nature Immunology*, *15*(7), 602–611. DOI: 10.1038/ni.2921 PMID: 24940954

Nhantumbo, A. A., Gudo, E. S., Caierão, J., Munguambe, A. M., Comé, C. E., Zimba, T. F., Moraes, M. O., Dias, C., & Cantarelli, V. V. (2016). Serotype distribution and antimicrobial resistance of Streptococcus pneumoniae in children with acute bacterial meningitis in Mozambique: Implications for a national immunization strategy. *BMC Microbiology*, *16*(1), 1–9. DOI: 10.1186/s12866-016-0747-y PMID: 27357587

Noah, N. D. (1987). *Epidemiology of bacterial meningitis*. Bacterial Meninggitis.

Nudelman, Y., & Tunkel, A. R. (2009). Bacterial meningitis: Epidemiology, pathogenesis and management update. *Drugs*, *69*(18), 2577–2596. DOI: 10.2165/11530590-000000000-00000 PMID: 19943708

Organization, W. H. (1995). Meningococcal meningitis. *Weekly Epidemiological Record= Relevé Épidémiologique Hebdomadaire, 70*(15), 105–107.

Peltola, H. (2000). Worldwide Haemophilus influenzae type b disease at the beginning of the 21st century: Global analysis of the disease burden 25 years after the use of the polysaccharide vaccine and a decade after the advent of conjugates. *Clinical Microbiology Reviews, 13*(2), 302–317. DOI: 10.1128/CMR.13.2.302 PMID: 10756001

Principi, N., Caironi, M., Venturini, F., Pani, L., & Esposito, S. (2015). Daptomycin in paediatrics: Current knowledge and the need for future research. *The Journal of Antimicrobial Chemotherapy*, *70*(3), 643–648. DOI: 10.1093/jac/dku453 PMID: 25406298

Principi, N., & Esposito, S. (2020). Bacterial meningitis: New treatment options to reduce the risk of brain damage. *Expert Opinion on Pharmacotherapy*, *21*(1), 97–105. DOI: 10.1080/14656566.2019.1685497 PMID: 31675255

Ricci, S., Grandgirard, D., Wenzel, M., Braccini, T., Salvatore, P., Oggioni, M. R., Leib, S. L., & Koedel, U. (2014). Inhibition of matrix metalloproteinases attenuates brain damage in experimental meningococcal meningitis. *BMC Infectious Diseases*, *14*(1), 1–10. DOI: 10.1186/s12879-014-0726-6 PMID: 25551808

Roos, K. L., Tunkel, A. R., Van De Beek, D., & Scheld, W. M. (2014). Acute bacterial meningitis. In *Infections of the Central Nervous System: Fourth Edition* (Tenth Edit). Elsevier Inc. DOI: 10.2310/IM.1270

Sáez-Llorens, X., Ramilo, O., Mustafa, M. M., Mertsold, J., & McCracken, G. H.Jr. (1990). Molecular pathophysiology of bacterial meningitis: Current concepts and therapeutic implications. *The Journal of Pediatrics*, *116*(5), 671–684. DOI: 10.1016/S0022-3476(05)82647-2 PMID: 2184210

Salazar, L., & Hasbun, R. (2017). Cranial imaging before lumbar puncture in adults with community-acquired meningitis: Clinical utility and adherence to the Infectious Diseases Society of America guidelines. *Clinical Infectious Diseases*, *64*(12), 1657–1662. DOI: 10.1093/cid/cix240 PMID: 28369295

Salomon, A., Berry, I., Tuite, A. R., Drews, S., Hatchette, T., Jamieson, F., Johnson, C., Kwong, J., Lina, B., Lojo, J., Mosnier, A., Ng, V., Vanhems, P., & Fisman, D. N. (2020). Influenza increases invasive meningococcal disease risk in temperate countries. *Clinical Microbiology and Infection*, *26*(9), 1257–e1. DOI: 10.1016/j.cmi.2020.01.004 PMID: 31935565

Scarborough, M., & Thwaites, G. E. (2008). The diagnosis and management of acute bacterial meningitis in resource-poor settings. *Lancet Neurology*, *7*(7), 637–648. DOI: 10.1016/S1474-4422(08)70139-X PMID: 18565457

Schuchat, A., Robinson, K., Wenger, J. D., Harrison, L. H., Farley, M., Reingold, A. L., Lefkowitz, L., & Perkins, B. A. (1997). Bacterial meningitis in the United States in 1995. *The New England Journal of Medicine*, *337*(14), 970–976. DOI: 10.1056/NEJM199710023371404 PMID: 9395430

Shapiro, S., Miller, A., Lahat, N., Sobel, E., & Lerner, A. (2003). Expression of matrix metalloproteinases, sICAM-1 and IL-8 in CSF from children with meningitis. *Journal of the Neurological Sciences*, *206*(1), 43–48. DOI: 10.1016/S0022-510X(02)00317-9 PMID: 12480084

Tenforde, M. W., Mokomane, M., Leeme, T. B., Tlhako, N., Tsholo, K., Chebani, T., Stephenson, A., Hutton, J., Mitchell, H. K., Patel, R. K. K., Hurt, W. J., Pilatwe, T., Masupe, T., Molefi, M., Guthrie, B. L., Farquhar, C., Mine, M., & Jarvis, J. N. (2019). Mortality in adult patients with culture-positive and culture-negative meningitis in the Botswana national meningitis survey: A prevalent cohort study. *The Lancet. Infectious Diseases*, *19*(7), 740–749. DOI: 10.1016/S1473-3099(19)30066-0 PMID: 31250824

Thigpen, M. C., Whitney, C. G., Messonnier, N. E., Zell, E. R., Lynfield, R., Hadler, J. L., Harrison, L. H., Farley, M. M., Reingold, A., Bennett, N. M., Craig, A. S., Schaffner, W., Thomas, A., Lewis, M. M., Scallan, E., & Schuchat, A. (2011). Bacterial meningitis in the United States, 1998–2007. *The New England Journal of Medicine*, *364*(21), 2016–2025. DOI: 10.1056/NEJMoa1005384 PMID: 21612470

Thomas, R., Le Tulzo, Y., & Bellissant, E. (1996). Place des corticoïdes dans le traitement des méningites purulentes chez l'adulte. *Medecine et Maladies Infectieuses*, *26*, 1119–1124. DOI: 10.1016/S0399-077X(96)80026-6

Thwaites, G. E., Bang, N. D., Dung, N. H., Quy, H. T., Oanh, D. T. T., Thoa, N. T. C., Hien, N. Q., Thuc, N. T., Hai, N. N., Lan, N. T. N., Lan, N. N., Duc, N. H., Tuan, V. N., Hiep, C. H., Chau, T. T. H., Mai, P. P., Dung, N. T., Stepniewska, K., White, N. J., & Farrar, J. J. (2004). Dexamethasone for the treatment of tuberculous meningitis in adolescents and adults. *The New England Journal of Medicine*, *351*(17), 1741–1751. DOI: 10.1056/NEJMoa040573 PMID: 15496623

Tsai, H., Shi, M., Lee, S., Wann, S., Tai, M., & Chen, Y. (2011). Expression of matrix metalloproteinases and their tissue inhibitors in the serum and cerebrospinal fluid of patients with meningitis. *Clinical Microbiology and Infection*, *17*(5), 780–784. DOI: 10.1111/j.1469-0691.2010.03393.x PMID: 21521415

Tunkel, A. R., Hartman, B. J., Kaplan, S. L., Kaufman, B. A., Roos, K. L., Scheld, W. M., & Whitley, R. J. (2004). Practice guidelines for the management of bacterial meningitis. *Clinical Infectious Diseases*, *39*(9), 1267–1284. DOI: 10.1086/425368 PMID: 15494903

Tunkel, A. R., & Scheld, W. M. (1993). Pathogenesis and pathophysiology of bacterial meningitis. *Clinical Microbiology Reviews*, *6*(2), 118–136. DOI: 10.1128/CMR.6.2.118 PMID: 8472245

Van de Beek, D., Brouwer, M. C., Thwaites, G. E., & Tunkel, A. R. (2012). Advances in treatment of bacterial meningitis. *Lancet*, *380*(9854), 1693–1702. DOI: 10.1016/S0140-6736(12)61186-6 PMID: 23141618

Wall, E. C., Chan, J. M., Gil, E., & Heyderman, R. S. (2021). Acute bacterial meningitis. *Current Opinion in Neurology, 35*(3), 386–395. DOI: 10.1097/WCO.0000000000000934 PMID: 33767093

Wehrli, W., & Staehelin, M. (1971). Actions of the rifamycins. *Bacteriological Reviews, 35*(3), 290–309. DOI: 10.1128/br.35.3.290-309.1971 PMID: 5001420

Weight, C. M., Venturini, C., Pojar, S., Jochems, S. P., Reiné, J., Nikolaou, E., Solórzano, C., Noursadeghi, M., Brown, J. S., Ferreira, D. M., & Heyderman, R. S. (2019). Microinvasion by Streptococcus pneumoniae induces epithelial innate immunity during colonisation at the human mucosal surface. *Nature Communications, 10*(1), 3060. DOI: 10.1038/s41467-019-11005-2 PMID: 31311921

Wen, S., Feng, D., Chen, D., Yang, L., & Xu, Z. (2020). Molecular epidemiology and evolution of Haemophilus influenzae. *Infection, Genetics and Evolution, 80*, 104205. DOI: 10.1016/j.meegid.2020.104205 PMID: 31981610

Wilson, M. R., Sample, H. A., Zorn, K. C., Arevalo, S., Yu, G., Neuhaus, J., Federman, S., Stryke, D., Briggs, B., Langelier, C., Berger, A., Douglas, V., Josephson, S. A., Chow, F. C., Fulton, B. D., DeRisi, J. L., Gelfand, J. M., Naccache, S. N., Bender, J., & Chiu, C. Y. (2019). Clinical metagenomic sequencing for diagnosis of meningitis and encephalitis. *The New England Journal of Medicine, 380*(24), 2327–2340. DOI: 10.1056/NEJMoa1803396 PMID: 31189036

Woodard, J. L., & Berman, D. M. (2006). Prevention of meningococcal disease. *Fetal and Pediatric Pathology, 25*(6), 311–319. DOI: 10.1080/15513810701209538 PMID: 17696042

Yushchenko, M., Weber, F., Mäder, M., Schöll, U., Maliszewska, M., Tumani, H., Felgenhauer, K., & Beuche, W. (2000). Matrix metalloproteinase-9 (MMP-9) in human cerebrospinal fluid (CSF): Elevated levels are primarily related to CSF cell count. *Journal of Neuroimmunology, 110*(1–2), 244–251. DOI: 10.1016/S0165-5728(00)00339-8 PMID: 11024556

Zender, H. O., Olivier, P., & Genné, D. (2009). Méningites bactériennes communautaires aiguës chez l'adulte. *Revue Medicale Suisse, 5*(220), 1968–1974. DOI: 10.53738/REVMED.2009.5.220.1968 PMID: 19908635

Chapter 3
Insights Into the Pathogenesis, Diagnosis, and Treatment of Neurosyphilis

Hanane El Fatimi
Mohammed VI University of Health Sciences, Morocco

Loubna Khalki
https://orcid.org/0000-0001-8612-8432
Mohammed VI University of Health Sciences, Morocco

Bilal El-Mansoury
https://orcid.org/0000-0002-2583-7515
Faculty of Sciences, Chouaib Doukkali University, Morocco & Royal College of Surgeons in Ireland (RCSI), Ireland

ABSTRACT

Neurosyphilis is a severe complication of syphilis that appears when the bacterium Treponema pallidum invades the central nervous system (CNS). The pathogenesis of this condition is complex, due to Treponema pallidum that infiltrates the CNS at any stage of infection, which leads to diverse neurological manifestations, ranging from asymptomatic forms to severe neuropsychiatric disorders. Moreover, the diagnosis remains challenging due to the variability of symptoms and typically requires a combination of serological tests and cerebrospinal fluid analysis for accurate confirmation. Penicillin remains the most effective treatment for neurosyphilis. This chapter will explore the importance of early intervention and ongoing research in improving both treatment outcomes and diagnostic accuracy.

DOI: 10.4018/979-8-3693-4070-7.ch003

INTRODUCTION

Treponema pallidum subspecies *pallidum*, the pathogen that causes syphilis, spreads throughout the body hours to days after inoculation (Buitrago-Garcia et al., 2019; Lin et al., 2016). It is believed that in the majority of syphilis cases, the central nervous system (CNS) is affected early on, even if this does not always result in overt clinical involvement (Ghanem, 2010). Therefore, it should come as no surprise that syphilis can cause neurological symptoms at any point in the illness, leading to neurosyphilis.

Neurosyphilis is a potentially severe and debilitating complication of syphilis, which is a sexually transmitted infection caused by the bacterium *Treponema pallidum*. It arises when the pathogen breaches the protective barriers of the CNS, leading to infection of the brain and spinal cord. Neurosyphilis may occur at any stage following syphilis infection and can resolve on its own, remain asymptomatic, or result in either short-term or chronic meningitis (Brown & Frank, 2003; Marra, 2015). Neurosyphilis can manifest in five different ways: as meningeal, meningovascular, asymptomatic, general paresis, and tabes dorsalis (Forrestel et al., 2020; Ghanem, 2010). The predominant type of neurosyphilis is asymptomatic, and patients are frequently unaware that they have the disease. Asymptomatic neurosyphilis is characterized by positive syphilis serology, abnormal findings in the cerebrospinal fluid (CSF), and the absence of any neurological signs or symptoms (Ghanem, 2010).

Recently, women and children whose mothers were infected have been documented, although men initially accounted for the majority of new cases (Ghanem, 2010). After penicillin was developed in the 1940s, the percentage of neurosyphilis cases dramatically decreased (Ghanem, 2010). A study conducted in Denmark found that between 1971 and 1979, only 50 cases were reported to the national health system. Many of these were likely individuals who had been reinfected following adequate penicillin treatment but did not receive subsequent therapy (Perdrup et al., 1981).

Hence, this chapter aims to provide an overview of neurosyphilis, covering its underlying pathophysiology, clinical presentation, and current strategies for diagnosis and therapies.

Epidemiology

Despite the true incidence of neurosyphilis remaining uncertain, as it is often not reportable in many national surveillance systems, and even where syphilis is tracked, insufficient data may hinder accurate classification of cases progressing to the neurological stage (Marra, 2015; Tuddenham & Ghanem, 2016). In recent years, the incidence of infectious syphilis has increased significantly, with most high-income countries reporting increases primarily among men who have sex with men (MSM) (Choudhri et al., 2018; King et al., 2022; Prevention, 2019)

In the pre-antibiotic era, early neurosyphilis affected 0.3% of patients who were not treated for syphilis, as opposed to 2-3% of those who had insufficient or incomplete treatment.

This implies that, possibly through changing the immune response, insufficient treatment may raise the chance of developing neurosyphilis at an early age. Additionally, it has been noted that about 30% of all instances of syphilis progressed to neurosyphilis, with 30% of those cases remaining asymptomatic. Additionally, 9.5% of patients with untreated early syphilis went on to acquire late neurosyphilis, according to the Oslo study (Singh, 2020).

Moreover, people living with HIV (PLWH) have around twice the neurosyphilis rate as the immunocompetent group (Workowski, 2021). This higher rate is caused by several risk factors, such as being male, MSM, older (≥45 years), not receiving combined antiretroviral therapy in PLWH, drug use disorders, not receiving anti-syphilitic therapy, reinfection following a prior syphilis infection, and patients in a serofast condition (Li et al., 2019; Pintado Maury et al., 2019; Salado-Rasmussen et al., 2019). Neurological symptoms may get worse if there are elevated serum and CSF rapid plasma reagin (RPR) titers, elevated CSF protein concentration, and a larger burden of cerebral small vessel disorders (Li et al., 2019; Tan et al., 2020; Xiang et al., 2021). Certain subtypes of T. pallidum, such as subtype 14d in China, are more likely to develop neurosyphilis (Dai et al., 2012). Additionally, susceptibility to neurosyphilis is influenced by host genetic factors, including single nucleotide polymorphisms in Toll-like receptors (TLR) 1, TLR2, TLR6, and the promoter region of interleukin 10 (IL-10) (Marra et al., 2014; Pastuszczak et al., 2015).

It is believed that the most prevalent forms of neurosyphilis are asymptomatic neurosyphilis and meningoencephalitis, although some cohort studies have reported meningovascular syphilis as having the highest incidence (Kissani et al., 2021). Neurosyphilis symptoms, including dementia paralytica, gummatous neurosyphilis, and tabes dorsalis, which were common before the use of antibiotics, have significantly decreased in frequency. Due to the prompt identification and treatment of syphilis, which shortens the illness course, as well as the broad use of antibiotics for other conditions, which may incidentally treat neurosyphilis, these numbers have decreased (Landry et al., 2019). On the other hand, otosyphilis and ocular syphilis incidence rates have increased, according to current research. Little proof of a particular type causing ocular syphilis has been found through molecular typing, indicating that this increase may just be the result of a comeback in syphilis infections overall (Zhou et al., 2022). As a result of inconsistencies in neurological screening and CSF evaluation, the true prevalence of neurosyphilis is likely underestimated (Gonzalez et al., 2019). Male sex has been identified as a significant epidemiological risk factor for neurosyphilis (S. Wu et al., 2024). The risk of neurosyphilis is estimated to be 2 to 3 times higher in Whites than in Blacks, despite Blacks having a fivefold higher incidence of other forms of syphilis. Neurosyphilis is also found to be twice as prevalent in men as in women. It is estimated that 3% to 5% with syphilis will develop neurological, ocular, or auditory complications in the United States population (Ha et al., 2024).

Indeed, recent studies from southern India have reported an increase in syphilis cases, particularly among high-risk groups, with latent syphilis being the most common presentation (Reddy et al., 2022; Solaimalai et al., 2022). In a study, 2.8% of patients with syphilis had a history of psychiatric disorders, and 28.7% had a history of substance use. While another study found that 29% of patients had both (Ouwens et al., 2019). Furthermore, compared to 75% in a study carried out in northeast India, 13.6% of neurosyphilis patients had high-risk sexual practices (Kayal et al., 2011). Sexually transmitted illnesses are also linked to impulsivity and risky behaviors, which are frequently linked to substance misuse (Arends et al., 2019). Substance abuse must therefore be addressed as a crucial component of syphilis treatment (Kanakaraj et al., 2024).

Pathogenesis and Histopathology of Neurosyphilis

In gross pathology, the lateral ventricles dilate and the frontal and temporal lobes atrophy while the sensorimotor and occipital cortex are spared. The atrophic regions are where chronic meningitis is most noticeable. Spirochetes are microscopically present in microglial cells, endothelial cells, and grey matter. Spirochetes do not exist in the white matter (Ha et al., 2024). Microscopic analysis, nerve loss is accompanied by perivascular infiltration of lymphocytes and plasma cells. It is possible to see endothelial swelling leading to endarteritis obliterans when vasculitis is present. Demyelination of the posterior spinal column and dorsal roots will be visible in the tabes dorsalis (Ha et al., 2024).

Experts have been debating the importance of the spirochete's direct invasion of the CNS and the involvement of immune responses to this invasion for decades (Hamill et al., 2024). Perivascular lymphocytic and plasma cell infiltration, along with nerve cell death, are among the histopathological alterations associated with neurosyphilis (Hamill et al., 2024). Endothelial cell edema in vasculitis develops into endarteritis obliterans. The posterior spinal column and dorsal roots in tabes dorsalis are demyelinated (Carlson et al., 2011). These could be the result of severe humoral responses, neutrophil hyperactivation, cytotoxic T-cell activation, or immunological dysregulation linked to delayed onset hypersensitivity reactions mediated by antibody–antigen complexes (Carlson et al., 2011).

It is highly established that *T. pallidum* can move across the blood-brain barrier (BBB) via intercellular connections, and inflammatory factors are crucial in controlling the junctions between BBB cells. Thus, cytokines such as IL-17 and IFN-γ cause endothelial contraction and compromise tight junction occludins, further increasing BBB permeability (Huppert et al., 2010). The *T. pallidum* adhesion protein Tp0751 affects the expression of tight junction proteins by inducing apoptosis and promoting IL-6 release, hence enabling BBB translocation (Lu et al., 2022). Furthermore, *T. pallidum* enhances chemotaxis in human microvascular endothelial cells by upregulating the chemokines CXCL6, CXCL8, and CXCL10 (WU et al., 2018). Following CNS invasion, T. *pallidum* directly causes vascular inflammation, tissue damage, and the release of cytokines. Some pathogenic proteins, such as Tp0751, Tp0965, as well as Tp0326, contribute to these processes by their separate mechanisms of endothelial permeability enhancement, adhesion promotion, and metabolic proliferation (Zhang et al., 2014). Insufficient Treg cells to prevent T-cell-mediated inflammation and intrathecal antibody production are indicated by elevated levels of CXCL13 and IFN-γ in the CSF of neurosyphilis patients (Drago et al., 2016). Moreover, via modulating IFN-γ production, lncRNA-ENST00000421645 enhances T-cell death, aggravating CNS injury by inducing inflammatory responses (K.-X. Wu et al., 2021). Hence, the activation of microglial cells and the autoimmune CNS response lead to promoting intercellular immune regulation and neuronal survival (Du et al., 2023). More research is needed to understand the mechanisms underlying microglial activation and functional alterations following neuronal damage in neurosyphilis. Genetic factors of the host also affect susceptibility; polymorphisms in the TLR1, TLR2, TLR6, and IL-10 promoters are linked to higher risk (Marra et al., 2014; Pastuszczak et al., 2015). The pathogenetic processes of neurosyphilis are still unknown despite advancements in the field, hence requiring additional research on the pathogens, host factors, and their interactions, as well as the etiological basis of clinical symptoms.

CLINICAL MANIFESTATIONS OF NEUROSYPHILIS

Asymptomatic Neurosyphilis

The bacterium *T.pallidum*, which causes syphilis, spreads swiftly and can infect the CNS within a few days *(Fig.1)* (Ghanem et al., 2020; Lukehart, 2008). Neuroinvasion occurs in up to 30% of individuals during the early phase of syphilis and often remains without symptoms; it can also be seen in the later stages of the disease (Ghanem et al., 2020; Lukehart, 2008). Asymptomatic neurosyphilis is identified by abnormal CSF findings in patients who have positive syphilis serology but do not exhibit any neurological signs or symptoms (Keidel & Moore, 1921). Both early and late stages of syphilis can have asymptomatic neurosyphilis. Additionally, two studies reported that 13.5% of individuals with early or latent syphilis showed CSF abnormalities indicative of asymptomatic neurosyphilis, with the highest incidence observed between 12 and 18 months following initial infection (MOORE & Faupel, 1928; O'LEARY et al., 1937). In addition, a seminal study by Moore et al. found that the degree of baseline CSF abnormalities determined the likelihood of developing late neurosyphilis (Moore, 1945). Asymptomatic syndromes have increased in frequency during the antibiotic era and account for one-third of clinically diagnosed cases of neurosyphilis (Hooshmand et al., 1972; Hotson, 1981; Simon, 1985).

Another study was taken from 58 individuals, including 16 PWH (Lukehart et al., 1988), 30% of patients with primary and secondary syphilis had *T. pallidum* found in their CSF. Indeed, *T. pallidum* was isolated from 50% (3 of 6) and 26% (7 of 27) of patients with and without neurological signs or symptoms among those who had secondary syphilis, respectively. Among those with *T. pallidum*-positive CSF, more than 30% (4 of 12) did not have any aberrant CSF results (Lukehart et al., 1988). In another investigation, *T. pallidum*-positive CSF was found in 15%–27% of individuals with early-stage syphilis who did not have CSF abnormalities (Chesney & Kemp, 1924). Thus, neuroinvasion is probably required but not the same as the CSF abnormalities that characterise asymptomatic neurosyphilis. It is unclear what percentage of people have chronic neuroinvasion and how it relates to early vs late asymptomatic neurosyphilis (Figure1). Asymptomatic neurosyphilis was reported in 25–35% of cases of early syphilis (O'LEARY et al., 1937) and 13.5% of cases of late syphilis in the pre-antibiotic era (MOORE & Faupel, 1928).

Asymptomatic neurosyphilis may not have any clinically significant consequences in the age of antibiotics. Although there is limited evidence supporting improved outcomes from CSF analysis in these groups, current national guidelines still recommend performing CSF evaluations to diagnose asymptomatic neurosyphilis in patients with tertiary syphilis, as well as in certain individuals who exhibit serological nonresponse or treatment failure (Workowski, 2021).

Symptomatic Neurosyphilis

Within a year after infection, early symptomatic neurosyphilis typically presents as acute meningitis, frequently basilar. Meningeal inflammation has been linked to cerebral vascular thrombosis, arteritis, and disorders involving the cranial nerves. There have also been reports of hydrocephalus accompanied by elevated intracranial pressure. The two most common tertiary forms of symptomatic neurosyphilis are parenchymatous, which usually appears more than 15 years after infection, or meningovascular, which generally manifests 5–12 years after infection (Hamill et al., 2024). Depending on where the infarct is located, endarteritis of the CNS blood arteries in meningovascular syphilis can cause thrombosis with infarction, which can result in stroke and its related symptoms. There is also a chance of developing spinal vascular infarct syndromes or spinal meningomyelitis (Ghanem, 2010; Ghanem et al., 2020; Swartz et al., 1999). Parenchymatous neurosyphilis usually develops at a later stage and manifests as either general paresis, typically 15–20 years after infection, or tabes dorsalis, which generally appears 20–25 years post-infection (Ghanem, 2010; Sparling, 1999).

Moreover, meningoencephalitis is a chronic disease that progresses slowly and causes general paresis. The symptoms could start slowly and include emotional instability, dementia, and a variety of other mental problems. Chronic degeneration of the spinal cord's posterior roots and columns causes tabetic neurosyphilis, which presents with a variety of symptoms (Ghanem, 2010; Sparling, 1999; Swartz et al., 1999). Gummas, or tumor-like masses made of granulomatous inflammation surrounding an infection site, can sporadically develop in the brain and spinal cord as a result of tertiary syphilis (Ghanem, 2010; Swartz et al., 1999).

Finally, though the symptoms may not entirely overlap, ocular and otic syphilis are thought to be subsets of neurosyphilis. Ocular and otic manifestations can coexist with any type of neurosyphilis and can appear at any phase of the disease. Therefore, signs and symptoms related to the eyes, ears, and nervous system should be evaluated at any stage of syphilis. Ocular syphilis can affect any component of one or both eyes, and particular portions of the eye may develop differently from the CNS. Because of this, there are differences in the clinical presentations (Tuddenham & Ghanem, 2016; Woolston et al., 2016). While conductive hearing loss is also possible in people with otosyphilis, sensorineural hearing loss is the most common type. 50% of cases of hearing loss may be bilateral. Additionally, people may have vestibular abnormalities such as vertigo, imbalance problems, or unstable gait (Ghanem et al., 2020; Yimtae et al., 2007).

Diagnosis of Neurosyphilis

The diagnosis of neurosyphilis can be made either clinical or laboratory criteria. Serum and CSF tests are typically used to diagnose neurosyphilis, and they are divided into treponemal and nontreponemal testing (Du et al., 2023). The venereal disease research laboratory (VDRL), the most used nontreponemal serum test, is the gold standard for specificity when blood contamination is not present. However, there is disagreement over its sensitivity, its operation is complicated, and there is a lack of reagent availability (Zhu et al., 2014).

The primary treponemal serum tests include the *T. pallidum* particle agglutination assay (TPPA), enzyme immunoassay (TP-EIA), chemiluminescence immunoassay, and fluorescent treponemal antibody absorption (FTA-ABS) test (Du et al., 2023). While these assays are very sensitive, they have low specificity (Park et al., 2020). Therefore, it is important that appropriate diagnostic biomarkers must be found. Due to its poor sensitivity and specificity, PCR detection of *T. pallidum* in the CSF has been temporarily stopped (Marks et al., 2018). Neurosyphilis could be predicted by elevated CSF/serum ratios of CXCL13, CXCL8, and CXCL10 chemokine concentrations, especially CXCL13 (Marra et al., 2010). Additionally, neurosyphilis was predicted by levels of serum IL-26, peripheral blood CD8+IFN-γ+ cells, macrophage migration inhibition factor in the CSF, and antibody index (AI) for intrathecal synthesis of particular anti-treponemal IgG (Alberto et al., 2022; Lin et al., 2016; Liu et al., 2019; Shen et al., 2022). On the other hand, aberrant expression of mir-570-3p, mir-570-5p, mir-570-5p, and mir-21-5p in CSF and serum may be another indicator of neurosyphilis (Chen et al., 2019). All these biomarkers lack validation and large sample size evaluation, and their specificity and sensitivity have not been assessed; hence, none of them are used for clinical diagnosis. Patients with neurosyphilis must attend follow-up appointments every three to six months for more than three years following their diagnosis.

Low follow-up rates result from lumbar punctures, an invasive examination for which patients are frequently uncooperative. In follow-up assessments, CSF white blood cell (WBC) counts are commonly used as a key laboratory indicator; However, these values can differ significantly between individuals (Marra et al., 2004), and their sensitivity and accuracy as a prognostic indicator are insufficient. Thus, establishing diagnostic standards and follow-up obligations for neurosyphilis should prioritise the validation of novel biomarkers with increased sensitivity and accuracy. Establishing diagnostic standards and follow-up obligations for neurosyphilis based on excellent evidence-based medicine continues to be a significant challenge (Du et al., 2023).

Treatment and Antibiotic Resistance of Neurosyphilis

Effective treatment of neurosyphilis depends on maintaining therapeutic concentrations of a treponemicidal antibiotic in the CSF over an adequate duration (Clement et al., 2014). Long-acting benzathine penicillin G is not recommended, as it fails to achieve sufficient CSF levels in later-stage syphilis. The preferred therapy is intravenous aqueous penicillin G, which reliably penetrates the CSF (Mohr et al., 1976). Recommended regimens include aqueous crystalline penicillin G at 18–24 million units per day, administered as 3–4 million units every four hours or by continuous infusion for 10–14 days, or procaine penicillin G (2.4 million units intramuscularly once daily) combined with probenecid (500 mg orally four times daily) for the same duration (Workowski et al., 2015). Furthermore, daily 2g of Ceftriaxone intramuscularly or intravenously for 10–14 days is an alternative (Singh, 2020).

A recent review reports that the authors could not establish a difference between ceftriaxone and penicillin G treatments due to the poor quality of the available data (Buitrago-Garcia et al., 2019). In cohort research conducted between 1997 and 2017, 208 individuals with neurosyphilis were included. The findings showed that 88% of the ceftriaxone group and 82% of the penicillin G group had serological cure rates (Bettuzzi et al., 2021). Conversely, another study demonstrates that the clinical cure rates for the ceftriaxone group were only 44%, and for the penicillin G group, they were only 18% (Buitrago-Garcia et al., 2019). In the meantime, 41.8% of the neurosyphilis patients had neurological sequelae (Ozturk-Engin et al., 2019). Intravenous penicillin G therapy was linked with a higher failure rate in patients with co-infection with neurosyphilis (Gordon et al., 1994; Marra et al., 1996). To date, Penicillin is the medicine of choice for treating neurosyphilis, and there is no evidence that *T. pallidum* is resistant to it (Peermohamed et al., 2020). While erythromycin and chloramphenicol have been shown to cause intestinal dysbiosis and irreversible aplastic anemia, respectively, tetracycline, erythromycin, and chloramphenicol have all been used to treat syphilis (Buitrago-Garcia et al., 2019). Penicillin and doxycycline both had comparable therapeutic outcomes in some studies (Girometti et al., 2021). However, doxycycline is not allowed for use in pregnant women despite being less expensive.

Parenteral penicillin G is the sole recognized treatment option for syphilis in pregnant women. Probenecid is frequently given in addition to antibiotics while treating neurosyphilis. A recent study proved that oral amoxicillin with probenecid could elevate the drug level in CSF (Janier et al., 2021).

However, in HIV-positive MSM, the combination of oral probenecid and intramuscular (IM) procaine penicillin should be taken with caution (Richardson & Goldmeier, 2021). The Jarisch-Herxheimer reaction (JHR) can develop within the first 24 hours after initiating neurosyphilis treatment. It is characterized by symptoms such as headache, fever, chills, muscle aches, and skin rashes, although its underlying mechanism remains poorly understood (Butler, 2017). JHR may result from the use of common antibiotics such as levofloxacin, penicillin, erythromycin, azithromycin, tetracyclines, and clarithromycin (Tsai et al., 2014).

JHR typically affects patients who have early syphilis; the risk of JHR rises by 19% for every twofold increase in RPR titer, indicating that a larger spirochete load may be a major contributing factor to the increased risk of JHR (Kapila & Schwartz, 2021). JHR may be more severe for PLWH, especially those who have encephalitis (Spelber & Lahijani, 2020). Prednisolone and other steroids are frequently used to prevent JHR; acetaminophen and TNF-α antibodies have also been utilized in certain situations (Cui et al., 2020).

Even if the CSF examination is normal, ocular syphilis and otologic syphilis should be treated similarly to neurosyphilis, in cooperation with an ophthalmologist or otologist (Gonzalez et al., 2019). While systemic steroids for otologic syphilis and topical or systemic steroids for ocular syphilis are frequently utilized, no controlled research has been done to date to show their effectiveness (Gonzalez et al., 2019). It is unclear how corticosteroids are used to control the level of inflammation. Adding corticosteroid may help prevent a Jarisch-Herxheimer reaction, which is an inflammatory response that frequently occurs when antimicrobial treatment for syphilis is started and can worsen uveitis (Fathilah & Choo, 2003). A recent study conducted by the International Ocular Syphilis Study Group's ophthalmologists revealed that most of them were recommending systemic corticosteroid therapy as an adjuvant, starting after the commencement of antibiotic treatment (Ramchandani et al., 2020). Usually, a month after starting penicillin therapy, the inflammation goes down and the patient's vision improves (National Center for Sexually Transmitted Disease Control et al., 2020), Fig1.

Figure 1. Recommended treatments for neurosyphilis.

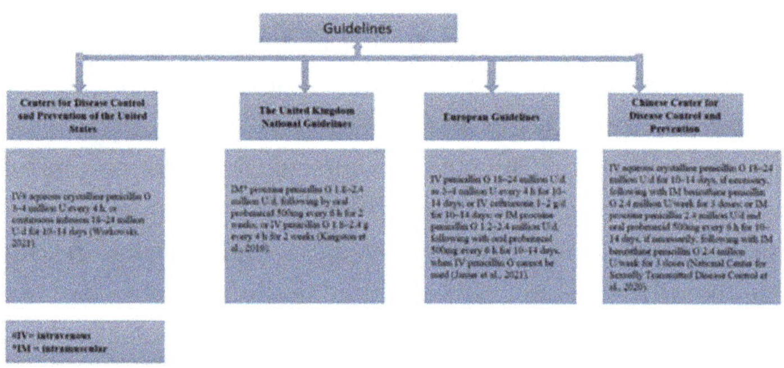

Adapted from Zhou et al. (2022).

CONCLUSION

Neurosyphilis is a serious complication of syphilis in which the central nervous system becomes involved, potentially resulting in significant neurological impairment. This condition can present with different symptoms, which pose challenges in diagnosis. The prevalence of neurosyphilis has declined with the advent of antibiotic therapy, particularly penicillin, which may prevent the progression of this disease and improve outcomes. More research is needed to understand its pathophysiology deeply and improve treatment and prevention strategies.

REFERENCES

Alberto, C., Deffert, C., Lambeng, N., Breville, G., Gayet-Ageron, A., Lalive, P., Toutous Trellu, L., & Fontao, L. (2022). Intrathecal synthesis index of specific anti-treponema IgG: A new tool for the diagnosis of neurosyphilis. *Microbiology Spectrum, 10*(1), e01477–e21. DOI: 10.1128/spectrum.01477-21 PMID: 35138118

Arends, R. M., Nelwan, E. J., Soediro, R., van Crevel, R., Alisjahbana, B., Pohan, H. T., von Borries, A. K. L., Schene, A. H., van der Ven, A. J. A. M., & Schellekens, A. F. A. (2019). Associations between impulsivity, risk behavior and HIV, HBV, HCV and syphilis seroprevalence among female prisoners in Indonesia: A cross-sectional study. *PLoS One*, *14*(2), e0207970. DOI: 10.1371/journal.pone.0207970 PMID: 30768609

Bettuzzi, T., Jourdes, A., Robineau, O., Alcaraz, I., Manda, V., Molina, J. M., Mehlen, M., Cazanave, C., Tattevin, P., Mensi, S., Terrier, B., Régent, A., Ghosn, J., Charlier, C., Martin-Blondel, G., & Dupin, N. (2021). Ceftriaxone compared with benzylpenicillin in the treatment of neurosyphilis in France: A retrospective multicentre study. *The Lancet. Infectious Diseases*, *21*(10), 1441–1447. DOI: 10.1016/S1473-3099(20)30857-4 PMID: 34051142

Brown, D. L., & Frank, J. E. (2003). Diagnosis and management of syphilis. *American Family Physician*, *68*(2), 283–290. PMID: 12892348

Buitrago-Garcia, D., Martí-Carvajal, A. J., Jimenez, A., Conterno, L. O., & Pardo, R. (2019). Antibiotic therapy for adults with neurosyphilis. *Cochrane Database of Systematic Reviews*, 5. PMID: 31132142

Butler, T. (2017). The Jarisch–Herxheimer reaction after antibiotic treatment of spirochetal infections: A review of recent cases and our understanding of pathogenesis. *The American Journal of Tropical Medicine and Hygiene*, *96*(1), 46–52. DOI: 10.4269/ajtmh.16-0434 PMID: 28077740

Carlson, J. A., Dabiri, G., Cribier, B., & Sell, S. (2011). The immunopathobiology of syphilis: The manifestations and course of syphilis are determined by the level of delayed-type hypersensitivity. *The American Journal of Dermatopathology*, *33*(5), 433–460. DOI: 10.1097/DAD.0b013e3181e8b587 PMID: 21694502

Chen, H., Zhou, Y., Wang, Z.-Y., Yan, B.-X., Zhou, W.-F., Wang, T.-T., Zheng, M., & Man, X.-Y. (2019). Exosomal microRNA profiles from serum and cerebrospinal fluid in neurosyphilis. *Sexually Transmitted Infections*, *95*(4), 246–250. DOI: 10.1136/sextrans-2018-053813 PMID: 30926713

Chesney, A. M., & Kemp, J. E. (1924). Incidence of Spirochaeta pallida in cerebrospinal fluid during early stage of syphilis. *Journal of the American Medical Association, 83*(22), 1725–1728. DOI: 10.1001/jama.1924.02660220001001

Choudhri, Y., Miller, J., Sandhu, J., Leon, A., & Aho, J. (2018). Sexually transmitted infections: Infectious and congenital syphilis in Canada, 2010–2015. *Canada Communicable Disease Report = Relevé des Maladies Transmissibles au Canada, 44*(2), 43. PMID: 29770098

Clement, M. E., Okeke, N. L., & Hicks, C. B. (2014). Treatment of syphilis: A systematic review. *Journal of the American Medical Association, 312*(18), 1905–1917. DOI: 10.1001/jama.2014.13259 PMID: 25387188

Cui, L., Xu, Z., & Hou, H. (2020). Diagnosis and treatment of spinal syphilitic gumma: A case report. *Frontiers in Neurology, 10*, 490958. DOI: 10.3389/fneur.2019.01352 PMID: 32010040

Dai, T., Li, K., Lu, H., Gu, X., Wang, Q., & Zhou, P. (2012). Molecular typing of Treponema pallidum: A 5-year surveillance in Shanghai, China. *Journal of Clinical Microbiology, 50*(11), 3674–3677. DOI: 10.1128/JCM.01195-12 PMID: 22972832

Drago, F., Javor, S., & Parodi, A. (2016). Neurosyphilis: From infection to autoinflammation? []. SAGE Publications Sage UK: London, England.]. *International Journal of STD & AIDS, 27*(4), 327–328. DOI: 10.1177/0956462415590710 PMID: 26873161

Du, F. Z., Zhang, X., Zhang, R. L., & Wang, Q. Q. (2023). CARE-NS, a research strategy for neurosyphilis. *Frontiers in Medicine, 9*(January), 1–7. DOI: 10.3389/fmed.2022.1040133 PMID: 36687428

Fathilah, J., & Choo, M. M. (2003). The Jarisch-Herxheimer reaction in ocular syphilis. *The Medical Journal of Malaysia, 58*(3), 437–439. PMID: 14750386

Forrestel, A. K., Kovarik, C. L., & Katz, K. A. (2020). Sexually acquired syphilis: Historical aspects, microbiology, epidemiology, and clinical manifestations. *Journal of the American Academy of Dermatology, 82*(1), 1–14. DOI: 10.1016/j.jaad.2019.02.073 PMID: 30986477

Ghanem, K. G. (2010). Neurosyphilis: A historical perspective and review. *CNS Neuroscience & Therapeutics, 16*(5), e157–e168. DOI: 10.1111/j.1755-5949.2010.00183.x PMID: 20626434

Ghanem, K. G., Ram, S., & Rice, P. A. (2020). The modern epidemic of syphilis. *The New England Journal of Medicine, 382*(9), 845–854. DOI: 10.1056/NEJMra1901593 PMID: 32101666

Ghani, S., Murthy, P., Jain, S., & Sarin, A. (2018). Syphilis and psychiatry at the Mysore Government Mental Hospital (NIMHANS) in the early 20th century. *Indian Journal of Psychiatry*, *60*(6, Suppl 2), S270–S276. DOI: 10.4103/psychiatry.IndianJPsychiatry_449_17 PMID: 29527060

Girometti, N., Junejo, M. H., Nugent, D., McOwan, A., Whitlock, G., Gedela, K., Patel, S., Suchak, T., & Tittle, V. (2021). Clinical and serological outcomes in patients treated with oral doxycycline for early neurosyphilis. *The Journal of Antimicrobial Chemotherapy*, *76*(7), 1916–1919. DOI: 10.1093/jac/dkab100 PMID: 33783506

Gonzalez, H., Koralnik, I. J., & Marra, C. M. (2019). Neurosyphilis. *Seminars in Neurology*, *39*(4), 448–455. DOI: 10.1055/s-0039-1688942 PMID: 31533185

Gordon, S. M., Eaton, M. E., George, R., Larsen, S., Lukehart, S. A., Kuypers, J., Marra, C. M., & Thompson, S. (1994). The response of symptomatic neurosyphilis to high-dose intravenous penicillin G in patients with human immunodeficiency virus infection. *The New England Journal of Medicine*, *331*(22), 1469–1473. DOI: 10.1056/NEJM199412013312201 PMID: 7969296

Ha, T., Tadi, P., Leslie, S., & Dubensky, L. (2024). *Neurosyphilis*. StatPearls.

Hamill, M. M., Ghanem, K. G., & Tuddenham, S. (2024). State-of-the-Art Review: Neurosyphilis. *Clinical Infectious Diseases*, *78*(5), e57–e68. DOI: 10.1093/cid/ciad437 PMID: 37593890

Hooshmand, H., Escobar, M. R., & Kopf, S. W. (1972). Neurosyphilis: A study of 241 patients. *Journal of the American Medical Association*, *219*(6), 726–729. DOI: 10.1001/jama.1972.03190320032011 PMID: 5066697

Hotson, J. R. (1981). Modern neurosyphilis: A partially treated chronic meningitis. *The Western Journal of Medicine*, *135*(3), 191. PMID: 7340118

Huppert, J., Closhen, D., Croxford, A., White, R., Kulig, P., Pietrowski, E., Bechmann, I., Becher, B., Luhmann, H. J., Waisman, A., & Kuhlmann, C. R. W. (2010). Cellular mechanisms of IL-17-induced blood-brain barrier disruption. *The FASEB Journal*, *24*(4), 1023–1034. DOI: 10.1096/fj.09-141978 PMID: 19940258

Janier, M., Unemo, M., Dupin, N., Tiplica, G. S., Potočnik, M., & Patel, R. (2021). 2020 European guideline on the management of syphilis. *Journal of the European Academy of Dermatology and Venereology*, *35*(3), 574–588. DOI: 10.1111/jdv.16946 PMID: 33094521

Kanakaraj, L., Mamtani, H., Dahale, A. B., Netravathi, M., Nagarathna, S., Sinha, S., & Thippeswamy, H. (2024). Psychiatric manifestations of neurosyphilis over past two decades: Findings from a tertiary care neuropsychiatric hospital in south India. *Asian Journal of Psychiatry*, *94*, 103952. DOI: 10.1016/j.ajp.2024.103952 PMID: 38364749

Kapila, R., & Schwartz, R. A. (2021). Neurosyphilis and the Jarisch-Herxheimer reaction: A therapy concern with HIV disease. *Dermatologic Therapy*, *34*(2), e14839. DOI: 10.1111/dth.14839 PMID: 33527658

Kayal, A. K., Goswami, M., Das, M., & Paul, B. (2011). Clinical spectrum of neurosyphilis in North East India. *Neurology India*, *59*(3), 344–350. DOI: 10.4103/0028-3886.82719 PMID: 21743160

Keidel, A. (1921). Studies in asymptomatic neurosyphilis: I. A tentative classification of early asymptomatic neurosyphilis. *Archives of Neurology and Psychiatry*, *6*(3), 286–291. DOI: 10.1001/archneurpsyc.1921.02190030033004

King, J., McManus, H., Gray, R., & McGregor, S. (2022). *HIV, viral hepatitis and sexually transmissible infections in Australia Annual surveillance report 2021.*

Kissani, N., Nafia, S., Zahlane, S., & Louhab, N. (2021). Neurosyphilis: A series of 178 cases at the 3rd-level hospital of Marrakesh (Morocco). *European Journal of Clinical Microbiology & Infectious Diseases*, *40*(10), 2129–2135. DOI: 10.1007/s10096-021-04253-y PMID: 33942164

Landry, T., Smyczek, P., Cooper, R., Gratrix, J., Bertholet, L., Read, R., Romanowski, B., & Singh, A. E. (2019). Retrospective review of tertiary and neurosyphilis cases in Alberta, 1973–2017. *BMJ Open*, *9*(6), e025995. DOI: 10.1136/bmjopen-2018-025995 PMID: 31230001

Li, W., Jiang, M., Xu, D., Kou, C., Zhang, L., Gao, J., Qin, K., Wu, W., & Zhang, X. (2019). Clinical and Laboratory Characteristics of Symptomatic and Asymptomatic Neurosyphilis in HIV-Negative Patients: A Retrospective Study of 264 Cases. *BioMed Research International*, *2019*(1), 2426313. DOI: 10.1155/2019/2426313 PMID: 31198783

Lin, L.-R., Lin, D.-H., Tong, M.-L., Liu, L.-L., Fan, J.-Y., Zhu, X.-Z., Gao, K., Chen, M.-J., Zheng, W.-H., Zhang, H.-L., Li, S.-L., Lin, H.-L., Lin, Z.-F., Niu, J.-J., & Yang, T.-C. (2016). Macrophage migration inhibitory factor as a novel cerebrospinal fluid marker for neurosyphilis among HIV-negative patients. *Clinica Chimica Acta*, *463*, 103–108. DOI: 10.1016/j.cca.2016.10.018 PMID: 27751728

Liu, L.-L., Liu, W.-N., Jiang, X.-Y., Chen, M.-H., Liu, Z.-J., Lin, Y., Zhu, S.-G., Lin, L.-R., Zheng, W.-H., & Yan, J.-H. (2019). Changes of T lymphocyte subsets in patients with HIV-negative symptomatic neurosyphilis. *Microbial Pathogenesis*, *130*, 213–218. DOI: 10.1016/j.micpath.2019.03.008 PMID: 30862559

Lu, S., Wang, J., He, Z., He, S., Zheng, K., Xu, M., Yuan, S., & Wu, Y. (2022). Treponema pallidum Tp0751 alters the expression of tight junction proteins by promoting bEnd3 cell apoptosis and IL-6 secretion. *International Journal of Medical Microbiology*, *312*(4), 151553. DOI: 10.1016/j.ijmm.2022.151553 PMID: 35358795

Lukehart, S. A. (2008). Biology of treponemes. *Sexually Transmitted Diseases*, *4*, 647–659.

Lukehart, S. A., Hook, E. W.III, Baker-Zander, S. A., Collier, A. C., Critchlow, C. W., & Handsfield, H. H. (1988). Invasion of the central nervous system by Treponema pallidum: Implications for diagnosis and treatment. *Annals of Internal Medicine*, *109*(11), 855–862. DOI: 10.7326/0003-4819-109-11-855 PMID: 3056164

Marks, M., Lawrence, D., Kositz, C., & Mabey, D. (2018). Diagnostic performance of PCR assays for the diagnosis of neurosyphilis: A systematic review. *Sexually Transmitted Infections*, *94*(8), 585–588. DOI: 10.1136/sextrans-2018-053666 PMID: 30061192

Marra, C. M. (2015). Neurosyphilis. *Continuum (Minneapolis, Minn.)*, *21*(6), 1714–1728. DOI: 10.1212/CON.0000000000000250 PMID: 26633785

Marra, C. M., Longstreth, W. T.Jr, Maxwell, C. L., & Lukehart, S. A. (1996). Resolution of serum and cerebrospinal fluid abnormalities after treatment of neurosyphilis: Influence of concomitant human immunodeficiency virus infection. *Sexually Transmitted Diseases*, *23*(3), 184–189. DOI: 10.1097/00007435-199605000-00005 PMID: 8724507

Marra, C. M., Maxwell, C. L., Tantalo, L., Eaton, M., Rompalo, A. M., Raines, C., Stoner, B. P., Corbett, J. J., Augenbraun, M., Zajackowski, M., Kee, R., & Lukehart, S. A. (2004). Normalization of cerebrospinal fluid abnormalities after neurosyphilis therapy: Does HIV status matter? *Clinical Infectious Diseases*, *38*(7), 1001–1006. DOI: 10.1086/382532 PMID: 15034833

Marra, C. M., Sahi, S. K., Tantalo, L. C., Ho, E. L., Dunaway, S. B., Jones, T., & Hawn, T. R. (2014). Toll-like receptor polymorphisms are associated with increased neurosyphilis risk. *Sexually Transmitted Diseases*, *41*(7), 440–446. DOI: 10.1097/OLQ.0000000000000149 PMID: 24922103

Marra, C. M., Tantalo, L. C., Sahi, S. K., Maxwell, C. L., & Lukehart, S. A. (2010). CXCL13 as a cerebrospinal fluid marker for neurosyphilis in HIV-infected patients with syphilis. *Sexually Transmitted Diseases*, *37*(5), 283–287. DOI: 10.1097/OLQ.0b013e3181d877a1 PMID: 20393380

Mohr, J. A., Griffiths, W., Jackson, R., Saadah, H., Bird, P., & Riddle, J. (1976). Neurosyphilis and penicillin levels in cerebrospinal fluid. *Journal of the American Medical Association*, *236*(19), 2208–2209. DOI: 10.1001/jama.1976.03270200046031 PMID: 989815

Moore, J. E. (1945). The chemotherapy of syphilis. *Bulletin of the New York Academy of Medicine*, *21*(1), 3. PMID: 19312421

Moore, J. E.MOORE. (1928). Asymptomatic neurosyphilis: V. A comparison of early and late asymptomatic neurosyphilis. *Archives of Dermatology and Syphilology*, *18*(1), 99–108. DOI: 10.1001/archderm.1928.02380130102009

National Center for Sexually Transmitted Disease Control, C. C. for D. C. and P., Committee of Sexually Transmitted Disease Chinese Medical Association, B. of D., & Committee of Sexually Transmitted Disease Chinese Medical Doctor Association, B. of D. (2020). (2019). Chinese expert consensus statement on diagnosis and treatment of syphilis. *Chinese Medical Journal*, *133*(19), 2335–2337. PMID: 32852386

O'Leary, P. A. (1937). Cooperative clinical studies in the treatment of syphilis: Asymptomatic neurosyphilis. *Archives of Dermatology*, *35*(3), 387–401. DOI: 10.1001/archderm.1937.01470210013002

Ouwens, I. M. D., Ott, A., Fiolet, A., Koehler, P. J., Vos, M., Oldhoff, J. M., & Verhoeven, W. M. A. (2019). Clinical presentation of laboratory confirmed neurosyphilis in a recent cases series. *Clinical Neuropsychiatry*, *16*(1), 17. PMID: 34908934

Ozturk-Engin, D., Erdem, H., Hasbun, R., Wang, S.-H., Tireli, H., Tattevin, P., Argemi, X., Ouamara-Digue, E., Gombos, A., Lakatos, B., Sırmatel, F., Cag, Y., Pekok, A. U., Senbayrak, S., Balkan, I. I., Gheno, M., Uzun, N., Kaya, S., Cicek-Senturk, G., & Vahaboglu, H. (2019). Predictors of unfavorable outcome in neurosyphilis: Multicenter ID-IRI Study. *European Journal of Clinical Microbiology & Infectious Diseases*, *38*(1), 125–134. DOI: 10.1007/s10096-018-3403-7 PMID: 30368740

Park, I. U., Tran, A., Pereira, L., & Fakile, Y. (2020). Sensitivity and specificity of treponemal-specific tests for the diagnosis of syphilis. *Clinical Infectious Diseases*, *71*(Supplement_1), S13–S20. DOI: 10.1093/cid/ciaa349 PMID: 32578866

Pastuszczak, M., Jakiela, B., Jaworek, A. K., Wypasek, E., Zeman, J., & Wojas-Pelc, A. (2015). Association of Interleukin-10 promoter polymorphisms with neurosyphilis. *Human Immunology, 76*(7), 469–472. DOI: 10.1016/j.humimm.2015.06.010 PMID: 26100683

Peermohamed, S., Kogilwaimath, S., & Sanche, S. (2020). Neurosyphilis. *Canadian Medical Association Journal, 192*(29), E844–E844. DOI: 10.1503/cmaj.200189 PMID: 32690559

Perdrup, A., Jørgensen, B. B., & Pedersen, N. S. (1981). The profile of neurosyphilis in Denmark A clinical and serological study of all patients in Denmark with neurosyphilis disclosed in the years 1971-1979 incl. by Wassermann reaction (CWRM) in the cerebrospinal fluid. *Acta Dermato-Venereologica. Supplementum, 96*, 1–14. PMID: 6953720

Pintado Maury, I., Alves, M., & Fonseca, T. (2019). Neurosyphilis prevalence at a Portuguese stroke unit care. *Aging Clinical and Experimental Research, 31*(8), 1155–1161. DOI: 10.1007/s40520-018-1052-4 PMID: 30343380

Prevention, C. for D. C. and. (2019). Sexually transmitted disease surveillance 2018. *Atlanta: US Department of Health and Human Services, 10.*

Ramchandani, M. S., Litvack, J. R., & Marra, C. M. (2020). Otosyphilis: A review of the literature. *Sexually Transmitted Diseases, 47*(5), 296–300. DOI: 10.1097/OLQ.0000000000001155 PMID: 32149965

Reddy, A. B., Pinto, M., Hegde, S. P., Iqbal, A. A. M., Bejai, V., & Shenoy, M. M. (2022). A retrospective study on seroprevalence and clinical spectrum of syphilis from a tertiary care Center in South India. *APIK Journal of Internal Medicine, 10*(3), 169–173. DOI: 10.4103/ajim.ajim_58_21

Richardson, D., & Goldmeier, D. (2021). Probenecid in the treatment of neurosyphilis in men who have sex with men: A commentary. *Sexually Transmitted Infections.* PMID: 34510007

Salado-Rasmussen, K., Wessman, M., Cowan, S. A., Gerstoft, J., & Katzenstein, T. L. (2019). Syphilitic hepatitis and neurosyphilis: An observational study of Danish HIV-infected individuals during a 13-year period. *Sexually Transmitted Infections, 95*(6), 416–418. DOI: 10.1136/sextrans-2018-053921 PMID: 30923165

Shen, Y., Dong, X., Liu, J., Lv, H., & Ge, Y. (2022). Serum interleukin-26 is a potential biomarker for the differential diagnosis of neurosyphilis and syphilis at other stages. *Infection and Drug Resistance, 15*, 3693–3702. DOI: 10.2147/IDR.S366308 PMID: 35859909

Simon, R. P. (1985). Neurosyphilis. *Archives of Neurology*, *42*(6), 606–613. DOI: 10.1001/archneur.1985.04060060112021 PMID: 3890813

Singh, A. E. (2020). Ocular and neurosyphilis: Epidemiology and approach to management. *Current Opinion in Infectious Diseases*, *33*(1), 66–72. DOI: 10.1097/QCO.0000000000000617 PMID: 31789673

Solaimalai, D., Gupta, A., George, L., Manesh, A., Karthik, R., Sathishkumar, D., Peter, C. V. D., Varghese, G. M., Pulimood, S. A., Kannangai, R., & Prakash, J. A. J. (2022). Upward trends of syphilis in the non-pregnant adults: A six-year report on clinical and epidemiological profile of syphilis from a tertiary care center, India. *Frontiers in Public Health*, *10*, 908591. DOI: 10.3389/fpubh.2022.908591 PMID: 35958862

Sparling, P. F. (1999). *Natural history of syphilis. Sexually Transmitted Diseases* (3rd ed.). McGraw-Hill.

Spelber, D., & Lahijani, S. (2020). Neurosyphilis presenting as mania and psychosis after incidental treatment with cephalexin: A case report and literature review of Jarisch-Herxheimer reactions. *Psychosomatics*, *61*(2), 177–180. DOI: 10.1016/j.psym.2019.06.001 PMID: 31331661

Swartz, M. N., Healy, B. P., & Musher, D. M. (1999). Late syphilis. *Sexually Transmitted Diseases*, 487–509.

Tan, X., Zhang, J., Li, J., Yue, X., & Gong, X. (2020). The prevalence of asymptomatic neurosyphilis among HIV-negative serofast patients in China: A meta-analysis. *PLoS One*, *15*(11), e0241572. DOI: 10.1371/journal.pone.0241572 PMID: 33147295

Tsai, M., Yang, C., Lee, N., Hsieh, S., Lin, Y., Sun, H., Sheng, W., Lee, K., Yang, S., & Liu, W. (2014). Jarisch-Herxheimer reaction among HIV-positive patients with early syphilis: Azithromycin versus benzathine penicillin G therapy. *African Journal of Reproduction and Gynaecological Endoscopy*, *17*(1). PMID: 25174641

Tuddenham, S., & Ghanem, K. G. (2016). Ocular syphilis: Opportunities to address important unanswered questions. *Sexually Transmitted Infections*, *92*(8), 563–565. DOI: 10.1136/sextrans-2016-052570 PMID: 27116973

Woolston, S. L., Dhanireddy, S., & Marrazzo, J. (2016). Ocular syphilis: A clinical review. *Current Infectious Disease Reports*, *18*(11), 1–6. DOI: 10.1007/s11908-016-0542-9 PMID: 27686678

Workowski, K. A. (2021). Sexually transmitted infections treatment guidelines, 2021. *MMWR. Recommendations and Reports*, 70. PMID: 34292926

Workowski, K. A., Bolan, G. A., & Prevention, C. for D. C. and. (2015). *Sexually transmitted diseases treatment guidelines, 2015.*

Wu, F., Hu, W., Xu, B., & Wang, Q. (2018). Effects of Treponema pallidum on the expression of chemokine ligand 6, 8, 10 in human brain microvascular endothelial cells. *Zhonghua Pifuke Zazhi*, 358–362.

Wu, K.-X., Wang, X.-T., Hu, X.-L., Jiang, X.-Y., Zhuang, J.-C., Xu, Y.-Z., Lin, L.-R., Tong, M.-L., Yang, T.-C., & Liu, L.-L. (2021). LncRNA-ENST00000421645 upregulates kank1 to inhibit IFN-γ expression and promote T cell apoptosis in neurosyphilis. *Frontiers in Microbiology*, *12*, 749171. DOI: 10.3389/fmicb.2021.749171 PMID: 34917045

Wu, S., Ye, F., Wang, Y., & Li, D. (2024). Neurosyphilis: Insights into its pathogenesis, susceptibility, diagnosis, treatment, and prevention. *Frontiers in Neurology*, *14*, 1340321. DOI: 10.3389/fneur.2023.1340321 PMID: 38274871

Xiang, L., Zhang, T., Zhang, B., Zhang, C., Hou, S., & Yue, W. (2021). The associations of increased cerebral small vessel disease with cognitive impairment in neurosyphilis presenting with ischemic stroke. *Brain and Behavior*, *11*(6), e02187. DOI: 10.1002/brb3.2187 PMID: 33998172

Yimtae, K., Srirompotong, S., & Lertsukprasert, K. (2007). Otosyphilis: A review of 85 cases. *Otolaryngology - Head and Neck Surgery*, *136*(1), 67–71. DOI: 10.1016/j.otohns.2006.08.026 PMID: 17210336

Zhang, R.-L., Zhang, J.-P., & Wang, Q.-Q. (2014). Recombinant Treponema pallidum protein Tp0965 activates endothelial cells and increases the permeability of endothelial cell monolayer. *PLoS One*, *9*(12), e115134. DOI: 10.1371/journal.pone.0115134 PMID: 25514584

Zhou, J., Zhang, H., Tang, K., Liu, R., & Li, J. (2022). An Updated Review of Recent Advances in Neurosyphilis. *Frontiers in Medicine*, *9*(September), 1–10. DOI: 10.3389/fmed.2022.800383 PMID: 36203756

Zhu, L., Gu, X., Peng, R.-R., Wang, C., Gao, Z., Zhou, P., Gao, Y., Shi, M., Guan, Z., & Seña, A. C. (2014). Comparison of the cerebrospinal fluid (CSF) toluidine red unheated serum test and the CSF rapid plasma reagin test with the CSF venereal disease research laboratory test for diagnosis of neurosyphilis among HIV-negative syphilis patients in China. *Journal of Clinical Microbiology*, *52*(3), 736–740. DOI: 10.1128/JCM.02522-13 PMID: 24335955

Chapter 4
Insights Into the Pathogenesis, Diagnosis, and Treatment of Tubercular Meningitis

Bhavya Sharda
All India Institute of Medical Sciences, Bhopal, India

Anand Kumar Maurya
All India Institute of Medical Sciences, Bhopal, India

ABSTRACT

The cause of tuberculosis (TB) is Mycobacterium tuberculosis. It remains a global health burden in developing and developed countries. TB meningitis (TBM) can occur when M. tuberculosis spreads to other organs, such as the brain and meninges, despite its primary role as a respiratory infection. The most serious type of tuberculosis is called tuberculous meningitis (TBM). One of the most severe clinical signs of tuberculosis (TB) is the involvement of the central nervous system (CNS), which occurs in 5–10% of extrapulmonary TB patients and makes up around 1% of all TB case. TBM has a significant death rate (20–50%) even when it is identified early and treated with the right antibiotics. Traditional techniques, like the culture of cerebrospinal fluid (CSF) and acid-fast bacilli (AFB) on smears, remain the gold standard for diagnosing TBM.

DOI: 10.4018/979-8-3693-4070-7.ch004

1. INTRODUCTION

The cause of tuberculosis [TB] is *Mycobacterium tuberculosis*. It remains a global health burden in both developing and developed countries. TB meningitis [TBM] can occur when *M. tuberculosis* spreads to other organs, such as the brain and meninges, despite its primary role as a respiratory infection (Spatola et al., 2024). The most serious type of tuberculosis is called tuberculous meningitis [TBM] (Kimuda et al., 2023). A significant clinical manifestation of tuberculosis is central nervous system involvement, which accounts for 5–10% of total extrapulmonary involvement. It constitutes around 1% of all total tuberculosis cases (Cherian & Thomas, 2011). TBM has a significant death rate [20–50%] even when it is identified early and treated with the right antibiotics. Traditional techniques, like the culture of cerebrospinal fluid [CSF] and acid-fast staining demonstrating acid-fast bacilli [AFB] on smears, remain the gold standard for diagnosing TBM. These techniques are inexpensive and popular in environments with limited resources (Lan et al., 2020). However, the small number of bacilli in CSF reduces the sensitivity of microscopy. Clinical decision-making is frequently delayed by the 42-day turnaround time of liquid culture method, even though culture is more sensitive (Stewart, 1953). The tuberculin skin test [TST] is also frequently employed in underdeveloped nations (Johnston et al., 2017). It is still challenging to find very sensitive diagnostic assays for TB meningitis. Improving existing diagnostic methods or creating fresh, creative strategies are urgently needed. Studies on novel biomarkers, such as tryptophan and neuromarkers of brain injury, provide fresh perspectives on the pathophysiology of tuberculosis meningitis. There are still significant knowledge gaps. Accurately diagnosing TBM is difficult since its clinical signs resemble those of other fungal, bacterial, or viral CNS infections and non-infectious CNS illnesses (Spatola et al., 2024). Understanding the pathophysiology underlying the disease's progression will help in developing new diagnostic methods (Spatola et al., 2024). Despite the extensive research, it may not always be easy to diagnose tuberculous meningitis early and distinguish it from pyogenic meningitis, particularly the partially treated kind. Pyogenic and tuberculous meningitis are a significant category of neurological conditions linked to substantial morbidity and mortality (Shekhar et al., 2013). Survivors are also at high risk for long-term neurological sequelae and CNS problems (Cherian & Thomas, 2011). Furthermore, TBM is most likely to develop in children and individuals with HIV, and it can be very deadly in these susceptible groups (Harausz et al., 2018).

2. EPIDEMIOLOGY

The majority of newly diagnosed active cases of tuberculosis occur in poor and underdeveloped nations, indicating that the disease continues to be a global burden (World Health Organization, 2007). The global epidemic is primarily caused by demographic variables like overcrowding, poverty, and malnutrition. In sub-Saharan Africa, 80% of new tuberculosis cases are associated with an immunocompromised state, whereas HIV is responsible for another 20% of infections (World Health Organization, 2007). According to pooled estimates, the percentage of TBM in HIV-negative individuals is 1.3% to 1.8% and 3.6% to 6.8% of people living with HIV (Dodd et al., 2021). Many TBM instances go undetected due to poor diagnostic test performance and availability. The global burden of TBM is very vague (Seddon et al., 2019). Five to ten percent of extrapulmonary TB cases in the United States had CNS involvement, according to a comprehensive epidemiological analysis of the disease (Rieder et al., 1990). One to two percent of people with active TB have been documented to have CNS-TB (Gupta et al., 2024). Five to eight percent of extrapulmonary tuberculosis [EPTB] cases in immunocompetent individuals are caused by CNS-TB. TBM is present in about 70–80% of CNS-TB patients (Gupta et al., 2024). Underdeveloped nations are found to have more no of cases of CNS-TB, according to studies done in industrialised countries (Bidstrup, Andersen, Skinhøj, & Andersen, 2002).

2.1 Worldwide TBM Prevalence:

In 2023, 45% of cases were reported in the WHO Southeast Asia Region, followed by the African Region [24%] and the Western Pacific Region [17%] (World Health Organization, 2024a). A total of 3,179 extrapulmonary illness locations were identified in the US region in 2023. Out of them, only 5.7% represent the TBM cases (Centers for Disease Control and Prevention, 2024). Vietnam accounts for a 4% prevalence of TBM (Dodd et al., 2021). One study in Brazil states that TBM accounts for a total of 6% of extrapulmonary tuberculosis (Gomes et al., 2014), while one study in Texas found this proportion up to 2.7% (Nguyen et al., 2019).

2.2 Prevalence of TBM in India

The incidence of tuberculosis in 2022 was 196, compared to 225 in 2015, while the fatality rate was 23 and 27, respectively, per one million (Mandal et al., 2023). Research shows that among those with tuberculosis, the prevalence of TBM might reach 55.3%. The estimated incidence of TBM in India is approximately 1.5 cases per 100,000 people (Kumar et al., 2023). According to reports, there were 195 tuberculosis cases per 100,000 people in India as of 2023. This indicates continued efforts to control the condition, as it shows a decline from prior years (Press Information Bureau, Government of India, 2024).

3. PATHOGENESIS OF TUBERCULOSIS OF CNS

M. tuberculosis is an acid-fast bacillus [AFB] that is aerobic, nonmotile, and does not generate spores. Standard Lowenstein-Jensen media takes several weeks to support bacterial growth. *M. tuberculosis* can be distinguished from other AFB using Field's biochemical and RNA/DNA-based techniques (Rock et al., 2008). An *M. tuberculosis* infection is contracted by breathing droplet nuclei, which ultimately results in lung alveolar deposition (Rock et al., 2008). Therefore, TBM starts as a lung infection and then spreads hematogenously to the brain. Aerosol droplet inhalation containing tubercular bacilli triggers a localised lung infection, activating antigen-presenting cells that emit various inflammatory markers (Davis, Rohlwink, Proust, Figaji, & Wilkinson, 2019). Under the influence of markers, infected dendritic cell structure migrate to local draining lymph node to promote the development of T-helper 1 cells. T helper one cells activate dendritic cells and macrophages to generate antimicrobial peptides and cytokines to confine the infection. They release cytokines at the injection site (O'Garra et al., 2013). Finally, a granuloma develops, having bacilli in the latent phase (Manyelo, Solomons, Walzl, & Chegou, 2021). One of the following two mechanisms may result in hematogenous spread to other organ systems, including the central nervous system: [i] Prior to granuloma formation, during primary TB infection, *M. tuberculosis* is filtered into the local lymph nodes which may lead to brief bacteraemia or [ii] Lung tissue destruction may happen from the latent infection stage developing into active TB disease due to a lapse or decline in the immunity, especially in the very young, elderly, or immunodeficient ones(Davis, Rohlwink, Proust, Figaji, & Wilkinson, 2019).*M. tuberculosis* bacilli avoid the alveolar epithelium through infected phagocytes or as free bacteria. The following hypothesised pathways could allow TB bacilli to cross the blood-CSF barrier [BCSFB] and the blood-brain barrier [BBB]: [i] *M. tuberculosis* pknD mediates invasion of the brain parenchyma or [ii] "Trojan horse," where tubercular bacilli uses macrophages and infecting neutrophils to get around the obstacles (Be et al., 2012). The tubercular bacilli in the brain cause lesions [called Rich foci] to form in subependymal surface, subpial or meninges (Isabel & Rogelio, 2014). Tubercular bacilli are then discharged into the ventricular system or subarachnoid region upon rupture of these lesions, causing meningeal inflammation and granulomatous infection (Press Information Bureau, Government of India, 2024). In 75% of children, TBM develops less than a year after the initial infection (Thwaites, Chau,

Mai, Drobniewski, McAdam, & Farrar, 2000). Host inflammatory responses cause formation and accumulation of thick inflammatory fluid [exudate] at the base of the brain, leading to poor results in TBM. By creating adhesions and obstructing the basal subarachnoid cisterns, the dense basal inflammatory fluid [exudate] causes hydrocephalus and increased intracranial pressure. According to one study, mycobacterial infections cause immunosuppressive effects on microglial cells, which are more noticeable when the strains are more virulent. These findings have led to the identification of microglia as crucial cells for comprehending the neuropathophysiology of tuberculosis (Curto et al., 2004).

Figure 1. Schematic diagram of the route of inhalation to the formation of TBM

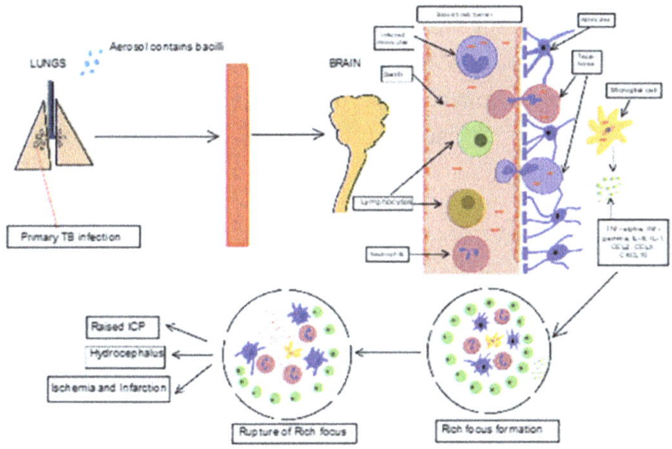

4. PATHOLOGY

4.1 Tubercular Meningitis

This thick gellike exudate, which is most florid in the interpeduncular fossa and suprasellar region anteriorly, can spread over the prepontine cistern and encircle the spinal cord after tubercle bacilli are released from granulomatous-like lesions into the subarachnoid space. Hydrocephalus results from obstruction at the level of the tentorial aperture caused by this thick inflammatory fluid, which envelops cranial nerves and arteries. Neutrophils, lymphocytes, Erythrocytes, and macrophages, are present in more developed thick inflammatory fluid (Rock et al., 2008). A collar of exudate surrounds the midbrain, and the passage of CSF around the upper brain stem is blocked when exudative material extends into the basal cisterns. Additionally, exudate may build up around the third and fourth ventricles' cerebral aqueducts, obstructing the CSF's passage through the ventricular system. Consequently, 75–80% of TBM patients experience hydrocephalus (Rohlwink et al., 2016; Thwaites et al., 2007). Increased intracranial pressure can seriously impair cerebral blood flow, and the pressure of growing ventricles and the opposing pressure of brain oedema brought on by pathologic processes can have a detrimental effect on the grey and white matter, resulting in pallor and generalised myelin loss (Dastur et al., 1995).

The Rich foci are seen in the brain parenchyma and meninges, usually following the vascular pattern. Notably, the basilar areas in the CNS, which are usually where the thick inflammatory fluid is found, do not have a preferential distribution of Rich foci. It is assumed that the tuberculous exudate's localisation to the basilar region is just the consequence of the CSF's typical flow pattern (Davis, Rohlwink, Proust, Figaji, & Wilkinson, 2019). The appearance of vasculitis in vertebrobasilar system, the circle of Willis arteries, and more perforating segments of middle cerebral artery, which leads to infarctions. It causes a severe effect in their distribution, which is seen most severely in TBM.

4.2 Tuberculoma

Tuberculomas are caused by brain parenchymal tubercles that proliferate instead of bursting into the subarachnoid space. As a result, they frequently happen without TBM but likely occur in conjunction with it. Multiple tuberculomas are observed, although they typically appear as solitary lesions. Around a central region of caseating necrosis, brain tuberculomas exhibit a characteristic granulomatous reaction consisting of large cells and epithelioid cells mixed with primary lymphocytes. Instead of pus, liquefaction of the central necrotic area includes a transparent or straw-coloured fluid (Kumar et al., 2002). Tuberculomas are believed to arise from increasing tubercles in the parenchyma and can occur independently or in conjunction with TBM. These lesions are usually granulomatous, with a necrotic core encircled by lymphocytes, astrocytes, and epithelioid cells [which can combine to produce Langhans giant cells]. They are linked to peripheral oedema and vascular growth (Rock et al., 2008); as time passes, the tubercles become clearly defined and encircled by reticulin fibre connective tissue, improving contrasted brain imaging. They can appear in the brainstem, cerebellum, and cerebrum, among other brain parts (Rock et al., 2008; Rohlwink et al., 2016).

4.3 Tuberculous Brain Abscess

Although rare, TB brain abscesses can develop independently or in conjunction with TBM (Kumar et al., 2002). Tubercular bacilli are found in confined collections of pus called abscesses without the epithelioid, giant, and mononuclear cell infiltrates characteristic of TB granulomas (Kumar et al., 2002). Single or multiple (Rock et al., 2008) abscesses have been seen in the cerebrum (Kumar et al., 2002) and posterior fossa (Saini et al., 2011). They are rare in the brain stem. The tubercular abscess wall is significantly thicker than seen in a pyogenic brain abscess, both grossly and radiographically (Kumar et al., 2002). Histopathological findings indicate that vascular tissue with granulation, which includes bacilli, acute and chronic inflammatory cells present in the pus or abscess wall (Whitener, 1978). Even though tuberculous meningitis and tuberculomas are common signs of CNS tuberculosis, TB brain abscesses are uncommon (Vijayakumar et al., 2012).

5. CLINICAL MANIFESTATIONS AND COMPLICATIONS

Age [children > adults], HIV co-infection, malnourishment, recent childhood measles, alcoholism, cancer, adult immunosuppressive medication usage, and disease incidence in the community are risk factors for CNS tuberculosis (Bidstrup, Andersen, Skinhøj, & Andersen, 2002). As a subacute illness, mild fever, lethargy, drowsiness, nausea, vomiting, personality changes, and pulmonary TB symptoms that typically appear for many days or sometimes up to weeks [an average of 6 to 30 days] in TBM. [like a cough] (Daniel, Grace, & Natrajan, 2019; Marx & Chan, 2011). Cranial neurological disorders, brain swelling, seizures, impaired mental status, and more intense headaches are some of the symptoms that patients with advanced illness may exhibit (Marx & Chan, 2011). Clinical symptoms in adults can include unconsciousness, confusion, palsy of various cranial nerves [cranial nerves III, IV, VI, and VIII], and a stiff neck (Manyelo, Solomons, Walzl, & Chegou, 2021). About 10% to 20% of instances result in clinical motor impairments, such as paraplegia, hemiplegia, or monoplegia (Thwaites, Chau, Mai, Drobniewski, McAdam, & Farrar, 2000). If TBM is not treated, death is always inevitable.

Clinical symptoms in children can include localised neurological indications, evidence of elevated pressure inside the brain [such as palsy of abducens nerve], and early apathy or agitation that develops into meningism (Manyelo, Solomons, Walzl, & Chegou, 2021). Children with TBM frequently have a high fever, neck pain, seizures and digestive issues such nausea and vomiting. Headaches are not so common in children (Cherian & Thomas, 2011). According to the stage of presentation, neurological manifestations may vary from irritability and drowsiness to comatose. Seizures are more common in children and are apt to occur early in the illness (Leonard, 2017). In children, TBM often appears three months after the initial TB infection (Cherian & Thomas, 2011). There seems to be a strong correlation between disseminated [military] TB and older children, in particular. Some have hypothesised that robust hematogenous spread raises the risk of a Rich focus developing and eventually rupturing (Donald et al., 2005). Children with TBM typically experience symptoms more quickly, and need medical help within few hours of the onset. Given this population's vulnerability to both TBM and disseminated TB, as well as the challenge of clinically assessing newborns for TBM, a number of pediatric experts recommend lumbar punctures for all children younger than 12 months. Even while it may be claimed that other high-risk, challenging to assess persons, like those who have severe HIV coinfection, also undergo lumbar punctures when diagnosed with tuberculosis, CNS symptoms typically prompt the doctor to include a lumbar puncture as part of the workup (Rock et al., 2008). The location of a tuberculoma or abscess greatly influences its clinical findings; patients may experience papilledema, dizziness, seizures, or other signs of high pressure in the brain. With tuberculomas, the rate at which symptoms appear is often monitored for weeks to months. Fever, headaches, and localised neurological impairments are common symptoms of brain abscesses, which occur more acutely within 1 week to 2 months but more slowly than bacterial brain abscesses (Kumar et al., 2002).

Atypical presentations: A few per cent of individuals arrive without the above-mentioned subacute course and distinctive prodrome. TBM occasionally manifests in adults as a slowly developing dementia that lasts for several months and is characterised by memory impairments, social disengagement, and personality changes (Leonard, 2017).

Complications: Patients with TBM may experience a variety of spinal issues, including tuberculous radiculomyelitis, an inflammation that affects the spinal cord and nerve roots; spinal tuberculomas, which are isolated lesions in the spinal cord; and syringomyelia, which is a cystic growth in the spinal cord and Infection of the vertebrae that frequently result in structural abnormalities is known as vertebral tuberculosis (Garg et al., 2023; Tai et al., 2017). Modifications to the Medical Research Council [MRC] staging system make it simple to determine the extent of clinical symptoms in TBM patients, as mentioned in Table 1 (Medical Research Council, 1948).

Table 1. Tubercular meningitis severity grading according to MRC

I	Patients who have no pareses, minimal or no meningitis symptoms, and nonspecific symptoms are generally well and fully cognizant. CSF examination was used to establish the diagnosis.
III	Individuals who are gravely unwell, profoundly unconscious, or have severe pareses
II	Individuals who fall between the first two groupings

In clinical practices, it is more beneficial to have a Glasgow Coma Scale [GCS] score-based grading, as shown in Table 2 (Heemskerk et al., 2011).

Table 2. Medical council grading system for TBM

Grade	Diagnostic standards
Grade 1	GCS 15 with zero focal neurology
Grade 2	GCS 15 along focused neurology or GCS of 11–14
Grade 3	GCS $\leq$ 10

Two scoring systems are used to diagnose TBM, i.e. "Thwaites' scoring" and "The Lancet consensus grading", as shown in Tables 3 and 4, respectively (Sulaiman et al., 2020).

Table 3. Thwaites' scoring

Criteria	Score
Age[years] More than or equal to 36 Less than 36	2 0
WBC[10^3 /ml] More than or equal to 15,000 Less than 15,000	4 0
History of illness[days] More than or equal to 6 Less than 6	5 0
CSF total WBC [10^3 /ml] More than or equal to 900 Less than 900	3 0
CSF % neutrophils More than or equal to 75 Less than 75	4 0

Table 4. Lancet Grading

Criteria	Score
Clinical guidelines:	[Maximum category score=6]
• Duration of symptoms more than 5 days	4
• TB-related general symptoms, including one or more of the following: Night sweats, a persistent cough that lasts longer than two weeks, or weight loss	2
• A positive TST or IGRA [only found in children below 10 years old] or a history of close association with an individual who has pulmonary tuberculosis during the past year.	2
• Focal neurological impairment [apart from cranial nerve palsies]	1
• Palsy of Cranial nerve	1
• Altered sensorium	1
CSF biochemistry	[Maximum category score = 4]
• Clear look	1
• Cells: 10–500 per microliter	1
• Lymphocytic dominance [> 50%]	1
• Protein content greater than 1 g/L	1
• A cerebral spinal fluid sugar level below 2·2 mmol/L or a CSF to plasma sugar ratio below 50%;	1
Criteria for brain imaging	[Maximum category score = 6]
• Enlarged ventricles	1
• Basal meningeal enlargement	2
• Tuberculoma in CNS	2
• Infarct	1
• Pre-contrast basal hyperdensity	2
Evidence of tuberculosis elsewhere	[Maximum category score = 4]
• Active TB is suggested by a chest radiograph with symptoms of pulmonary TB = 2 and military pulmonary TB = 4	2/4
• CT/ MRI/ sonography evidence for tuberculosis other than CNS	2
• Smear positive identified or culture positive from the sample other than CSF like sputum, lymph node aspirate, gastric aspirate, urine, blood	4
• Positive commercial *M tuberculosis* NAAT from sample other than CNS specimen	4

6. DIAGNOSIS

6.1 Traditional Csf Examination

CSF from individuals with CNS tuberculosis typically shows substantially raised protein levels, hypoglycaemia [low glucose], and mild lymphocytic pleocytosis (Luo et al., 2018; Shekhar et al., 2013; Wang et al., n.d.). As a result, it resembles to other various infectious and non-infectious CNS diseases. According to one study of adult CNS TB cases in Turkey that were not HIV-infected, 85% of patients had CSF lymphocytes, 15% had neutrophils, 77% had high protein levels, 67.2% had hypoglycaemia, and 54% had raised opening pressure (Sütlaş et al., 2003). Even though hypoglycaemia is widespread in both TBM and bacterial meningitis, its presence may offer a useful distinguishing characteristic that sets these aetiologies apart from other reasons of meningoencephalitis, particularly when considering empirical antibiotics (Thwaites et al., 2002). In certain instances, the preponderance of neutrophils probably indicates an early stage of infection that will eventually change to a primarily lymphocytic profile over days to weeks (Cao et al., 2022). In rare cases, patients with TBM have been shown to have expected CSF results (Chohan et al., 2012). It has been noted that antituberculosis treatment can cause the CSF to shift to neutrophil predominance momentarily (Sütlaş et al., 2003). The formation of tuberculomas during treatment has been linked in at least one retrospective series to this "paradoxical response," which has been hypothesised to be caused by a hypersensitivity brought on by tubercular protein secretion during antituberculosis treatment (Sütlaş et al., 2003).

6.2 Microbiological Analysis

Mycobacterium tuberculosis detection and diagnostic confirmation of TBM are hampered by low bacterial counts in cerebrospinal fluid [CSF], especially in children where it might be challenging to obtain sufficient CSF quantities (Donovan & Thwaites, 2020).

6.2.1 Acid-Fast Bacilli [AFB] Smear

Finding AFB in the CSF through smear and culture methods remains the most important and widely available way to diagnose CNS tuberculosis. Approximately 100 AFB/ml of CSF can be detected using standard staining techniques as Ziehl and Neelsen staining, the Kinyoun method, or auramine-rhodamine staining (Verdon et al., 1996). The sensitivity of staining CSF smears for AFB bacilli is low [between 10% to 15%] (Bahr, Meintjes, & Boulware, 2019). As a result, smear microscopy cannot accurately diagnose TBM. The World Health Organisation [WHO] advises using mycobacterial culture, the gold standard for TB diagnosis, for TBM in adults and children.

6.2.2 Culture

Lowenstein-Jensen [L-J] and Ogawa are examples of traditional solid media. Furthermore, the sensitivity of L-J culture is between 50 and 70 percent of the case definitions (Thwaites, Chau, & Farrar, 2004). The liquid culture system includes BACTEC and Mycobacteria growth indicator tube [MGIT 960]. MGIT tubes are incubated for 42 days until MGIT equipment automatically recognises them as positive (Chen et al., 2022). Traditional L-J culture has gradually been superseded by liquid culture, because of their higher sensitivity, quicker turnaround times, and capacity to support a larger variety of isolates, including those from specimens with low bacilli counts and those that are difficult to cultivate on solid media. Getting a culture is essential because MTB growth in culture enables drug sensitivity testing, which can significantly influence prognosis and appropriate therapy selection (Cherian & Thomas, 2011). Compared to other TB tests, culture has a higher sensitivity [approximately 50%] for diagnosing tuberculosis; nevertheless, one disadvantage is its turnaround time, which can reach eight weeks with solid media like Lowenstein-Jensen (Bahr, Meintjes, & Boulware, 2019; Thwaites, Chau, Mai, Drobniewski, McAdam, & Farrar, 2000).

6.2.3 MPT64 AG

MPT64 is an antigen test that distinguishes the *M. tuberculosis complex* from mycobacteria other than TB species, a large culture filtrate protein [24 kDa] (Nagai et al., 1991; Yamaguchi et al., 1989) encoded by the RD2 region genes (Fu et al., 2009). It is based on a quick immunochromatographic assay and is straightforward. All culture-positive isolates are tested for presumptive identification (Arora et al., 2015). A 0.1ml of positive liquid culture is put into the sample well. The test cassette strips are then incubated at room temperature for 15-30 minutes. The pink band in the 'C' region confirms the test validity. An additional pink band in the 'T' region confirms the positivity for TBM (Arora et al., 2015).

6.2.4 Drug Susceptibility Testing [DST]

Drug sensitivity tests come in various forms and are frequently employed in underdeveloped nations as a handy way to direct the selection of therapeutic anti-tuberculosis medications. This approach is time-consuming; results can be obtained in two to three weeks, and medication susceptibility can be demonstrated in at least three to four weeks (Caviedes et al., 2000). The MODS[Microscopic observation drug susceptibility] assay is a test for susceptibility to drugs based on microscopic inspection and the MGIT culture approach. This assay is dependable, affordable, and capable of quickly detecting medication susceptibility while cultivating MTB. MODS is more practical than other methods in diagnosing clinically suspected TBM. With a sensitivity of 92.7% and specificity of 99.3%, MODS is a quick and accurate tool that has been created in recent years to rapidly identify pyrazinoic acid, a reduced form of pyrazinamide [PZA], in order to assess PZA resistance. In nations with TB burden and limited resources, there will be a sizable market for this assay, which shows great promise (Alcántara et al., 2019). This is used in the management of Tubercular Meningitis.

6.3 Biochemical Analysis

6.3.1 ADA Levels

ADA deaminates adenosine irreversibly, an essential enzyme in purine metabolism, turning it into inosine. ADA is a sign of cell-mediated immunity and linked to lymphocyte differentiation and proliferation (Rock et al., 2008). ADA1 and ADA2 are the two distinct isoforms of ADA. Although ADA1 is found in various organs, it has a key role in the activity of lymphocytes along with macrophages. ADA2 is predominantly expressed across macrophages and increases in several infections and diseases associated with the immune system. The ADA measures of the CSF are to enhance the TBM detection, which has been assessed in several studies (Choi et al., 2002; Coovadia et al., 1986; Mishra, 1996). While some studies have demonstrated differentiation between bacterial meningitis and TBM using only ADA, others may not (Gambhir et al., 1999), and other study found that ADA wasn't that much effective to differentiate TBM associated with HIV-infected individuals (Corral et al., 2004). The practical application of this assay is further complicated by the lack of recognised conventional cut-offs of ADA values for diagnosing TBM. ADA values in CSF help to predict poor neurological outcomes in paediatric TBM patients (Jakka et al., 2005). For the detection of TBM, this test has 89% sensitivity and a 91% specificity (Prasad et al., 2023).

6.3.2 Tuberculostearic Acid

Several types of gas chromatography have identified Tuberculostearic acid, a fatty acid constituent of the cell wall. It is present in the cerebrospinal fluid of patients with tuberculous meningitis (Brooks et al., 1990; Fong et al., 2023). The clinical application of this technique has been restricted due to the need for costly equipment and significant skill, even though it has demonstrated good sensitivity and specificity in limited investigations (Rock et al., 2008).

6.4 Molecular Diagnostic Techniques

6.4.1 Nucleic Acid Amplification Tests

Microbiological techniques like AFB staining and culture are restricted because there aren't many bacteria in the CSF with TBM; however, molecular biology approaches are beneficial by using NAATs to identify the MTB genome, the molecular detection of pathogens in CSF aids in the diagnosis of TB and anti-TB medication resistance. These are considerably more accurate tests than smear screening. Therefore, it requires a shorter period of diagnosis as compared to culture procedures (Pormohammad et al., 2019). Additionally, even after brief anti-TB treatment [5–15 days], NAATs can identify TB DNA (Thwaites, Caws, Chau et al, 2004).

a. Xpert MTB/RIF

Cepheid [United States] created the Xpert MTB/RIF. It is a completely automated, real-time, heminested PCR assay. Xpert may concurrently identify rifampicin resistance and tubercular bacilli in CSF and other clinical specimens using the rpoB gene (World Health Organization, 2011). Rapidly producing results in two hours, Xpert is highly automated, has a reduced risk of cross-contamination compared to culture, and is safer than smear microscopy (Cresswell et al., 2018). In clinical practice, Xpert sensitivity is relatively low despite its high specificity for identifying TBM. It is seen mostly in specimens with negative smear results and in HIV-associated individuals. Centrifuging CSF samples can increase sensitivity, but to improve the early identification of TBM, it must be used in conjunction with other extremely sensitive detection methods. This test has a high specificity, whereas its sensitivity is low for diagnosing TBM (Chen et al., 2020).

b. Xpert MTB/RIF Ultra

Cepheid [United States] has created an advanced-generation level of Xpert assay dubbed Xpert MTB/RIF Ultra, that doubles specimen capacity while utilising the previous reaction system and equipment to lessen the constraints. Semi-nested PCR is replaced with nested PCR as the detection method. Two targets of DNA [IS6110 and IS1081] are introduced concurrently (Bahr, Meintjes, & Boulware, 2019) for more precise MTB and RIF resistance detection. According to specific research, Xpert MTB/RIF Ultra has a lesser LOD [16 colony forming units/mL] than Xpert [114 cfu/mL] (Chakravorty et al., 2017). This is used in TBM Identification. Xpert MTB/RIF Ultra is superior to other traditional microbiological techniques. Although its sensitivity is not that much good (Bahr et al., 2016; Chen et al., 2020). This test has a 68% sensitivity and 100% specificity (Chen et al., 2020) for diagnosing TBM.

c. LAMP [Loop-Mediated Isothermal Amplification] Test

It is a NAAT that uses DNA primers and polymerases that bind to target DNA and are subsequently amplified. LAMP has also been used to diagnose TBM. LAMP may be more appropriate for environments with limited resources because it can lamp up DNA in a single tube at a consistent temperature under 60-65 minutes (Poplin et al., 2020). Compared to traditional PCR, LAMP-based assays have 88–96% sensitivity, while traditional in-house PCR has a sensitivity of 53% (Poplin et al., 2020).

d. TruNAAT

The automated, battery-powered, portable Truenat MTB test is intended for use in locations with limited infrastructure, such as mobility vans or outlying health centres (World Health Organization, 2024b). A detection limit is to be set according to manufacture kit. The assay detects the nrdZ gene, that encodes the cobalamin-dependent protein. Additionally, this recognises the gene sequence of IS6110. It takes about 40 minutes to extract DNA and identify MTB. If the results came positive, the same extracted DNA will now be placed onto its Rif chip and examined for rifampicin resistance (World Health Organization, 2024b). This can be used to change the treatment plan of tubercular meningitis patients.

e. Line Probe Assays

The line probe assay [LPA] has been recommended by the WHO, Geneva. It is also recommended by the Foundation for Innovative New Diagnostics [FIND] for directly identifying MDR-TB from cultures (World Health Organization, 2016). It is used to identify mutations in the sites of the rpoB, inhA, and katG genes, as well as deletions found in the wild-type gene sites. This test uses reverse hybridization after multiplex PCR (World Health Organization, 2016).

The MTBDRplus LPA [Hain Lifesciences, Germany] (World Health Organization, 2022) is used to confirm Xpert-detected cases of rifampin resistance using DNA from a flagged MGIT culture. The cetyltrimethylammonium bromide [CTAB] method extracts DNA from positive MGIT cultures (Honoré-Bouakline et al., 2003). The purified DNA is subsequently utilized for this test in accordance with the manufacturer's instructions. Diagnosing TBM as soon as possible and identifying treatment resistance quickly to manage this medical issue effectively and promptly is ideal. The effectiveness of a commercially available LPA [Genotype® MTBDR plus test] on culture isolates and direct CSF samples of TBM patients is there (Gupta et al., 2015).

6.4.2 Assays Based on PCR

Multiplex PCR enables the simultaneous amplification of many target fragments of DNA in just one test. Multiplex PCR may help in differentiating MTB in CSF samples and non-tuberculous mycobacterial species (Kumar et al., 2014). Three primers are used in this PCR: IS6110, protein b, along with MPT64. TBM achieved

94.4% sensitivity and 100% specificity, respectively (Poplin et al., 2020). This is also one of the methods used in TBM identification.

6.5 Immunological Tests

a. Lipid Antigen Detection

A glycolipid called lipoarabinomannan is a component of the cell wall of mycobacteria (Patel et al., 2009). The lipoarabinomannan component of bacteria in the CSF is also being used. LAM antigen has 64% sensitivity and a 69% specificity for detection of TBM (Patel et al., 2009).

b. Cy-Tb Test

Recently, *Mycobacterium tuberculosis* antigen-based skin tests [TBST] have used particular TB antigens, like the Cy-Tb. This particular TBST may provide a cost-effective substitute and is more accurate than the Tuberculin Skin Test. It is a purified protein derivative-based skin test. The next-generation skin test for TB infection [TBI] detection is Cy-Tb (Pai et al., 2008). The *Mycobacterium tuberculosis complex* [MTBC] releases cell filtrate protein 10 [CFP-10] and early secretory antigen 6 [ESAT-6]. These are two distinct antigens found in Cy-Tb in a 1:1 ratio. It is used to identify MTB in TBM patients.

c. Interferon-Gamma Release Assays [IGRAs]

The emergence of T-cell-based interferon-gamma release assays [IGRA] has significantly advanced in recent years. Compared to the pure protein derivative [PPD], IGRAs are in vitro tests that are more sensitive to MTB. These depend on the release of interferon-γ [IFN-γ] after antigens [such as culture filtrate protein 10 [CFP10] and early secreted antigenic target 6 [ESAT6]] activate T cells. Strong proof that the BCG vaccination has no effect on IGRAs' reasonable specificity has been revealed by systematic reviews (Menzies et al., 2007; Pai et al., 2008). Blood IGRA and CSF IGRA can be good diagnostic studies for detecting TBM (Shi et al., 2022).

6.6 Newer Methods

a. MALDI TOF

Matrix-assisted laser desorption-ionisation time of flight mass spectrometry [MALDI-TOF-MS] is taking the place of traditional techniques for identifying mycobacteria in medical laboratories. Numerous obstacles in identifying bacteria are addressed by this relatively straightforward method. Identifying species with similar behavioural, genetic, and biochemical features was previously unattainable, until technology developed, and databases holding full spectra of known organisms grew. Mass-to-charge ratio of particles determines how they are ionized and separated in the analytical technique known as MALDI-TOF MS. It tracks how long it takes to reach a detector at the end of a time-of-flight tube. The created spectrum, which has mass-to-charge ratios along the x-axis and intensity along the y-axis, is compared to a database of spectra via identified mycobacteria (Rychert, 2019). This technique is used to identify the organism at the species level in TBM cases.

b. Next-Generation Sequencing [NGS]

The necessity for a quicker and more precise diagnostic approach to support early treatment is highlighted by the traditional use of classical microbiological techniques for TBM diagnosis, which have produced poor and frequently delayed results.

NGS is a method for concurrently sequencing multiple genes at high throughput, to be compared to reference sequence libraries later. Two examples of NGS applications are whole-genome sequencing [WGS] and target NGS. The former is helpful when researching acquired resistance in bacteria since it makes it possible to sequence specific genome regions, focusing on genes of interest. In the second instance, the complete genome has been sequenced, which is highly beneficial for TB research and epidemiological surveillance, to name just two applications. Both methods can be carried out on the same sequencer using DNA extracts from clinical samples or bacterial cultures. Targeted NGS can produce positive results in these situations, but sensitivity is significantly decreased when a significant amount of human DNA is present (Beviere et al., 2023). The *Mycobacterium tuberculosis* genome may be quickly and efficiently sequenced using NGS, which enables comprehensive genetic diversity analysis, treatment resistance detection, and possibly earlier, more precise diagnosis. However, particularly in environments with limited resources, its high cost, technical complexity, and requirement for strong bioinformatics pipelines may prevent its broad implementation (Beviere et al., 2023).

6.7 Radiological Assessment

Although the diagnosis accuracy of TBM and tuberculomas has significantly increased with the introduction of brain scanning methods such as CT scan [computerized tomography scans] and MRI [magnetic resonance imaging], no set of radiographic abnormalities is pathognomonic for CNS TB. A recent review of the use of neuroradiographic methods in assessing CNS TB was conducted elsewhere

(Bernaerts, Vanhoenacker, Parizel, Van Goethem, van Altena, & Laridon, 2003). Basal meningeal hypertrophy, increased pressure in brain, arterial ruptures in the brain stem, and supratentorial parenchymal proliferation of brain are frequently recognised neuroradiological characteristics of TBM (Bernaerts, Vanhoenacker, Parizel, Van Goethem, van Altena, & Laridon, 2003). The potential of brain scanning techniques to detect its symptoms in HIV-associated individuals has raised some concerns as they can't distinguish whether it is because of TB or because of HIV infection (Villoria et al., 1995). CT found basal meningeal hypertrophy, enlargement of ventricles, tuberculoma, and rupture of various arteries, which helped distinguish CNS tuberculosis and bacterial meningitis. It also suggested that basal meningeal hypertrophy, tuberculoma, or both are highly sensitive and highly specific for TBM (Przybojewski et al., 2006). In general, MRI is more effective as compare to CT scans in evaluating CNS TB (Rock et al., 2008). But its availability is limited globally, and there is also a need of general anaesthesia in younger children, which indicates its influence on TBM diagnosis is limited (Andronikou, Wieselthaler, Smith, Douis, Fieggen, & van Toorn, 2005). It isn't easy to radiographically assess therapy response in TBM because of the response's unpredictability. Even with adequate therapy, some individuals may show a persistent increase in basal meningeal expansion, while others may show an initial increase, and healing may be viewed as lacking basal meningovascular enhancement. Meningeal calcium deposits and certain areas of degeneration are possible long-term effects of TBM (Bernaerts, Vanhoenacker, Parizel, Van Goethem, van Altena, & Laridon, 2003). Either high or low density, circular, lobulated masses with uneven walls that exhibit homogeneous or ring enhancement following contrast administration are commonly referred to as tuberculomas (Katti, 2004). They are usually located in the frontal and parietal lobes and manifest as single or multiple nodules. Calcifications, local atrophy, or the absence of any lingering radiological anomalies are examples of late radiographic alterations in tuberculomas. Tuberculous brain abscesses typically require surgery for microbiological diagnosis because they cannot be reliably distinguished radiographically from pyogenic abscesses (Katti, 2004).

7. TREATMENT

7.1 Antitubercular Therapy

Clinical methods such as the "Thwaites' scoring" and the "Lancet grading" are used in diagnosing tuberculous meningitis [TBM]. They aid in distinguishing bacterial meningitis in particular from other forms of meningitis. For the first 18 to 24 months, a patient should take at least five medications, including fluoroquinolone and another injectable agent, according to the WHO (Davis et al., 2018). The conventional chemotherapy plan, commonly referred to as the RIPE protocol, consists of a lengthy "continuation phase" with two medications and an "intensive phase" with four drugs. It is specifically composed of 25 mg/kg per day of pyrazinamide [PZE], 5 mg/kg per day of isoniazid [INH], 10 mg/kg per day of rifampicin [RMP], and 15 mg/kg per day of streptomycin [SM]/ethambutol [ETB] for atleast two months, followed by isoniazid and rifampicin for atleast seven to ten months (Dawi et al., 2024; Nahid et al., 2016).

The same dosages are used to treat pulmonary TB and CNS-TB [strong recommendation, low level of evidence]. A 6-month intensive program [6HRZEto] may be modified to a 12-month program [2HRZE/10HR] for children and adolescents with TB meningitis that has been clinically or bacteriologically diagnosed [without any indication or suspicion of MDR/RR-TB] [new: conditional recommendation, very low certainty of evidence] (World Health Organization, 2022).

Suppose the patient has a history of previous TB therapy. In that case, in contrast with a patient who has MDR-TB or a poor clinical response to first-line TB medication within two weeks despite a definitive diagnosis and satisfactory treatment adherence, MDR-TB therapy should be taken into consideration. Similar to how ordinary TBM is treated without controlled trials, MDR tubercular meningitis is primarily treated according to one's experience treating MDR pulmonary tuberculosis, which does not have enough evidence to back it (Rock et al., 2008). Second-line medications like aminoglycosides only cross the blood-brain barrier when meninges are inflamed, and fluoroquinolones can enter the central nervous system but have lower levels in CSF (DeVincenzo et al., 1999). When extremely drug-resistant tuberculosis [XDR-TB] [which is defined by resistance to rifampicin, isoniazid, fluoroquinolones, and either amikacin, capreomycin, or kanamycin] develops, even these second-line therapies will be ineffective. With their intense CNS penetration, second-line medications like cycloserine and ethionamide, which share structural similarities with isoniazid, may be the only ones available to start a treatment plan for XDR TBM (Rock et al., 2008).

Eliminating MTB and controlling host inflammatory reactions are key components of TBM therapy (Dawi et al., 2024). Eliminating inflammatory processes like ferroptosis is a key component of alternative treatment for TB meningitis caused by oxidative stress. Ferroptosis happens concurrently with the disease's progression. Because of this, scientists have looked into several potential treatments that specifically address the ferroptosis and oxidative stress mechanisms that underlie TB meningitis. One standard and ongoing treatment for ferroptosis is iron chelators. Deferoxamine, deferiprone, and deferasirox are three primary iron chelators—have received FDA approval for clinical use (Dawi et al., 2024).

7.2 Adjunctive Steroid Therapy

Corticosteroids are adjunctive agents to decrease inflammation in the subarachnoid region (O'Toole et al., 1969). The use of corticosteroids in this fashion has always been associated with concerns about the possible reduction of medication penetration into the central nervous system and the degradation of cellular defence against *M. tuberculosis*. There doesn't seem to be any difference between corticosteroid therapy and first-line antituberculosis therapy in terms of drug penetration into the CSF (O'Toole et al., 1969). Dexamethasone is prescribed in a starting dose of 8 mg per day for children under 25 kg and 12 mg per day for adults and children above 25 kg. The first dose is administered for three weeks, after which it is progressively reduced over the next three weeks (Donovan et al., 2018).

7.3 Surgical Therapy

Since the development of efficient antituberculosis therapy, surgery has mostly been utilized to treat the serious complication of retension of fluid in brain, reduce the mass effect of tuberculomas, and drain brain abscesses. Although the exact cause is unknown, hydrocephalus is believed to be caused by basal meningitis, in which the CSF flow is obstructed from the fourth ventricle's exit site to the arachnoid villi's site of absorption or perhaps the arachnoid villi themselves are destroyed (Paliwal & Garg, 2021). Ventriculoperitoneal shunts [VPS], osmotic medications, sequential lumbar punctures, external ventricular irrigation, or diuretics can all be used to treat hydrocephalus, a very prevalent side effect of CNS tuberculosis. The use of corticosteroids and traditional antituberculosis medication has largely overshadowed the function of surgery for tuberculomas, which is primarily reserved for treatment failures or situations where the diagnosis is unclear. Therapies available for tubercular abscesses include basic puncture, continuous draining, fractional drainage, periodic aspiration through a burr hole, stereotactic drainage, and total abscess excision (Rock et al., 2008). When VPS is used to treat TBM-associated hydrocephalus, success rates have varied from 40 to 50%, with a complication risk of roughly 30% (Agarwal et al., 2005). Recent encouraging results about the safety and efficacy of neuroendoscopy in treating hydrocephalus may reduce the need for VPS in all population (Baticulon & Dewan, 2021; Husain et al., 2005).

8. PROGNOSIS

The mortality rate ranged from 5% to 23%. Between 14 and 52 percent of children with TBM experienced neurological aftereffects after treatment. In 2014, a systematic evaluation of the treatment results for childhood TBM examined 1636 children and 19 studies. The chances of surviving without handicaps were 36.7%, whereas the probability of dying even with treatment was 19.3% (Daniel, Grace, & Natrajan, 2019). Close monitoring is frequently required after the start of antituberculosis medication because the development of sequelae, such as hydrocephalus, may also be delayed. It has been demonstrated that in children with CNS TB, weekly and monthly follow-up CT scans following the initial scan are especially crucial for identifying significant diagnostic findings and adverse sequelae (Andronikou, Wieselthaler, Smith, Douis, Fieggen, & van Toorn, 2005). About 20 to 30 percent of TBM survivors suffer from some neurological damage. These disabilities include hemiparesis, blindness, deafness, mental retardation, visual impairment, epilepsy, palsies of cranial nerve, and neuropathy. The presenting stage of the disease can also predict poor neurological outcomes (Donovan et al., 2018; Girgis et al., 1998).

9. PREVENTION

According to several studies, BCG has an effectiveness of 75 to 85% in preventing TBM (Filho et al., n.d.; Miceli et al., 1988). BCG immunisation also prevents TBM, according to two recent meta-analyses. BCG's effectiveness lasts ten years following newborn vaccination (Syggelou et al., 2020). In areas where tuberculosis is very endemic, the BCG vaccine is often effective enough to justify ongoing immunisation efforts. It even appears to lower the severity of the disease when it does arise. However, a prior BCG immunization does not undermine the need to investigate TBM in the proper medical settings, as efficacy is not 100% as with all immunisations (Rock et al., 2008).

10. SUMMARY

This chapter includes TBM's clinical characteristics, aetiology, and epidemiology, highlighting the most serious form of tuberculosis.These indicate the challenges associated with the diagnosis and therapy of TBM. This chapter concludes that TBM-related issues urgently need better monitoring, and treatment methods are required. Future studies should focus on improving TBM through newer diagnostic techniques, investigating novel therapy combinations of antitubercular drugs, and assessing the efficacy and safety of complementary medicines.Improving existing diagnostic methods or creating fresh, creative strategies for diagnosing TBM are urgently needed. Despite improvements in diagnostic technology and efficient treatment alternatives, it still presents significant management issues. 20%-40% of those affected die despite anti-TB chemotherapy, and many of those who survive have severe neurological impairments (Kurien et al., 2013).

REFERENCES

Agarwal, D., Gupta, A., & Mehta, V. S. (2005). Role of shunt surgery in pediatric tubercular meningitis with hydrocephalus. *Indian Pediatrics*, *42*(7), 245–249. https://www.indianpediatrics.net/july2005/735.pdf

Alcántara, R., Fuentes, P., Antiparra, R., Santos, M., Gilman, R. H., & Kirwan, D. E. (2019). MODS-Wayne, a colorimetric adaptation of the microscopic-observation drug susceptibility (MODS) assay for detection of Mycobacterium tuberculosis pyrazinamide resistance from sputum samples. *Journal of Clinical Microbiology*, *57*(2), e01162–e18. https://www.ncbi.nlm.nih.gov/pmc/articles/PMC6355525/

Andronikou, S., Wieselthaler, N., Smith, B., Douis, H., Fieggen, A. G., & van Toorn, R. (2005). Value of early follow-up CT in paediatric tuberculous meningitis. *Pediatric Radiology*, *35*(11), 1092–1099. DOI: 10.1007/s00247-005-1549-9

Arora, J., Kumar, G., Verma, A. K., Bhalla, M., Sarin, R., & Myneedu, V. P. (2015). Utility of MPT64 antigen detection for rapid confirmation of Mycobacterium tuberculosis complex. *Journal of Global Infectious Diseases*, *7*(2), 66–69. https://www.ncbi.nlm.nih.gov/pmc/articles/PMC4448327/

Bahr, N. C., Marais, S., Caws, M., van Crevel, R., Wilkinson, R. J., & Tyagi, J. S. (2016). GeneXpert MTB/RIF to diagnose tuberculous meningitis: Perhaps the first test but not the last. *Clinical Infectious Diseases*, *62*(9), 1133–1135. https://www.ncbi.nlm.nih.gov/pmc/articles/PMC4826457/

Bahr, N. C., Meintjes, G., & Boulware, D. R. (2019). Inadequate diagnostics: The case to move beyond the bacilli for detection of meningitis due to Mycobacterium tuberculosis. *Journal of Medical Microbiology*, *68*(5), 755–760. https://www.ncbi.nlm.nih.gov/pmc/articles/PMC7176281/

Bahr, N. C., Meintjes, G., & Boulware, D. R. (2019). Inadequate diagnostics: The case to move beyond the bacilli for detection of meningitis due to Mycobacterium tuberculosis. *Journal of Medical Microbiology*, *68*(5), 755–760. https://www.microbiologyresearch.org/content/journal/jmm/10.1099/jmm.0.000975

Baticulon, R. E., & Dewan, M. C. (2021). Endoscopic third ventriculostomy and choroid plexus coagulation in infants: Current concepts and illustrative cases. Neurology India, 69(Suppl. 2). https://journals.lww.com/neur/fulltext/2021/69002/endoscopic_third_ventriculostomy_and_choroid.38.aspx

Be, N. A., Bishai, W. R., & Jain, S. K. (2012). Role of Mycobacterium tuberculosis pknD in the pathogenesis of central nervous system tuberculosis. *BMC Microbiology*, *12*, 7. https://www.ncbi.nlm.nih.gov/pmc/articles/PMC3322341/

Bernaerts, A., Vanhoenacker, F. M., Parizel, P. M., Van Goethem, J. W. M., van Altena, R., & Laridon, A. (2003). Tuberculosis of the central nervous system: Overview of neuroradiological findings. *European Radiology*, *13*(8), 1876–1890. DOI: 10.1007/s00330-002-1608-7
Bernaerts, A., Vanhoenacker, F. M., Parizel, P. M., Van Goethem, J. W. M., van Altena, R., & Laridon, A. (2003). Tuberculosis of the central nervous system: Overview of neuroradiological findings. *European Radiology*, *13*(8), 1876–1890. DOI: 10.1007/s00330-002-1608-7
Beviere, M., Reissier, S., Penven, M., Dejoies, L., Guerin, F., & Cattoir, V. (2023). The role of next-generation sequencing (NGS) in the management of tuberculosis: Practical review for implementation in routine. *Pathogens (Basel, Switzerland)*, *12*(8), 978. https://www.ncbi.nlm.nih.gov/pmc/articles/PMC10459500/

Bidstrup, C., Andersen, P. H., Skinhøj, P., & Andersen, Å. B. (2002). Tuberculous meningitis in a country with a low incidence of tuberculosis: Still a serious disease and a diagnostic challenge. *Scandinavian Journal of Infectious Diseases*, *34*(11), 811–814. DOI: 10.1080/0036554021000026938

Brooks, J. B., Daneshvar, M. I., Haberberger, R. L., & Mikhail, I. A. (1990). Rapid diagnosis of tuberculous meningitis by frequency-pulsed electron-capture gas-liquid chromatography detection of carboxylic acids in cerebrospinal fluid. *Journal of Clinical Microbiology*, *28*(5), 989–997. https://www.ncbi.nlm.nih.gov/pmc/articles/PMC267852/

Cao, D., Wang, T., Wang, Y., & Han, J. (2022). Analysis of cases with cerebrospinal fluid characteristics similar to tuberculous meningitis. *BioMed Research International, 2022*, 9692804. https://www.ncbi.nlm.nih.gov/pmc/articles/PMC9825210/

Caviedes, L., Lee, T. S., Gilman, R. H., Sheen, P., Spellman, E., & Lee, E. H. (2000). Rapid, efficient detection and drug susceptibility testing of Mycobacterium tuberculosis in sputum by microscopic observation of broth cultures. *Journal of Clinical Microbiology*, *38*(3), 1203–1208. https://www.ncbi.nlm.nih.gov/pmc/articles/PMC86377/

Centers for Disease Control and Prevention. (2024). Tuberculosis (TB) disease in the United States, 1993–2023 [Slide set]. https://www.cdc.gov/tb-surveillance-report-2023/resources/slide-set.html

Chakravorty, S., Simmons, A. M., Rowneki, M., Parmar, H., Cao, Y., & Ryan, J. (2017). The new Xpert MTB/RIF Ultra: Improving detection of Mycobacterium tuberculosis and resistance to rifampin in an assay suitable for point-of-care testing. *mBio*, *8*(4), e00812–e00817. https://www.ncbi.nlm.nih.gov/pmc/articles/PMC5574709/

Chen, Y., Wang, Y., Liu, X., Li, W., Fu, H., & Liu, X. (2022). Comparative diagnostic utility of metagenomic next-generation sequencing, GeneXpert, modified Ziehl–Neelsen staining, and culture using cerebrospinal fluid for tuberculous meningitis: A multi-center, retrospective study in China. *Journal of Clinical Laboratory Analysis*, *36*(4), e24307. https://www.ncbi.nlm.nih.gov/pmc/articles/PMC8993600/

Chen, Y. Z., Sun, L. C., Wen, Y. H., Li, Z. W., Fan, S. J., & Tan, H. K. (2020). Pooled analysis of the Xpert MTB/RIF assay for diagnosing tuberculous meningitis. *Bioscience Reports*, *40*(1), BSR20191312. https://www.ncbi.nlm.nih.gov/pmc/articles/PMC6946622/

Cherian, A., & Thomas, S. (2011). Central nervous system tuberculosis. *African Health Sciences*, *11*(1), 116–127. https://www.ncbi.nlm.nih.gov/pmc/articles/PMC3092316/

Chohan, T., Jain, A., Saeed, M., & Saeed, S. A. (2012). Tuberculous meningitis, an unusual presentation in a young lady. *BMJ Case Reports*, *2012*, bcr1220115370. https://www.ncbi.nlm.nih.gov/pmc/articles/PMC3417028/

Choi, S. H., Kim, Y. S., Bae, I. G., Chung, J. W., Lee, M. S., & Kang, J. M. (2002). The possible role of cerebrospinal fluid adenosine deaminase activity in the diagnosis of tuberculous meningitis in adults. *Clinical Neurology and Neurosurgery*, *104*(1), 10–15. https://www.sciencedirect.com/science/article/pii/S0303846701001597

Coovadia, Y. M., Dawood, A., Ellis, M. E., Coovadia, H. M., & Daniel, T. M. (1986). Evaluation of adenosine deaminase activity and antibody to Mycobacterium tuberculosis antigen 5 in cerebrospinal fluid and the radioactive bromide partition test for the early diagnosis of tuberculosis meningitis. *Archives of Disease in Childhood*, *61*(5), 428–435. https://www.ncbi.nlm.nih.gov/pmc/articles/PMC1777799/

Corral, I., Quereda, C., Navas, E., Martín-Dávila, P., Pérez-Elías, M. J., & Casado, J. L. (2004). Adenosine deaminase activity in cerebrospinal fluid of HIV-infected patients: Limited value for diagnosis of tuberculous meningitis. *European Journal of Clinical Microbiology & Infectious Diseases*, *23*(6), 471–476. DOI: 10.1007/s10096-004-1110-z

Cresswell, F. V., Bangdiwala, A. S., Bahr, N. C., Trautner, E., Nuwagira, E., & Ellis, J. (2018). Tuberculous meningitis diagnosis and outcomes during the Xpert MTB/RIF era: A 6.5-year cohort study in Uganda. *Wellcome Open Research*, *3*, 64. https://www.ncbi.nlm.nih.gov/pmc/articles/PMC6039934/

Curto, M., Reali, C., Palmieri, G., Scintu, F., Schivo, M. L., & Sogos, V. (2004). Inhibition of cytokines expression in human microglia infected by virulent and non-virulent mycobacteria. *Neurochemistry International, 44*(6), 381–392. https://www.sciencedirect.com/science/article/pii/S0197018603002031

Daniel, B. D., Grace, G. A., & Natrajan, M. (2019). Tuberculous meningitis in children: Clinical management & outcome. *The Indian Journal of Medical Research, 150*(2), 117–130. https://www.ncbi.nlm.nih.gov/pmc/articles/PMC6829784/

Daniel, B. D., Grace, G. A., & Natrajan, M. (2019). Tuberculous meningitis in children: Clinical management & outcome. *The Indian Journal of Medical Research, 150*(2), 117–130. https://www.ncbi.nlm.nih.gov/pmc/articles/PMC6829784/

Dastur, D. K., Manghani, D. K., & Udani, P. M. (1995). Pathology and pathogenetic mechanisms in neurotuberculosis. *Radiologic Clinics of North America, 33*(4), 733–752.

Davis, A., Meintjes, G., & Wilkinson, R. J. (2018). Treatment of tuberculous meningitis and its complications in adults. *Current Treatment Options in Neurology, 20*(3), 5. Advance online publication. DOI: 10.1007/s11940-018-0490-9

Davis, A. G., Rohlwink, U. K., Proust, A., Figaji, A. A., & Wilkinson, R. J. (2019). The pathogenesis of tuberculous meningitis. *Journal of Leukocyte Biology, 105*(2), 267–280. https://www.ncbi.nlm.nih.gov/pmc/articles/PMC6355360/

Davis, A. G., Rohlwink, U. K., Proust, A., Figaji, A. A., & Wilkinson, R. J. (2019). The pathogenesis of tuberculous meningitis. *Journal of Leukocyte Biology, 105*(2), 267–280. https://academic.oup.com/jleukbio/article/105/2/267/6935402

Dawi, J., Mohan, A. S., Misakyan, Y., Affa, S., Gonzalez, E., & Hajjar, K. (2024). The role of oxidative stress in TB meningitis and therapeutic options. *Diseases (Basel, Switzerland), 12*(3), 50. https://www.mdpi.com/2079-9721/12/3/50

DeVincenzo, J. P., Berning, S. E., Peloquin, C. A., & Husson, R. N. (1999). Multidrug-resistant tuberculous meningitis: Clinical problems and concentrations of second-line antituberculous medications. *The Annals of Pharmacotherapy, 33*(11), 1184–1188. DOI: 10.1345/aph.19008

Dodd, P. J., Osman, M., Cresswell, F. V., Stadelman, A. M., Lan, N. H., & Thuong, N. T. T. (2021). The global burden of tuberculous meningitis in adults: A modelling study. *PLOS Global Public Health, 1*(12), e0000069. https://www.ncbi.nlm.nih.gov/pmc/articles/PMC10021871/

Donald, P. R., Schaaf, H. S., & Schoeman, J. F. (2005). Tuberculous meningitis and miliary tuberculosis: The Rich focus revisited. *The Journal of Infection*, *50*(3), 193–195. DOI: 10.1016/j.jinf.2004.02.010

Donovan, J., Phu, N. H., Mai, N. T. H., Dung, L. T., Imran, D., & Burhan, E. (2018). Adjunctive dexamethasone for the treatment of HIV-infected adults with tuberculous meningitis (ACT HIV): Study protocol for a randomised controlled trial. *Wellcome Open Research*, *3*, 31. https://www.ncbi.nlm.nih.gov/pmc/articles/PMC6143919/

Donovan, J., & Thwaites, G. E. (2020). Tuberculous meningitis: Where to from here? *Current Opinion in Infectious Diseases*, *33*(3), 259–266. https://www.ncbi.nlm.nih.gov/pmc/articles/PMC7259381/

Filho, V. W., de Castilho, E. A., Rodrigues, L. C., & Huttly, S. R. A. (n.d.). *Effectiveness of BCG vaccination against tuberculous meningitis: A case-control study in São Paulo*.

Fong, T. H., Shi, W., Ruan, G., Li, S., Liu, G., & Yang, L. (2023). Tuberculostearic acid incorporated predictive model contributes to the clinical diagnosis of tuberculous meningitis. *iScience*, *26*(10), 107858. https://www.ncbi.nlm.nih.gov/pmc/articles/PMC10520543/

Fu, R., Wang, C., Shi, C., Lu, M., Fang, Z., & Lu, J. (2009). An improved whole-blood gamma interferon assay based on the CFP21-MPT64 fusion protein. *Clinical and Vaccine Immunology; CVI*, *16*(5), 686–691. https://www.ncbi.nlm.nih.gov/pmc/articles/PMC2681596/

Gambhir, I. S., Mehta, M., Singh, D. S., & Khanna, H. D. (1999). Evaluation of CSF-adenosine deaminase activity in tubercular meningitis. *The Journal of the Association of Physicians of India*, *47*(2), 192–194.

Garg, D., Radhakrishnan, D. M., Agrawal, U., Vanjare, H. A., Gandham, E. J., & Manesh, A. (2023). Tuberculosis of the spinal cord. *Annals of Indian Academy of Neurology*, *26*(2). https://journals.lww.com/annalsofian/fulltext/2023/26020/tuberculosis_of_the_spinal_cord.5.aspx

Girgis, N. I., Sultan, Y., Farid, Z., Mansour, M. M., Erian, M. W., & Hanna, L. S. (1998). Tuberculosis meningitis, Abbassia Fever Hospital-Naval Medical Research Unit No. 3-Cairo, Egypt, from 1976 to 1996. *The American Journal of Tropical Medicine and Hygiene*, *58*(1), 28–34. https://www.ajtmh.org/view/journals/tpmd/58/1/article-p28.xml

Gomes, T., Reis-Santos, B., Bertolde, A., Johnson, J. L., Riley, L. W., & Maciel, E. L. (2014). Epidemiology of extrapulmonary tuberculosis in Brazil: A hierarchical model. *BMC Infectious Diseases*, *14*, 9. https://www.ncbi.nlm.nih.gov/pmc/articles/PMC3893400/

Gupta, M., Tobin, E. H., & Munakomi, S. (2024). CNS tuberculosis. In *StatPearls*. StatPearls Publishing. https://www.ncbi.nlm.nih.gov/books/NBK585138/

Gupta, R., Thakur, R., Gupta, P., Jalan, N., Kushwaha, S., & Gupta, M. (2015). Evaluation of GenoType MTBDRplus line probe assay for early detection of drug resistance in tuberculous meningitis patients in India. *Journal of Global Infectious Diseases*, *7*(1), 5–10. https://www.ncbi.nlm.nih.gov/pmc/articles/PMC4338458/

Harausz, E. P., Garcia-Prats, A. J., Law, S., Schaaf, H. S., Kredo, T., & Seddon, J. A. (2018). Treatment and outcomes in children with multidrug-resistant tuberculosis: A systematic review and individual patient data meta-analysis. *PLoS Medicine*, *15*(7), e1002591. https://www.ncbi.nlm.nih.gov/pmc/articles/PMC6040687/

Heemskerk, D., Day, J., Chau, T. T. H., Dung, N. H., Yen, N. T. B., & Bang, N. D. (2011). Intensified treatment with high dose rifampicin and levofloxacin compared to standard treatment for adult patients with tuberculous meningitis (TBM-IT): Protocol for a randomized controlled trial. *Trials*, *12*, 25. https://www.ncbi.nlm.nih.gov/pmc/articles/PMC3041687/

Honoré-Bouakline, S., Vincensini, J. P., Giacuzzo, V., Lagrange, P. H., & Herrmann, J. L. (2003). Rapid diagnosis of extrapulmonary tuberculosis by PCR: Impact of sample preparation and DNA extraction. *Journal of Clinical Microbiology*, *41*(6), 2323–2329. https://www.ncbi.nlm.nih.gov/pmc/articles/PMC156509/

Husain, M., Jha, D. K., Rastogi, M., Husain, N., & Gupta, R. K. (2005). Role of neuroendoscopy in the management of patients with tuberculous meningitis hydrocephalus. *Neurosurgical Review*, *28*(4), 278–283. DOI: 10.1007/s10143-005-0397-2

Isabel, B. E., & Rogelio, H. P. (2014). Pathogenesis and immune response in tuberculous meningitis. *The Malaysian Journal of Medical Sciences : MJMS*, *21*(1), 4–10. https://www.ncbi.nlm.nih.gov/pmc/articles/PMC3952336/

Jakka, S., Veena, S., Rao, A. R. M., & Eisenhut, M. (2005). Cerebrospinal fluid adenosine deaminase levels and adverse neurological outcome in pediatric tuberculous meningitis. *Infection*, *33*(4), 264–266. DOI: 10.1007/s15010-005-5005-4

Johnston, J. C., Chiang, L., & Elwood, K. (2017). Mycobacterium kansasii. *Microbiology Spectrum*, *5*(1). Advance online publication. DOI: 10.1128/microbiolspec.TNMI7-0011-2016

Katti, M. K. (2004). Pathogenesis, diagnosis, treatment, and outcome aspects of cerebral tuberculosis. *Medical Science Monitor*, *10*(9), RA215–RA229. www.medscimonit.com/abstract/index/idArt/11749

Kimuda, S., Kasozi, D., Namombwe, S., Gakuru, J., Mugabi, T., & Kagimu, E. (2023). Advancing diagnosis and treatment in people living with HIV and tuberculosis meningitis. *Current HIV/AIDS Reports*, *20*(6), 379–393. https://www.ncbi.nlm.nih.gov/pmc/articles/PMC10719136/

Kumar, A., Mudassir, S., Ranjan, A., Wankhade, B., Rai, A. K., & Kumar, S. (2023). Clinical profile and mortality predictors in hospitalised patients of tuberculous meningitis. *Neurology Asia*, *28*(1), 149–157. http://www.neurology-asia.org/articles/neuroasia-2023-28(1)-149.pdf

Kumar, P., Benny, P., Jain, M., & Singh, S. (2014). Comparison of an in-house multiplex PCR with two commercial immuno-chromatographic tests for rapid identification and differentiation of MTB from NTM isolates. *International Journal of Mycobacteriology*, *3*(1), 50–56. https://www.sciencedirect.com/science/article/pii/S2212553114000028

Kumar, R., Pandey, C., Bose, N., & Sahay, S. (2002). Tuberculous brain abscess: Clinical presentation, pathophysiology and treatment (in children). *Child's Nervous System*, *18*(3), 118–123. DOI: 10.1007/s00381-002-0575-2

Kurien, R., & Sudarsanam, T. D. S., & Thomas, K. (2013). Tuberculous meningitis: A comparison of scoring systems for diagnosis. Oman Medical Journal, 28(3), 163–166. http://www.omjournal.org/fultext_PDF.aspx?DetailsID=372&type=fultext

Lan, Y., Chen, W., Yan, Q., & Liu, W. (2020). Interferon-γ release assays for tuberculous meningitis diagnosis: A meta-analysis. *Archives of Medical Science : AMS*, *17*(5), 1241–1250. https://www.ncbi.nlm.nih.gov/pmc/articles/PMC8425237/

Leonard, J. M. (2017). Central nervous system tuberculosis. *Microbiology Spectrum*, *5*(2). Advance online publication. DOI: 10.1128/microbiolspec.TNMI7-0044-2017

Luo, M., Wang, W., Zeng, Q., Luo, Y., Yang, H., & Yang, X. (2018). Tuberculous meningitis diagnosis and treatment in adults: A series of 189 suspected cases. *Experimental and Therapeutic Medicine*, *16*(3), 2770–2776. https://www.ncbi.nlm.nih.gov/pmc/articles/PMC6122581/

Mandal, S., Rao, R., & Joshi, R. (2023). Estimating the burden of tuberculosis in India: A modelling study. *Indian Journal of Community Medicine : Official Publication of Indian Association of Preventive & Social Medicine*, *48*(3), 436–442. https://www.ncbi.nlm.nih.gov/pmc/articles/PMC10353668/

Manyelo, C. M., Solomons, R. S., Walzl, G., & Chegou, N. N. (2021). Tuberculous meningitis: Pathogenesis, immune responses, diagnostic challenges, and the potential of biomarker-based approaches. *Journal of Clinical Microbiology*, *59*(3), e01771–e20. https://www.ncbi.nlm.nih.gov/pmc/articles/PMC8106718/

Marx, G. E., & Chan, E. D. (2011). Tuberculous meningitis: Diagnosis and treatment overview. *Tuberculosis Research and Treatment*, *2011*, 798764. https://www.ncbi.nlm.nih.gov/pmc/articles/PMC3335590/

Medical Research Council. (1948). Streptomycin treatment of tuberculous meningitis. *Lancet*, *251*(6503), 582–596. https://linkinghub.elsevier.com/retrieve/pii/S0140673648920030

Menzies, D., Pai, M., & Comstock, G. (2007). Meta-analysis: New tests for the diagnosis of latent tuberculosis infection: Areas of uncertainty and recommendations for research. *Annals of Internal Medicine*, *146*(5), 340–354. https://www.acpjournals.org/doi/abs/10.7326/0003-4819-146-5-200703060-00006

Miceli, I., de Kantor, I. N., Colaiácovo, D., Peluffo, G., Cutillo, I., & Gorra, R. (1988). Evaluation of the effectiveness of BCG vaccination using the case control method in Buenos Aires, Argentina. *International Journal of Epidemiology*, *17*(3), 629–634. DOI: 10.1093/ije/17.3.629

Mishra, O. (1996). Cerebrospinal fluid adenosine deaminase activity for the diagnosis of tuberculous meningitis in children. *Journal of Tropical Pediatrics*, *42*(3), 129–132. https://academic.oup.com/tropej/article-lookup/doi/10.1093/tropej/42.3.129

Nagai, S., Wiker, H. G., Harboe, M., & Kinomoto, M. (1991). Isolation and partial characterization of major protein antigens in the culture fluid of Mycobacterium tuberculosis. *Infection and Immunity*, *59*(1), 372–382. https://www.ncbi.nlm.nih.gov/pmc/articles/PMC257751/

Nahid, P., Dorman, S. E., Alipanah, N., Barry, P. M., Brozek, J. L., & Cattamanchi, A. (2016). Official American Thoracic Society/Centers for Disease Control and Prevention/Infectious Diseases Society of America clinical practice guidelines: Treatment of drug-susceptible tuberculosis. *Clinical Infectious Diseases*, *63*(7), e147–e195. https://academic.oup.com/cid/article/63/7/e147/2196792

Nguyen, D. T., Agarwal, S., & Graviss, E. A. (2019). Trends of tuberculosis meningitis and associated mortality in Texas, 2010-2017, a large population-based analysis. *PLoS One*, *14*(2), e0212729. https://www.ncbi.nlm.nih.gov/pmc/articles/PMC6395025/

O'Garra, A., Redford, P. S., McNab, F. W., Bloom, C. I., Wilkinson, R. J., & Berry, M. P. R. (2013). The immune response in tuberculosis. *Annual Review of Immunology, 31*(1), 475–527. https://www.annualreviews.org/doi/10.1146/annurev-immunol-032712-095939

O'Toole, R. D., Thornton, G. F., Mukherjee, M. K., & Nath, R. L. (1969). Dexamethasone in tuberculous meningitis. *Annals of Internal Medicine*, *70*(1), 39–48. https://www.acpjournals.org/doi/abs/10.7326/0003-4819-70-1-39

Pai, M., Zwerling, A., & Menzies, D. (2008). Systematic review: T-cell–based assays for the diagnosis of latent tuberculosis infection: An update. *Annals of Internal Medicine*, *149*(3), 177–184. https://www.ncbi.nlm.nih.gov/pmc/articles/PMC2951987/

Paliwal, V. K., & Garg, R. K. (2021). Hydrocephalus in tuberculous meningitis - Pearls and nuances. Neurology India, 69(Suppl. 2). https://journals.lww.com/neur/fulltext/2021/69002/hydrocephalus_in_tuberculous_meningitis___pearls.12.aspx

Patel, V. B., Bhigjee, A. I., Paruk, H. F., Singh, R., Meldau, R., & Connolly, C. (2009). Utility of a novel lipoarabinomannan assay for the diagnosis of tuberculous meningitis in a resource-poor high-HIV prevalence setting. *Cerebrospinal Fluid Research*, *6*, 13. https://www.ncbi.nlm.nih.gov/pmc/articles/PMC2777116/

Poplin, V., Boulware, D. R., & Bahr, N. C. (2020). Methods for rapid diagnosis of meningitis etiology in adults. *Biomarkers in Medicine*, *14*(6), 459–479. https://www.ncbi.nlm.nih.gov/pmc/articles/PMC7248681/

Pormohammad, A., Nasiri, M. J., McHugh, T. D., Riahi, S. M., & Bahr, N. C. (2019). A systematic review and meta-analysis of the diagnostic accuracy of nucleic acid amplification tests for tuberculous meningitis. *Journal of Clinical Microbiology*, *57*(6), e01113–e01118. https://www.ncbi.nlm.nih.gov/pmc/articles/PMC6535607/

Prasad, M. K., Kumar, A., Nalini, N., Kumar, P., Mishra, B., & Lata, D. (2023). Diagnostic accuracy of cerebrospinal fluid (CSF) adenosine deaminase (ADA) for tuberculous meningitis (TBM) in adults: A systematic review and meta-analysis. *Cureus*, *15*(6), e39896. https://www.ncbi.nlm.nih.gov/pmc/articles/PMC10316459/

Press Information Bureau, Government of India. (2024, November). https://static.pib.gov.in/WriteReadData/specificdocs/documents/2024/nov/doc2024115429801.pdf

Przybojewski, S., Andronikou, S., & Wilmshurst, J. (2006). Objective CT criteria to determine the presence of abnormal basal enhancement in children with suspected tuberculous meningitis. *Pediatric Radiology*, *36*(7), 687–696. http://link.springer.com/10.1007/s00247-006-0160-z

Rieder, H. L., Snider, D. E., & Cauthen, G. M. (1990). Extrapulmonary tuberculosis in the United States. *The American Review of Respiratory Disease*, *141*(2), 347–351. http://www.atsjournals.org/doi/abs/10.1164/ajrccm/141.2.347

Rock, R. B., Olin, M., Baker, C. A., Molitor, T. W., & Peterson, P. K. (2008). Central nervous system tuberculosis: Pathogenesis and clinical aspects. *Clinical Microbiology Reviews*, *21*(2), 243–261. https://www.ncbi.nlm.nih.gov/pmc/articles/PMC2292571/

Rohlwink, U. K., Kilborn, T., Wieselthaler, N., Banderker, E., Zwane, E., & Figaji, A. A. (2016). Imaging features of the brain, cerebral vessels and spine in pediatric tuberculous meningitis with associated hydrocephalus. *The Pediatric Infectious Disease Journal*, *35*(10), e301–e310. https://www.ncbi.nlm.nih.gov/pmc/articles/PMC5024759/

Rychert, J. (2019). Benefits and limitations of MALDI-TOF mass spectrometry for the identification of microorganisms. Infectiology Journal, 2(4), 1–5. https://www.infectiologyjournal.com/articles/benefits-and-limitations-of-malditof-mass-spectrometry-for-the-identification-of-microorganisms.html

Saini, A. G., Dogra, S., Kumar, R., Nada, R., & Singh, M. (2011). Primary tuberculous cerebellar abscess: Case report. *Annals of Tropical Paediatrics*, *31*(4), 367–369. DOI: 10.1179/1465328111Y.0000000037

Seddon, J. A., Tugume, L., Solomons, R., Prasad, K., & Bahr, N. C. (2019). The current global situation for tuberculous meningitis: Epidemiology, diagnostics, treatment and outcomes. *Wellcome Open Research*, *4*, 167. https://www.ncbi.nlm.nih.gov/pmc/articles/PMC7029758/

Shekhar, R., Rao, J. R., Devi, K. A., & Rao, R. B. (2013). CSF proteins as discriminatory markers of tubercular and pyogenic meningitis. *Journal of Clinical and Diagnostic Research : JCDR*, *7*(8), 1586–1588. https://www.ncbi.nlm.nih.gov/pmc/articles/PMC3782903/

Shi, F., Qiu, X., Yu, M., & Huang, Y. (2022). Tuberculosis-specific antigen stimulated and unstimulated interferon-γ for tuberculous meningitis diagnosis: A systematic review and meta-analysis. *PLoS One*, *17*(8), e0273834. https://www.ncbi.nlm.nih.gov/pmc/articles/PMC9426936/

Spatola, M., Nziza, N., Irvine, E. B., Cizmeci, D., Jung, W., & Van, L. H. (2024). Distinctive antibody responses to Mycobacterium tuberculosis in pulmonary and brain infection. *Brain*, *147*(9), 3247–3260. https://www.ncbi.nlm.nih.gov/pmc/articles/PMC11370789/

Stewart, S. M. (1953). The bacteriological diagnosis of tuberculous meningitis. *Journal of Clinical Pathology*, *6*(3), 241–242. https://www.ncbi.nlm.nih.gov/pmc/articles/PMC1023629/

Sulaiman, T., Medi, S., Erdem, H., Senbayrak, S., Ozturk-Engin, D., & Inan, A. (2020). The diagnostic utility of the "Thwaites' system" and "Lancet consensus scoring system" in tuberculous vs. non-tuberculous subacute and chronic meningitis: Multicenter analysis of 395 adult patients. *BMC Infectious Diseases*, *20*, 788. https://www.ncbi.nlm.nih.gov/pmc/articles/PMC7585215/

Sütlaş, P. N., Ünal, A., Forta, H., Şenol, S., & Kırbaş, D. (2003). Tuberculous meningitis in adults: Review of 61 cases. *Infection*, *31*(6), 387–391. DOI: 10.1007/s15010-003-3179-1

Syggelou, A., Spyridis, N., Benetatou, K., Kourkouni, E., Kourlaba, G., & Tsagaraki, M. (2020). BCG vaccine protection against TB infection among children older than 5 years in close contact with an infectious adult TB case. *Journal of Clinical Medicine*, *9*(10), 3224. https://www.mdpi.com/2077-0383/9/10/3224

Tai, M. L. S., Nor, H. M., Viswanathan, S., Rose, N., Zain, M., & Pow, Z. Y. (2017). Spinal tuberculous disease is common in tuberculous meningitis. *Neurology Asia*.

Thwaites, G., Chau, T., Mai, N., Drobniewski, F., McAdam, K., & Farrar, J. (2000). Tuberculous meningitis. *Journal of Neurology, Neurosurgery, and Psychiatry*, *68*(3), 289–299. https://www.ncbi.nlm.nih.gov/pmc/articles/PMC1736815/

Thwaites, G., Chau, T. T. H., Mai, N. T. H., Drobniewski, F., McAdam, K., & Farrar, J. (2000). Tuberculous meningitis. *Journal of Neurology, Neurosurgery, and Psychiatry*, *68*(3), 289–299. DOI: 10.1136/jnnp.68.3.289

Thwaites, G. E., Caws, M., Chau, T. T. H., Dung, N. T., Campbell, J. I., & Phu, N. H. (2004). Comparison of conventional bacteriology with nucleic acid amplification (amplified Mycobacterium direct test) for diagnosis of tuberculous meningitis before and after inception of antituberculosis chemotherapy. *Journal of Clinical Microbiology*, *42*(3), 996–1002. https://www.ncbi.nlm.nih.gov/pmc/articles/PMC356903/

Thwaites, G. E., Chau, T. T. H., & Farrar, J. J. (2004). Improving the bacteriological diagnosis of tuberculous meningitis. *Journal of Clinical Microbiology*, *42*(1), 378–379. https://www.ncbi.nlm.nih.gov/pmc/articles/PMC321694/

Thwaites, G. E., Chau, T. T. H., Stepniewska, K., Phu, N. H., Chuong, L. V., & Sinh, D. X. (2002). Diagnosis of adult tuberculous meningitis by use of clinical and laboratory features. *Lancet*, *360*(9342), 1287–1292. https://www.thelancet.com/journals/lancet/article/PIIS0140-6736(02)11318-3/fulltext

Thwaites, G. E., Macmullen-Price, J., Chau, T. T. H., Mai, P. P., Dung, N. T., & Simmons, C. P. (2007). Serial MRI to determine the effect of dexamethasone on the cerebral pathology of tuberculous meningitis: An observational study. *Lancet Neurology*, *6*(3), 230–236. https://www.ncbi.nlm.nih.gov/pmc/articles/PMC4333204/

Verdon, R., Chevret, S., Laissy, J. P., & Wolff, M. (1996). Tuberculous meningitis in adults: Review of 48 cases. *Clinical Infectious Diseases*, *22*(6), 982–988. DOI: 10.1093/clinids/22.6.982

Vijayakumar, B., Sarin, K., & Mohan, G. (2012). Tuberculous brain abscess and subdural empyema in an immunocompetent child: Significance of AFB staining in aspirated pus. *Annals of Indian Academy of Neurology*, *15*(2), 130–133. https://www.ncbi.nlm.nih.gov/pmc/articles/PMC3345591/

Villoria, M. F., Fortea, F., Moreno, S., Muñoz, L., Manero, M., & Benito, C. (1995). MR imaging and CT of central nervous system tuberculosis in the patient with AIDS. *Radiologic Clinics of North America*, *33*(4), 805–820.

Wang, J. L., Han, C., Yang, F. L., Wang, M. S., & He, Y. (n.d.). Normal cerebrospinal fluid protein and associated clinical characteristics in children with tuberculous meningitis. Annals of Medicine, 53(1), 885–889. https://www.ncbi.nlm.nih.gov/pmc/articles/PMC8205029/

Whitener, D. R. (1978). Tuberculous brain abscess: Report of a case and review of the literature. *Archives of Neurology*, *35*(3), 148–155. DOI: 10.1001/archneur.1978.00500270030007

World Health Organization. (2007). Global tuberculosis control: Surveillance, planning, financing (WHO/HTM/TB/2007.376). https://iris.who.int/bitstream/handle/10665/43629/9789241563141_eng.pdf?sequence=1

World Health Organization. (2011). Automated real-time nucleic acid amplification technology for rapid and simultaneous detection of tuberculosis and rifampicin resistance: Xpert MTB/RIF system (WHO/HTM/TB/2011.4).

World Health Organization. (2016). The use of molecular line probe assay for the detection of resistance to isoniazid and rifampicin: Policy update. Author. https://iris.who.int/handle/10665/250586

World Health Organization. (2022). *Line probe assays for detection of drug-resistant tuberculosis: Interpretation and reporting manual for laboratory staff and clinicians*. Author.

World Health Organization. (2022). *WHO consolidated guidelines on tuberculosis. Module 5: Management of tuberculosis in children and adolescents*. Author.

World Health Organization. (2024a). *Global Tuberculosis Report 2024.*

World Health Organization. (2024b). *WHO consolidated guidelines on tuberculosis: Module 3. Diagnosis—Rapid diagnostics for tuberculosis detection* (3rd ed.). Author.

Yamaguchi, R., Matsuo, K., Yamazaki, A., Abe, C., Nagai, S., & Terasaka, K. (1989). Cloning and characterization of the gene for immunogenic protein MPB64 of Mycobacterium bovis BCG. *Infection and Immunity*, *57*(1), 283–288. https://www.ncbi.nlm.nih.gov/pmc/articles/PMC313089/

Chapter 5
Viral Infections of Central Nervous System in Children:
Clinical Presentation, Diagnosis, and Treatment Modalities

Shikha Tewari
https://orcid.org/0000-0002-4140-6256
Medanta Hospital, Lucknow, India

Bhawana Jain
https://orcid.org/0000-0002-5319-4684
Medanta Hospital, Lucknow, India

ABSTRACT

Central Nervous System (CNS) infections are caused by a variety of pathogens including bacteria, virus, fungi, protozoa, and parasites. Viral CNS infections can present as meningitis, encephalitis, or localized abscesses. Such infections are challenging to diagnose and the blood brain barrier in the human body guards the entry of the pathogens into CNS. The CNS is also shielded by neuroanatomical barriers which may be blood CSF barrier or the blood brain barrier and the fibroblasts from olfactory nerve. Our immune cells enhance these barriers by activating T cells with protective function. Once invasion occurs, the viruses interact with various cell populations of CNS and can induce pro-inflammatory immune response that leads to development of pathologies like viral meningitis and encephalitis. Children have immature immune defenses and blood–brain barrier; hence, they are more vulnerable to viral CNS infections compared to adults. Viruses like enteroviruses account for more than 50% of CNS infections amongst children. Infections, either mild or

DOI: 10.4018/979-8-3693-4070-7.ch005

severe, severely impact the quality of life in developing children and chief cause of morbidities and mortality worldwide. This chapter aims to provide an overview on viral pathogens of nervous system, their pathogenesis, diagnosis, and treatment options available in the current scenario. The authors review various viral pathogens of CNS in children and describe their casual microbiological cause, clinical features, and provide an update on the classical and latest diagnostic approaches and treatment strategies available for them. Newly developed PCR-based methods that are efficiently capable of detecting and diagnosing the neurotropic viruses in almost all sample types are discussed. The chapter finds its importance in providing an overview for management approach of viral infections of the central nervous system in children from the point of clinical presentation, diagnosis, treatment, and complications.

1. INTRODUCTION

Infections of the central nervous system (CNS) are largely caused by viruses, and these infections can be life endangering in children (Autore et al., 2021). Incidence rate of CNS viral infections, in developed countries the ranges from 10 to 20 cases per 100,000 children per year. However the data in developing countries is still ambiguous and scarce, pertaining to recurring outbreaks and lost to follow-up cases. A recent study on meta-analysis reported the occurrence of CNS infections in low- and middle-income countries is about 726 and 299 cases per 100,000 population respectively, however rate is 11 cases per 100,000 population in high-income countries (Sheybani, F et al., 2023)

Viral infections occurring in the central nervous system have capacity to remerge. Re-emerging infections and the clinical range is primarily determined by on some factors, which comprise the geographical place of the viral vector, host immune status, genetic composition of virus, and some environmental aspects. Many a times, they are misdiagnosed and their etiology is often missed, at times due to a lack of appropriate diagnostic methods and sometime due to lack of experience in elucidating viral epidemiology and biology. (Abdullahi AM et al., 2020). The etiologic mediators of viral CNS infections also differ and alter depending on geographical settings. Herpes simplex viruses (HSVs) are one of the most prevalent pathogens isolated among children as well as in adults in the Australia, United States (US), and Italy. In some parts of India the enteroviruses (EVs) have been identified as the leading cause of viral encephalitis, but the most prevalent pathogen in eastern India among children and adults was HSVs (Leung AK et al., 2018). In Southern Vietnam, the most frequent cause of viral encephalitis among children is the Japanese encephalitis virus (JEV). Thus, exploring and studying the epidemiology of neurotropic viruses plays an important role in designing the targeted intervention and treatment of viral diseases of CNS.

Pathogenesis of Neurotropic Viruses

Neurotropic viruses take entry into CNS through various routes, interact with several cell populations of CNS, and thus induce several diseases. The CNS is protected by neuroanatomical barriers which include meningitis blood CSF barrier (BCSFB) the blood brain barrier (BBB) and the fibroblasts from olfactory nerve (Tumani H et al., 2018). Additionally, immune cells augment these barriers by stimulating T cells with defensive function in response to possibly neuro-invasive infection (Morseman et al., 2020). These make strong protection of CNS against intruding pathogens via olfactory nerves, CSF and haematogenous spread through neurons or immune cells. However neurotropic viruses have their own machineries to invade CNS interact with local cells and activate pro-inflammatory immune response that leads to development of diseases. When infection occurs microglia get activated and subsequently induce activation of innate immune response and also the adaptive immune response (Olson et al., 2001). Microglia also acts with astrocytes to initiate chemotaxsis of immune cells, as neutrophils. The pathogenesis of viral infection can be categorised into following:

A. ***Viral invasion in Mammalian host:*** Viruses can attack its mammalian host via any possible potential doorway of entry. Comprising direct contact through skin or mucous membrane, gastrointestinal tract, genitourinary tract and respiratory passage. Few viruses are inoculated by bite of mosquitoes or any other blood sucking vectors.
B. ***Entry into neuroCNS:*** Neurogenic Viruses can come in the central nervous system of host via following potentially different ways:
    a. Through olfactory Nerve or Choroid Plexus
    b. Via Haematogenous spread
    c. Through infected immune cells
    d. Direct crossing of Blood brain barrier
    e. Through neruve or dendritic cells
C. ***Replication of Virus in CNS:*** In extracellular space of CNS most viruses infect particular cellular elements which is decided by the diaspora of different cellular receptors
D. ***Virus Induced immune pathology:*** Following mechanism have been identified which causes pathology in CNS by viruses.
    a. Oxidative stress and apoptosis
    b. Neuro-inflammation

c. Autophagy and Mitophagy
d. Neurotransmission system
e. Neuronal Metabolism
f. Alzheimer's Drs pathology hallmark
g. Protein misfolding and aggregate

E. ***Persistent viral infections:*** Most viral infections are acute and are cleaned by host immune system within a span of few weeks or months. Yet there are number of lasting viral infections of CNS. Re-emergence of infection may occur and it is dependent on host defence ability to clear infection, genomic composition and virulence of virus and other geographical and environmental exposures to virus.
F. Sequeale and Complications:

The world-wide epidemiology of CNS viral infections is currently predisposed by the adoption of more reliable diagnostic techniques, initiation of vaccination programs, and the advent of new pathogens (Autore et al., 2021). Even though prognosis is often favourable, mortality rate and long-standing events due to viral encephalitis and meningitis can arise. The burden for public health systems, cost wise, to maintain such patients is high with a high associated hospitalization cost. However, viral meningitis and encephalitis represent a diagnostic challenge, and specific treatment options are still scarce.

CNS infections can present in form of meningitis, myelitis, abscess or encephalitis. Some of the factors which affect the kind of pathogens invading the CNS could be age, immune status, epidemiological trends and systemic infections. The spread of pathogens is commonly occurs through blood nevertheless it can also spread in additional ways such as sinus inflammation (sinusitis), inflammation in the ear (otitis), or in form of pus build-up in teeth and gum (dental abscess). Early identification of the CNS infection is of utmost importance to minimise the effect of the disease and to begin the right treatment at right time. While the gold standard for pathogenic infection diagnosis is still by culturing the causative organisms . In majority of cases of CNS infections the routine labs are not well equipped to culture these viruses which are expected to cause the disease.

Neurotropic viruses are the viruses with both neuroinvasive and neurovirulence properties that cause central nervous system (CNS) diseases. This book chapter aims to define a complete representation of different children neurotropic viruses, their genetic structure, viral replication geographical location and demographic profile. Neurotropic viruses Including: Entero virus, JE Virus, Dengue, Zika, WNV, Mumps, Measles, Nipah & Hendra, HSV, VZV, EBV, CMV, SARS CoV 2, Influenza and Adeno virus have been summarised in Table 1. The tables summarises mechanism involving mode of infection entry in host CNS, development of neuropathology and Clinical presentation. However on the basis of their characteristics they have been detailed as below

2. DETAILED CHARACTERISTICS AND EPIDEMIOLOGY

Nearly all organisms can infect the CNS; however there are distinct etiological alterations in different geographical regions and in different seasons. Some pathogens are endemic, others sporadic and yet others cause epidemics. Hence the precise epidemiology of CNS infections is difficult to determine; also in many cases there are difficulties in determining an exact microbiological identification predominantly in the resource limited countries. The paediatric patients are unable to communicate their problem and usually the diagnosis is late. Many times the viral infection are misdiagnosed as bacterial infections, which leads unnecessary medication and high fatality.

Geographical distribution also plays on important role on etiology of viral CNS infections. For example Herpes simplex viruses (HSVs) are common pathogen amid children and adults in the United States (US), Australia, and Italy, and in Southern Vietnam, the Japanese encephalitis virus (JEV) is common viral encephalitis among children. Similarly in some parts of India, enteroviruses (EVs) were the leading cause of viral encephalitis, and HSVs most prevalent pathogen in eastern India among children and adults (*Abdullahi et al., 2020*). Further in the chapter we will be discussing different neurotropic viruses their genotypic configuration, replication, geographic location and their demographic profile.

A. Picornaviruses

Picornaviridae is one of the largest virus families. Its members are small (approximately 30 nm), non-enveloped, single-stranded ribonucleic acid (RNA) viruses. The family contains 29 genera, with Enteroviruses (EVs) and Parechoviruses (PeVs) being significant human pathogens. The genus EV is distributed into 13 species (A-J) and Rhinoviruses (RVs) A-C. Only seven of these are pathogenic to humans; others infect only animals (1, 4-6). EVs are further sub-grouped into Polioviruses, Coxsackieviruses A and B, Echoviruses, numbered EVs, and RVs. The genus PeV is divided into two species, Parechovirus A and B. There are 16 subtypes of Parechovirus A species, containing 16 genotypes categorized as human Parechoviruses (HPeVs) 1-16 (*Rotbart, 2000; Van der Linden et al., 2015*). The EV genus consists of a simple viral capsid constructed from 60 repeating protomers, each containing four structural proteins (VP1-4) that together formulate the icosahedral shell of the virus (*Van der Linden et al., 2015*).

Enteroviruses

Enteroviruses (EVs) characterize the chief viral pathogens that causes meningitis in youngsters, comprising about 85% of meningitis cases. The serotypes of circulating nonpolio-EVs alter every year, however some EVs continue to show prevalence over time. Over 55 per cent of the viral infections of the central nervous system (CNS) among children, are accountable to them. A detailed study could help improve their diagnosis of the potentially life-threatening condition. Although enteroviruses are known as collection of viruses that usually pose a number of mild infections, however they may cause severe illness if they infect the CNS, (Mumbai-based iGenetic Diagnostics, study). The route of EVs is often predominantly fecal-oral transmission, and humans being lone reservoir of infection. In very sporadic cases, EV infection may be caused through the inhalation of droplets. Icubation period of EV infection ranges between three and six days. However pathogenesis of EV infection remains unclear. It is expected that specific receptors on enterocytes are probably attached by viral particles that replicate themselves in the Peyer's patches of the lamina propria (Principi & Esposito,2015; Knoester et al., 2019, Pérez-Vélez et al., 2007). Other viral elements across the nasopharynx spread to the lymphatic system of the respiratory region. EVs is carried to the spleen at the first viremic phase then to liver and heart, and in these organs, the virus rapidly replicates. Thus leading to another viremic phase with symptoms of infection. The CNS is expected to be involved during both phases of infection.

Enteroviruses (EVs) are the primary viral pathogens responsible for approximately 85% of meningitis cases in children. Although often associated with mild infections, they can cause life-threatening conditions if they invade the central nervous system (CNS), where they are responsible for over 55% of all viral infections in this region.

Primary Route: Transmission is predominantly fecal-oral, with humans serving as the sole natural reservoir. Secondary Route infection can also occur through respiratory droplets, though this is less common. Incubation Period typically ranges from 3 to 6 days before symptoms manifest. Pathogenesis and Disease Progression: The exact mechanisms of EV pathogenesis remain a subject of ongoing research, but the process generally follows these stages: 1.Gastrointestinal Attachment: Viral particles are believed to attach to specific receptors on enterocytes. 2. Primary replication occurs in the Peyer's patches of the lamina propria and in the lymphoid tissue of the nasopharynx (Principi & Esposito,2015; Knoester et al., 2019, Pérez-Vélez et al., 2007). First Viremic Phase: The virus spreads to the spleen, liver, and heart, where it undergoes rapid replication. Second Viremic Phase: A subsequent wave of viral spread leads to systemic symptoms. The CNS can become involved during either of these viremic phases. Detailed studies, such as those conducted by iGenetic Diagnostics, (Mumbai-based iGenetic Diagnostics, study), emphasize that rapid and accurate diagnosis is critical to managing these potentially severe infections

B. Arboviruses

Arboviruses (arthropod-borne viruses) comprise a diverse group of approximately 537 viruses distributed globally. Characterized by high genetic plasticity and rapid mutation rates, these primarily RNA-based viruses are transmitted to humans through arthropod vectors such as mosquitoes, ticks, and sandflies (Lindsey et al., 2014; David & Abraham, 2016). While horizontal transmission via vectors is most common, spread can also occur vertically (mother-to-child) or through nosocomial routes like blood transfusions and organ transplants. Environmental factors—including temperature, rainfall, and vegetation—heavily influence their year-round transmission cycles (Rizzo, 2016). Arboviruses of clinical significance are categorized into four primary groups: Togaviridae, Flaviviridae, Bunyavirales, and Reoviridae.

1. Togaviridae (Alphaviruses)

The genus Alphavirus consists of small, enveloped, single-stranded positive-sense RNA viruses categorized by geographic origin (Travassos da Rosa et al., 1998; Chen et al., 2018). Encephalitic alphaviruses circulate globally and are categorized by their geographic distribution into Old World and New World groups. New World alphaviruses, primarily found in the Americas, are highly neurotropic; this group includes the Venezuelan equine encephalitis virus (VEEV), Eastern equine encephalitis virus (EEEV), and Western equine encephalitis virus (WEEV) (Chen 2018). New World Alphaviruses are primarily neurotropic, causing encephalitis. Mortality rates vary significantly, from 1% (VEEV/WEEV) to as high as 75% (EEEV). Old World Alphaviruses: Found in Europe, Asia, and Africa, this group includes the Chikungunya (CHIKV), Mayaro, and Una viruses. While typically associated with fever and joint pain, CHIKV has re-emerged as a major epidemic threat in over 45 countries, causing severe neurological complications across all age groups (Chen et al., 2018).

Transmission and Mortality: The transmission cycles of these viruses vary by species:

- EEEV and WEEV: Typically circulate between mosquitoes and bird populations.
- VEEV: Cycles between mosquitoes and rodents (enzootic) or mosquitoes and horses (epizootic).

In humans, these infections can rapidly lead to encephalitis. Mortality rates are approximately 1% for VEEV and WEEV, but significantly higher for EEEV, ranging from 50% to 75% (Chen 2018).

Regional Impact and Emerging Threats: Amongst New World- VEEV is the most significant neurotropic alphavirus in this region, responsible for numerous outbreaks across North, Central, and South America. In Old World: Found across Europe, Asia, and Africa, most members of this group generally cause less severe disease, though certain viruses like Chikungunya (CHIKV) can cause neurological complications.

- **Chikungunya (CHIKV):** Recently re-emerged as a major epidemic, CHIKV has spread to over 45 countries. While vertebrate animals traditionally serve as reservoirs, humans have become the primary reservoirs in recent urban epidemics. It is now recognized for causing severe neurological issues across all age groups; notably, during outbreaks in the Caribbean and La Réunion Island, encephalitis rates reached 187 per 100,000 infants (Travassos da Rosa 1998; Chen 2018).

2. Flaviviridae

Flaviviruses are enveloped, single-stranded RNA viruses. The family is divided into two main transmission categories: Tick-Borne Flaviviruses- Including Tick-borne encephalitis virus (TBEV) and Powassan virus (POWV), these cause 10,000–15,000 human cases annually across Europe and Asia (Robertson 2009).

Mosquito-Borne Flaviviruses

1.Japanese Encephalitis Virus (JEV)

The leading cause of pediatric viral encephalitis in East Asia. JEV primarily affects children, with peak incidence during summer and autumn. Despite its high mortality and morbidity, vaccination efforts (such as those for mumps in the UK) have historically helped mitigate CNS infection rates, though improved PCR diagnostics have recently led to higher reported hospitalization rates (Amicizia 2018).In East Asia, JEV is the primary cause of acute childhood encephalitis. The disease follows a bimodal distribution, peaking in infants under one year old and again in children aged five and older (Amicizia 2018). Transmission is highest during summer and autumn, coinciding with peak arboviral activity. Notably, JEV frequently targets immunocompetent children; studies show that over 91% of pediatric viral CNS cases occurred in patients with no underlying health conditions (Amicizia 2018). While historical immunization (e.g., against mumps) reduced CNS infection rates in the late 20th century, hospitalization rates have risen since 2003, largely due to more sensitive PCR diagnostic testing.

2. Dengue Virus (DENV)

Dengue virus is globally distributed and currently endemic in approximately 100 countries. Its widespread expansion is driven by human migration, rapid urbanization, armed conflict, and deficiencies in waste, water, and vector management (Nonyong 2021). The virus is transmitted to humans through the bite of female Aedes mosquitoes, primarily Ae. aegypti and Ae. albopictus. DENV is classified into four genetically distinct but related serotypes (DENV 1–4) that circulate heavily in both urban and peri-urban environments (Nonyong 2021).

3. Yellow Fever Virus (YFV)

A major public health priority, YFV causes yellow fever and is prevalent across most continents, with the highest impact in Africa and the Americas. While West Africa experiences a higher infection frequency (approximately 50 cases per million people compared to 5 per million in South America), South America exhibits a higher mortality rate. This disparity in fatality rates is potentially attributed to genetic variations in the virus (Nonyong 2021).

Additional Viruses: This group also includes the West Nile Virus (WNV), Zika Virus (ZIKV), and St. Louis Encephalitis Virus (SLEV) (Holbrook 2017).

- **St. Louis Encephalitis Virus (SLEV):**SLEV is a significant mosquito-borne flavivirus found throughout North, Central, and South America. In North America, it remains one of the most prominent arboviral threats. It is particularly noted for its pediatric impact, accounting for 35% to 60% of all symptomatic cases of aseptic meningitis in children (Curren 2018).
- **Zika Virus (ZIKV):** Discovered in 1947, ZIKV emerged as a global health emergency in 2016. It has since spread to 48 countries across the Americas, with additional imported cases reported in Europe, Canada, and the United States (Gubler 2017; Gutiérrez-Bugallo 2019).
- **West Nile Virus (WNV):** Now globally widespread, WNV causes annual encephalitis outbreaks with mortality rates between 5% and 10% (Abdullahi 2020). While most infections are subclinical, approximately 1% of patients develop severe neurological complications, including meningoencephalitis (Gubler 2017). First identified in the West Nile sub-region of Uganda, West Nile virus (WNV) has since expanded its reach to temperate and tropical regions worldwide. As of 2025, it remains a global concern, causing annual

encephalitis outbreaks with reported mortality rates between 5% and 10% (Abdullahi 2020).

Vector and Spread: While primarily transmitted by ornithophilic (bird-feeding) mosquitoes, WNV can also be spread through blood transfusions, organ transplants, or transplacentally from mother to fetus (Gutiérrez-Bugallo 2019).

Outbreak History: The virus has caused sporadic epidemics across Africa, the Middle East, Asia, and Australia (Gubler 2017).The majority of WNV infections are subclinical (asymptomatic). However, fewer than 1% of infected individuals develop severe neuroinvasive disease, which can range from meningitis to encephalitis or meningoencephalitis (Gubler 2017).

Non-Vector Transmission: While primarily spread by mosquitoes, certain flaviviruses like JEV and WNV can also be transmitted via blood transfusions, organ transplants, or transplacentally from mother to fetus during pregnancy (Gutiérrez-Bugallo 2019).

3) **Bunyaviralis**: Members of this order are enveloped viruses measuring approximately 100 nm in diameter (Abdullahi AM et.al 2020). Their genome consists of negative-sense, single-stranded RNA organized into three distinct segments, each contained within its own nucleocapsid (a tripartite structure) (Abdullahi AM et.al 2020). Bunyaviralis comprises of three significant genera. Nairovirus which Includes Crimean-Congo hemorrhagic fever virus (CCHFV). Orthobunyavirus which Includes California encephalitis virus (CEV), Jamestown Canyon virus (JCV), and La Crosse virus (LACV). Phlebovirus that Includes Toscana virus (TOSV) and Rift Valley fever virus (RVFV).
4) **Reoviridae:** This family consists of non-enveloped viruses characterized by a segmented, double-stranded RNA (dsRNA) genome. The virion is typically divided into 10 to 12 segments, and each genus within the family employs unique strategies for host infection and replication. The family is categorized into two primary subfamilies:

Sedoreovirinae- Includes genera such as Orbivirus, Rotavirus, Cardoreovirus, and Phytoreovirus. **Spinareovirinae:** Comprises genera including Orthoreovirus, Aquareovirus, and Dinovernavirus. Among these, the genus Orbivirus is of significant clinical importance, notably including the Colorado tick fever virus (CTFV).

C. Paramyxoviruses

Members of the large Paramyxoviridae family cause various diseases in both humans and animals. Three genera within this family are particularly significant due to their ability to cause neurological diseases:

- **Rubulavirus**: This genus includes the mumps virus, a neurotropic pathogen that can cause complications such as meningitis and encephalitis in humans.
- **Morbillivirus:** This genus contains the measles virus, a clinically critical species that may lead to acute post-infectious encephalitis or subacute sclerosing panencephalitis.
- **Henipavirus:** This genus features highly neurotropic members, specifically the Nipah virus (NiV) and Hendra virus (HeV), both of which are known to cause severe, often fatal, acute encephalitis.

1) The Mumps Virus

Mumps Virus (MuV): Classified within the genus Orthorubulavirus of the family Paramyxoviridae, the mumps virus is a non-segmented, pleomorphic, enveloped, single-stranded RNA virus. Its structure includes an inner helical ribonucleoprotein core composed of the viral genome associated with two proteins that function as an RNA-dependent RNA polymerase. On its surface, two primary glycoproteins facilitate infection:

Hemagglutinin-neuraminidase (HN): Responsible for the adsorption of the virion to host cells by binding to sialic acid receptors.

Fusion (F) protein: Mediates the penetration of genetic material into the host cell through membrane fusion (Rubin S, et al., 2015)..

MuV primarily affects the central nervous system (CNS) and glandular tissues and can be isolated from saliva, cerebrospinal fluid (CSF), blood, breast milk, and urine. Transmission occurs through direct contact with infected saliva or respiratory secretions, as well as via contaminated fomites like bedding or doorknobs. While mumps is a major cause of encephalitis in unvaccinated populations (Rubin S, et al., 2015), cases of vaccine-associated meningitis have been reported, particularly with certain strains like Urabe Am9. For these strains, the frequency of meningitis is estimated at approximately one to 10 cases per 10,000 doses, typically manifesting 15 to 35 days post-vaccination. However, as noted by Campbell et al., there is currently no substantial evidence to prove that encephalitis observed in vaccinated children is directly caused by the mumps component of the vaccine (Crowley et al).

2) The Measles Virus

The measles virus (MV), a member of the Morbillivirus genus, it is an enveloped, pleomorphic, negative-sense, single-stranded RNA virus with a diameter of approximately 200 nm. Its non-segmented genome is about 16,000 nucleotides long, containing six genes that code for eight viral proteins (six structural and two non-structural).

The six structural proteins are- Hemagglutinin (H) protein, Fusion (F) protein, Nucleocapsid (N) protein, Phosphoprotein (P), Matrix (M) protein, Large (L) protein (Leung AK, 2018).. MV remains a leading cause of morbidity and mortality in developing countries. MV infection can lead to severe central nervous system (CNS) complications, affecting up to 30% of cases, with approximately one in 6,000 cases developing severe measles encephalitis. Transmission typically occurs via airborne droplets, small-particle aerosols that remain suspended in the air, or direct contact with infected secretions. Contact with contaminated fomites is a less frequent transmission route (Leung AK, 2018).

3) Henipaviruses,

This genus consists of enveloped, non-segmented, negative-sense, single-stranded RNA viruses. It includes two critical emerging zoonotic pathogens: Nipah virus (NiV) and Hendra virus (HeV). Both are capable of causing severe acute encephalitis and acute respiratory distress syndrome (ARDS) (Montgomery JM, et al., 2008). The natural reservoir for these viruses is fruit bats of the genus Pteropus. These bats carry the viruses asymptomatically, showing no clinical signs of illness. Transmission to domestic animals typically occurs when feed or grazing areas are contaminated with bat excreta, such as urine or feces. The pathways for human infection differ by virus:

Hendra virus (HeV): Human cases are almost exclusively linked to direct contact with infected horses.

Nipah virus (NiV): In regions like Bangladesh, transmission often occurs through the consumption of raw date palm sap contaminated by bat secretions. Additionally, NiV is notable for its documented capacity for human-to-human transmission.

D. Arenaviruses (Lymphocytic Choriomeningitis Viruses) (LCMV)

Virology and Structure: Lymphocytic choriomeningitis virus (LCMV) is the primary member of the Arenaviridae family known to cause human disease. This enveloped, single-stranded RNA virus possesses a genome divided into two segments: Small (S) and Large (L). The S segment encodes the nucleocapsid protein (NP) and the glycoprotein precursor (GPC), while the L segment encodes the viral RNA-dependent RNA polymerase (L) and the Z (zinc finger-like) protein. To date, over 30 strains have been identified, showcasing specialized enzymatic functions for viral transcription and replication (Montgomery JM, 2008).

Epidemiology: The house mouse (Mus musculus) serves as the primary reservoir for LCMV, though other rodents like hamsters, rats, and guinea pigs can also carry the virus. Humans typically contract the infection through contact with rodent excreta, with a higher incidence noted during winter months when rodents move indoors. High-risk groups include laboratory personnel, pet owners, and individuals living in unsanitary conditions across the Americas, Europe, Asia, and Africa. Seroprevalence studies indicate varying global exposure rates, such as 5% in the United States, 1.7% in Madrid, and as high as 36% on the Island of Vir in Croatia (Bonthius DJ, 2012).

Clinical Presentation: In children, LCMV infection primarily manifests as aseptic meningitis, occurring in approximately 15% of confirmed postnatal cases. While less common, more severe neurological presentations like meningoencephalitis and encephalitis have been documented. When the virus is transmitted congenitally, it can lead to severe teratogenic effects, including microencephaly and other developmental abnormalities (Abdullahi AM, 2020).

Diagnosis and Management: Diagnosis: Definitive diagnosis is achieved by detecting specific IgM or IgG antibodies using ELISA or indirect immunofluorescence assays. Additionally, PCR testing can be utilized to identify viral RNA in the blood or cerebrospinal fluid (CSF). While viral culture is possible for postnatal infections, it is less commonly used.

Management: There is currently no FDA-approved specific treatment for LCMV infections of the central nervous system; therefore, supportive care is the standard of practice. While antivirals such as Ribavirin and Favipiravir have shown potential in experimental settings, their clinical efficacy for LCMV remains under evaluation (Bonthius DJ, 2012).

Prognosis and Complications

Congenital LCMV infection carries a poor prognosis, with mortality rates reaching approximately 35%. Survivors often face long-term neurological challenges, including mental retardation, hydrocephalus, chorioretinitis, permanent visual impairment, and chronic seizure disorders (Abdullahi AM, 2020).

E. Herpes Family Viruses

The *Herpesviridae* family consists of enveloped, double-stranded DNA viruses known for their neurotropic nature and ability to establish lifelong latency within host neurons. Key members associated with neurological diseases include HSV-1, HSV-2, Varicella-Zoster Virus (VZV), Epstein-Barr Virus (EBV), and Cytomegalovirus (CMV). These viruses are characterized by complex genomes containing numerous open reading frames (ORFs) and microsatellites (short tandem repeats). All herpesvirus genomes have been known to comprise microsatellites that are multiple sites with short tandem repeats (STR regions) of one to six nucleotide motifs and homopolymers as numerous microsatellites class.

1. Herpes Simplex Virus Type 1 (HSV-1)

HSV-1 primarily infects epithelial surfaces before establishing a latent state in sensory neurons.

- **Structure:** Its large DNA genome is divided into "Long" and "Short" unique regions, flanked by inverted repeats. Approximately 84% of the genome codes for proteins across at least 74 ORFs.
- **Clinical Impact:** Reactivation can lead to severe meningitis or encephalitis, often resulting in significant developmental impairments or permanent neurological disability.

2. Varicella-Zoster Virus (VZV / HHV-3)

VZV is a human-specific virus with a genome of approximately 125,000 base pairs and 70 ORFs.

- **Pathogenesis:** Primary childhood infection causes *varicella (chickenpox)*, after which the virus becomes dormant in the cranial or spinal ganglia.
- **Reactivation:** If cellular immunity wanes due to age or immunosuppression, the virus reactivates as **herpes zoster (shingles)**.

3. Epstein-Barr Virus (EBV / HHV-4)

Identified in 1964, EBV is an enveloped virus containing a linear DNA genome with roughly 100 genes.

- **Structure:** The virion features a protein capsid surrounded by a "tegument" layer containing glycoproteins that dictate cell tropism and receptor binding. It is categorized into two subtypes based on nuclear antigen variations.
- **Transmission:** EBV is globally ubiquitous. In children, it spreads via saliva and respiratory secretions (often through shared toys or utensils). It can also be transmitted via blood transfusions, organ transplants, or transplacentally.
- **Risk Factors:** Overcrowding, low socioeconomic status, and immunocompromised states increase the risk of transmission.

4. Cytomegalovirus (CMV / HHV-5)

CMV possesses the largest genome among human herpesviruses (230–240 kb).

- **Structure:** The DNA core is protected by a 162-capsomere protein capsid, a tegument, and a lipid envelope, reaching a total diameter of up to 180 nm.
- **Epidemiology:** CMV is highly prevalent worldwide, with seroprevalence rates ranging from 30% to 100% depending on the region. In developed nations, congenital CMV affects approximately 0.6% to 0.7% of live births.
- **Transmission:** Routes include direct contact with bodily fluids, nosocomial spread, and transplacental transmission.
- **Clinical Significance:** Congenital CMV is a leading cause of non-hereditary birth defects and neurological impairment.

F. Influenza Viruses

Neurological complications have been reported in around 15% of youngsters infected with one or another strain of influenza. Additionally, influenza viruses comprise for about 2–11% of encephalitis cases in childhood. Neurological illness associated with influenza virus infection is often demarcated as influenza-associated encephalitis/encephalopathy (IAE). The term encephalopathy was chosen as influenza virus is seldom neuroinvasive. As direct CNS incursion by influenza virus is occasional, while viral RNAs in CSF have been identified in some infections. Infection of influenza could cause a extensive range of neurological indications, starting with a somewhat changed mental state, vertigo, febrile seizures, and demyelinating illness to status epilepticus, meningitis, and even stroke. A retrospective study by Mastrolia et al., emphasized that all youngsters showing severe neurological features in the influenza period must be assessed for influenza-associated CNS impediments albeit respiratory connection is slight. Moreover, the absence of underlying diseases or other risk factors is not protecting against influenza-associated neurological problems.

F. Lymphocytic Choriomeningitis Virus

Lymphocytic choriomeningitis virus (LCMV) is a rare source of human CNS infections in developed countries. The threat of harbouring LCMV infections is connected to cahnces of having contact with discharges from rodents, particularly during the months in winter.

G. Severe Acute Respiratory Syndrome Coronavirus 2 (SARS-CoV-2)

Studies have stated that the neuro-invasive possiblity of SARS-CoV-2 are supported by studies on neurological appearances in 36% of adult patients. A systematic review and meta analyses of studies involving approximately 3700 pediatric COVID-19 patients showed that 17% of them had common neurological disorders and 1% had signs and indications of severe brain association. In patients with multisystem inflammatory syndrome in children (MIS-C), the occurrence of irregular neurological conclusions has been stated in about 55% of cases . Providentially, in many children, neurological indicators, largely characterised by headache and anosmia, are minor, temporary and do not complicate the COVID-19 development. However, in some children that have SARS-CoV-2 disease, severe clinical complications connected with pertinent changes shown in neuroimaging, electroencephalography, nerve conduction testing and electromyography results can show.

3. CLINICAL PRESENTATION

A diagnosis of acute meningitis is established through a clinical evaluation identifying signs of meningeal inflammation. Key diagnostic indicators include: Physical Findings: The presence of fever, headache, and neck rigidity (nuchal rigidity), along with positive Kernig and Brudzinski signs. CSF Analysis: Confirmation typically requires identifying pleocytosis (elevated white blood cell count) in the cerebrospinal fluid. Pyogenic (bacterial) meningitis is generally characterized by a predominance of polymorphonuclear leukocytes. Viral, fungal, and tuberculous meningitis usually present with a majority of lymphocytes.

While viral meningitis is frequently self-limiting and resolves with supportive care, bacterial and fungal infections are medical emergencies. Without prompt treatment, they can progress rapidly to severe neurological dysfunction or death. In clinical scenarios where symptoms of both meningitis and encephalitis (inflammation of the brain parenchyma) occur simultaneously, the condition is classified as meningoencephalitis.

Picornaviruses Clinical presentation: The collective neurologic manifestation caused by HEVs is aseptic meningitis with chances life-threatening encephalitis wherein infants show symptoms of irritability, anorexia, fever, shock, limb stiffness and also seizures. In case of neonates, the distinctive clinical appearance is fever and prominent protuberant anterior fontanelle. CNS infection casued by Picornaviruses normally exhibits as meningitis and in case of infants presentation is with fever, loss of appetite, irritability and body feebleness, loss of cognizance or circulatory shock.

Arboviruses Clinical presentation: Arboviruses cause a widespread CNS ailments ranging from encephalomyelitis, neuritis, meningoencephalitis, meningitis, encephalitis, and myelitis. Nevertheless, encephalitis is the most common neurologic appearance. First symptoms in children including cough, catarrh (flu-like), fever and sore throat and then accompanied by vomiting, nausea and meningismus.

Togaviridae/Alphaviruses These have a small gestation period of 2-4 days with acute stage lasting for about 1-2 days that has symptoms of fever, sore throat and body pain. It is then followed by anorexia and extreme body weakness which normally last for about 2-3 weeks through advancement towards encephalitis in less than 4% cases. Members of this class comprise Venezuelan Equine, Western and Eastern Encephalitis viruses (VEEV, WEEV and EEEV respectively) that have symptoms of fever, convulsion, neck stiffness or coma . An additional member of this family is Chikungunya virus (CHIKV) which represents with fever, convulsions and may represent in multiorgan impairment.

Flaviviridae Members of this class frequently present through meningitis or meningoencephalitis displaying recurrent fever, body stiffness, body weakness, convulsions and signs of meningeal irritation .They include Japanese encephalitis virus (JEV), tick-borne encephalitis virus (TBEV), Powassan encephalitis virus (POWV), Dengue virus (DENV), Yellow fever virus (YFV), West Nile virus(WNV), St. Louis encephalitis virus (SLE) and Zika virus (ZIKV) which usually arise as congenital infection clinically displayed with microcephaly and showing signs of cognitive impairment.

Bunyaviridae generally represent as encephalitis displaying symptoms of fever, nausea, vomiting, abdominal distention, lethargy, convulsions and loss of consciousness with an development period of 7 -15 days. Other associates are Rift Valley Fever virus (RVFV) and Toscana virus (TOSV) which are generally asymptomatic, but once symptoms typically occur they present with meningitis or meningoencephalitis.

Reoviridae Clinically represents symptoms of fever, nausea, vomiting, abdominal distension, skin rashes and photophobia which is formerly accompanied by features of meningitis or meningoencephalitis

Paramyxoviruses Clinical presentation: An extensive range of CNS indicators from meningitis to meningoencephalitis and less common but fatal encephalitis. Category of thses viruses include Henipaviruses, Measles virus (MV) and Mumps virus (MuV), including of Nipah and Hendra viruses (NiV and HeV respectively). MuV can manifest as asymptomatic aseptic meningitis or further as symptomatic aseptic meningitis which is categorised by fever, nausea, vomiting, headache (in older children), neck stiffness and meningismus. The less common but severe manifestation is encephalitis which is caused in less than 0.5% of cases of mump infection. These are represented by fever, focal or generalized convulsions, signs of meningeal irritation, delirium and coma. Meningoencephalitis can happen concomitantly with meningitis which is both benign and self-limiting with no severe complications. The neurologic manifestation of MV ranges from Acute demyelinating encephalomyelitis (ADME) that is an severe inflammation of brain along with myelin damage. Measles inclusion body encephalitis (MIBE) which arises in patients with supressed immunity and Sub-acute sclerosing panencephalitis (SSPE) which arises as a complication about 4years after MV infection and thus less common in infants. The signs and symptoms comprise febrile convulsions, poor appetite, indications of meningeal irritation or unconsciousness. After a prodromal phase of fever and lethargy, Henipavirus infection results in relapsing encephalitis which is categorized by fever and convulsions, limb weakness, segmental myoclonus, dizziness, vomiting, impairment in spatial perception, changed consciousness, drowsiness, and anomalous plantar response that quickly progresses to coma within 48 hours.

Arenaviruses (Lymphocytic Choriomeningitis Virus) Clinical presentation: Lymphocytic Choriomeningitis Virus (LCMV) contagion in youngsters usually represent with symptoms of meningitis, and if counteracted post-natally, it is related with aseptic meningitis that is caused in around 15% of cases with established infections. Infrequently meningoencephalitis and encephalitis have been reported with severe impediments. Patients of congenital microencephaly and teratogenesis instigated by LCMV has also been reported in neonates.

Herpes Family Viruses Clinical presentation: HSV CNS infection has a broad spectrun of clinical representation involving of meningitis, encephalitis, and meningoencephalitis. Aseptic meningitis is the the main CNS manifestation representing with fever, convulsion, and loss of consciousness. Early diagnosis is also complicated as early indications are generally non-specific. Childhood HSE is principally instigated by HSV-1, while HSV-2 is usually secluded in neonates and infants as it is practically always attained from an infected maternal genital tract. The members of this family include VZV, EBV and CMV. Varicella-zoster virus (VZV) is a fellow of herpes viral family, and it is typically related with meningoencephalitis and postinfectious encephalopathy that represent with fever, vomiting, bulging of anterior fontanelle, downward gaze deviation, apathy, convulsions, loss of consciousness and focal neurologic deficit. Aseptic meningitis is rare with VZV infection . Additional member is Epstein Barr virus (EBV) which commonly cause encephalitis that clinically represent with fever, convulsions or loss of consciousness. CMV CNS infection also usually represent with encephalitis that primarily affects immunocompromised patients and the commonest manifestation in infants is congenital infection showing fever, convulsions, vomiting, poor appetite, signs of meningeal irritation and altered level of consciousness.

4. DIAGNOSIS

Timely management approach of viral infections of the CNS require accurate diagnosis of the disease and Pathogen. Detecting CNS infections are rare and once diagnosed, infections have to categorized either "viral" or "bacterial" to start the treatment modalities. (Erdem 2017). As per new microbiological molecular technology detection of an infectious agent is now promising using approaches such as polymerase chain reaction (PCR) and extremely sensitive protein based antibody- or antigen-detection systems (Johnson RT. 1996). ADEM can be identified by highly sensitive magnetic resonance imaging (MRI), and responds well to steroid treatment. Etiological data is also be supportive from a predictive viewpoint for the specific patient and from a public health point of view for the community, principally in the cases of enterovirus and arbovirus infections. Though numerous molecular methods have in recent times been established, the etiology of viral infections continue to be poorly understood. Besides, since maximum researches do not emphasis on the detection of viruses affecting only children, the frequency of these viral infections in children is still unknown. All viruses can be diagnosed by a single RT-PCR protocol and multiple primer pairs. Enzyme linked immunosorbent assay (ELISA) has also been used to successfully diagnosed arboviruses by identifying virus specific Ig M antibody. Another indispensable device for confirming diagnosis and evaluating extent of brain damage is Neuroimaging. Although both computed tomography (CT) scan and magnetic resonance imaging (MRI) are used for this purpose, but MRI has tendency to be more accurate in diagnosis. In molecular confirmation RT-PCR can tested on samples of blood, urine, CSF or breast milk. Diagnosis is also sustained by CSF pleocytosis and high proteins. Following are the different molecular methods which are currently in use to explore and diagnose the viral as well as bacterial infection, using the minimal amount of sample.

Real-Time PCR

Polymerase chain reaction (PCR) has undergone a lot of advancement since its invention in 1985 by Kary Mullis. Real time is one of its advancement where the real time monitoring of PCR reaction can be done. RT PCR has proven to be a power tool to diagnose and report viral infections, identifies and differentiates organism causing infection. It can be easily performed on almost all samples be it CSF, BAL, Blood, Stool, Urine, pus and blood samples. With minimal involvement of human interference many IVD approved assays have been developed by various vendor worldwide. These are called Cartilage Based Nucleic Acid Testing. These molecular methods performed on cerebrospinal fluid, are asserted to be the new "gold standard" for diagnosing CNS infections, offering higher sensitivity and specificity compared to conventional methods especially in case of pathogens which are otherwise difficult to detect. Commercial diagnostic platforms offer various singleplex and multiplex PCR assays for suitable and easy testing of targets that represent similar clinical illness.

Cartilage Based Nucleic Acid Testing (CBNAAT)

Many commercially available kits have cartilage based nucleic acid based (CB-NAAT) testing which can detected these pathogens in 2-3hours. Meningitis panel CBNAAT based Film array technique which uses multiplex PCR. It comprises of an automated nucleic acid test having nucleic acid extraction, reverse transcription, and nucleic acid amplification, with an average result turnaround time of 75 minutes per run and a handling time of less than five minutes. Approximately 200μL of CSF is used for the BioFire® FilmArray® meningitis/encephalitis panel PCR panel. Conveyance of clinical samples from collection services to the testing laboratory takes around 15 minutes. This PCR method identifies 14 pathogens: Varicella-zoster virus, Cryptococcus, Cytomegalovirus, Enterovirus, Parechovirus, neoformans/ gattii, Escherichia coli K1, Haemophilus influenzae, Herpes simplex virus (HSV) 1/2, HHV-6, Listeria monocytogenes, Neisseria meningitidis, Streptococcus pneumoniae and Streptococcus agalactiae. This method takes less than 4 hours to detect and identify the pathogen.

2. Chip-Based CBNAAT

Trunat is a Microchip based real-time PCR Test for Viran RNA /DNA for Herpes Simplex Virus 1 and Herpes Simplex Virus 2, CMV. These assays are based on Taqman chemistry, using higher primer sensitivity and specificity Minimal sample is requirement 6μL. In less than two hours results are read on screen and RT PCR is carried out on smart chip with pre-set data for quantitation of results. The assay are completely closed and free for carryover contamination.

3. Genexpert: Viral Load Detection and Follow Up, and Syndromic Testing

Cepheid's GeneXpert platform based molecular assays, including real-time PCR, to detect viral loads in specimens like cerebrospinal fluid (CSF). These assays offer rapid turnaround times, which is critical for apt diagnosis and managing of CNS infections. These molecular methods, are asserted to be the new "gold standard" for diagnosing CNS infections, offering higher sensitivity and specificity compared to conventional methods. Assays are available for specific viruses like HSV-1, HSV-2, VZV, and enterovirus, which are commonly associated with CNS infections. However assays are not available for all the pathogens of CNS infections. There are syndromic panels available for detecting multiple pathogens associated with specific clinical syndromes, like respiratory infections or meningitis. These provide effective and timely detection of CNS pathogen within two hours.

4. Next Generation Sequencing

The adption of newer molecular assays including next-generation sequencing have expanded diagnostic abilities for recognizing infectious like encephalitis or meningitis. PCR has emerged as an exceptional system to diagnose the known pathogens. Pan-omic molecular systems have potential for usage in this area. Molecular biology based approaches are anticipated to be widely used in diagnosing and monitoring CNS infections, however results produced by these approaches especially next generation sequencing platforms need to be cautiously deduced in relation to the clinical findings. Technical advancements in metagenomics and deep sequencing have plausible use for diagnosing of clinical infections. As the nature of BBB, CSF and brain biopsies is sterile hence they are ideal to be further explored by the use of molecular technology for pathogen detection and as well as for the discovery of newer pathogens.

Some other encouraging developments have been made in the sub fiels of molecular biology viz. transcriptomics, proteomics and metabolomics. Where in host and microbial microRNA (miRNA) profiles have been used for diagnosing and finding various inflammatory and infectious diseases markers (He T,et al. 2016). Two miRNAs, miR-155 and miRNA-29b, Potential biomarkers for JEV infection as well as therapeutic targets using the method for anti-JEV therapy have been reported. Using markers like host neural EGF2 (epidermal growth factor like 2) and APOB (apolipoprotein B) in samples of CSF the diagnosis of tuberculer meningitis is possible with 89% sensitivity and 92% specificity. Also the metabolite profiling of CSF from patient sample has been stated beneficial in classifying the organism, making diagnosis, describing its epidemiology, and deciding treatment assessment of CNS infections in HIV patients. Although lot of advancement has been made still here are some lacuna in development of fast, accurate, sensitive and specific molecular assays for a increasing list of evolving and re-emerging neurotropic viruses. Expansion of test list of options also has upcoming challenges in choosing suitable tests and deciding on correct analysis of test outcomes.

5. Treatment Modalities and Complications

Definitive treatment for neurotropic viruses has remained unelusive as the course of disease differs in individuals and is dependent on innate immunity of the individual. In most of the cases Antiviral drugs have been proved to be effective. Prevention through childhood vaccination, wherever available is the best management option. Early diagnosis and prompt treatment strategies are the key.

There are studies that report major long-term neurologic sequelae in children which rae having picornavirus CNS infection (deCrom SC, et al., 2016, Vergnano S, 2015) The symptoms may include occurrence of seizures, chronic myoclonic jerks, impaired cognitive function and other associated abnormal behavior, like late achievement of developmental milestones and autonomic dysfunction (Kadambari S, et al., 2019). Some Psychiatric disorders alike attention deficit hyperactivity disorder (ADHD) and schizophrenia have been reported in children having infection of enterovirus encephalitis (Thong WY, et al., 2017). In a similar way Chikungunya virus (CHIKV) which usually starts with symptoms of fever may represent convulsions and cause multiple organ damage. Viruses like West Nile virus(WNV), Powassan encephalitis virus (POWV), St. Louis encephalitis virus (SLE), Dengue virus (DENV), tick-borne encephalitis virus (TBEV), Japanese encephalitis virus (JEV), Yellow fever virus (YFV) and Zika virus (ZIKV) that frequently are found as congenital infections, at times clinically manifest with microcephaly and also cognitive disorders. Few systemic infectious diseases having their personal characteristic clinical features could sporadically present with brain function disorder. These disorders are caused may be due to incursion of the pathogens into CNS, as in dengue fever, chikungunya, scrub typhus and leptospirosis. These presentation in such illustrations, are labelled as a complication of the primary disease.

Universaly, CNS viruses are known to cause life-long neurologic illness at the rate of around 50 per million cases per year displaying neurocognitive sequelae in survivors for example deafness, mental retardation, emotional problem and hemiparesis. Obstructive hydrocephalus and severe axonal polyneuropathy are also being reported in some uncommon cases of mumps meningitis; however, the retrieval is rapid. In mump encephalitis death may occur in up to10- 20% of cases, while 33% of survivors show evidence of prolonged neurological sequelae (*Abdullahi AM, 2020*). Subacute sclerosing panencephalitis is a fatal, progressive degenerative central nervous system disease that usually presents within 10 years after the measles virus infection has been caused as virus is persistent in neurons and oligodendrocytes in case of viral infections. Similarly LCMV congenital infection also has a bad diagnosis with a high death rate of approximately 35%. Those who survive the disease generally pose high neurodebility with microcephaly, mental impedance, hydrocephalus, chorioretinitis, visual impairment and tendency of seizure. Nearly 70% of the cases which do not receive treatment lead to death or are left with a permanent neurologic insufficiency in almost all survivors. The outcome can be anything comprising microcephaly, hydrocephaly, porencephalic cysts, spasticity, chorioretinitis, blindness, deafness, learning disabilities and seizures. Inherited CMV is deciphered as the chief cause of nongenetic basis of sensorineural hearing loss (SNHL) in children and it's a main reason of delayed neurodevelopmental process in them.

CONCLUSION

Methods to manage and treat viral infections infecting central nervous system in children depending on their clinical presentation, diagnosis, treatment modalities and complications is very complex. As conclusive treatment is still unavailable, nevertheless still there are certain antiviral drugs available which have been proven to be effective. The best possible management option is prevention of the CNS viral diseases is by immunising the children by vaccinating them in childhood wherever available.

REFERENCES

Abdullahi, A. M., Sarmast, S. T., & Singh, R. (2020). Molecular biology and epidemiology of neurotropic viruses. *Cureus, 12*(8), e9674. Advance online publication. DOI: 10.7759/cureus.9674 PMID: 32923269

Amicizia, D., Zangrillo, F., Lai, P. L., Iovine, M., & Panatto, D. (2018). Overview of Japanese encephalitis disease and its prevention. Focus on IC51 vaccine (IXIARO®). *Journal of Preventive Medicine and Hygiene, 59*(1), E99–E107. DOI: 10.15167/2421-4248/jpmh2018.59.1.962 PMID: 29938245

Autore, G., Bernardi, L., Perrone, S., & Esposito, S. (2021). Update on viral infections involving the central nervous system in pediatric patients. *Children (Basel, Switzerland), 8*(9), 782. Advance online publication. DOI: 10.3390/children8090782 PMID: 34572214

Bonthius, D. J. (2012). Lymphocytic choriomeningitis virus: An underrecognized cause of neurologic disease in the fetus, child, and adult. *Seminars in Pediatric Neurology, 19*(3), 89–95. DOI: 10.1016/j.spen.2012.02.002 PMID: 22889536

Chen, R., Mukhopadhyay, S., Merits, A., Bolling, B., Nasar, F., Coffey, L. L., Powers, A., & Weaver, S. C.ICTV Report Consortium. (2018). ICTV virus taxonomy profile: Togaviridae. *The Journal of General Virology, 99*(6), 761–762. DOI: 10.1099/jgv.0.001072 PMID: 29745869

Curren, E. J., Lindsey, N. P., Fischer, M., & Hills, S. L. (2018). St. Louis encephalitis virus disease in the United States, 2003–2017. *The American Journal of Tropical Medicine and Hygiene, 99*(4), 1074–1079. DOI: 10.4269/ajtmh.18-0420 PMID: 30182919

Dando, S. J., Mackay-Sim, A., Norton, R., Currie, B. J., St John, J. A., Ekberg, J. A. K., Batzloff, M., Ulett, G. C., & Beacham, I. R. (2014). Pathogens penetrating the central nervous system: Infection pathways and the cellular and molecular mechanisms of invasion. *Clinical Microbiology Reviews, 27*(4), 691–726. DOI: 10.1128/CMR.00118-13 PMID: 25278572

David, S., & Abraham, A. (2016). Epidemiological and clinical aspects on West Nile virus, a globally emerging pathogen. *Infectious Diseases, 48*(8), 571–586. DOI: 10.3109/23744235.2016.1164890 PMID: 27207312

DeCrom, S. C., Rossen, J. W. A., van Furth, A. M., & Obihara, C. C. (2016). Enterovirus and parechovirus infection in children: A brief overview. *European Journal of Pediatrics, 175*(8), 1023–1029. DOI: 10.1007/s00431-016-2725-7 PMID: 27156106

Erdem, H., Inan, A., Guven, E., Hargreaves, S., Larsen, L., Shehata, G., Pernicova, E., Khan, E., Bastakova, L., Namani, S., Harxhi, A., Roganovic, T., Lakatos, B., Uysal, S., Sipahi, O. R., Crisan, A., Miftode, E., Stebel, R., Jegorovic, B., & Nassar, M. (2017). The burden and epidemiology of community-acquired central nervous system infections: A multinational study. *European Journal of Clinical Microbiology & Infectious Diseases*, *36*(9), 1595–1611. DOI: 10.1007/s10096-017-2973-0 PMID: 28397100

Gubler, D. J., Vasilakis, N., & Musso, D. (2017). History and emergence of Zika virus. *The Journal of Infectious Diseases*, *216*(Suppl. 10), S860–S867. DOI: 10.1093/infdis/jix451 PMID: 29267917

Gutiérrez-Bugallo, G., Piedra, L. A., Rodriguez, M., Bisset, J. A., Lourenço-de-Oliveira, R., Weaver, S. C., Vasilakis, N., & Vega-Rúa, A. (2019). Vector-borne transmission and evolution of Zika virus. *Nature Ecology & Evolution*, *3*(4), 561–569. DOI: 10.1038/s41559-019-0836-z PMID: 30886369

He, T., Kaplan, S., Kamboj, M., & Tang, Y.-W. (2016). Laboratory diagnosis of central nervous system infection. *Current Infectious Disease Reports*, *18*(11), 35. Advance online publication. DOI: 10.1007/s11908-016-0545-6 PMID: 27686677

Holbrook, M. R. (2017). Historical perspectives on flavivirus research. *Viruses*, *9*(5), 97. Advance online publication. DOI: 10.3390/v9050097 PMID: 28468299

Johnson, R. T. (1996). Acute encephalitis. *Clinical Infectious Diseases*, *23*(2), 219–226. DOI: 10.1093/clinids/23.2.219 PMID: 8842253

Kadambari, S., Braccio, S., Ribeiro, S., Allen, D. J., Pebody, R., Brown, D., Cunney, R., Sharland, M., & Ladhani, S. (2019). Enterovirus and parechovirus meningitis in infants younger than 90 days old in the UK and Republic of Ireland: A British Paediatric Surveillance Unit study. *Archives of Disease in Childhood*, *104*(6), 552–557. DOI: 10.1136/archdischild-2018-315643 PMID: 30530486

Knoester, M., Helfferich, J., Poelman, R., Van Leer-Buter, C., Brouwer, O. F., & Niesters, H. G. M. (2016). EV-D68 AFM Working Group. (2019). Twenty-nine cases of enterovirus-D68-associated acute flaccid myelitis in Europe 2016: A case series and epidemiologic overview. *The Pediatric Infectious Disease Journal*, *38*(1), 16–21. DOI: 10.1097/INF.0000000000002188 PMID: 30234793

Leung, A. K., Hon, K. L., Leong, K. F., & Sergi, C. M. (2018). Measles: A disease often forgotten but not gone. *Hong Kong Medical Journal*, *24*(5), 512–520. DOI: 10.12809/hkmj187470 PMID: 30245481

Lindsey, N. P., Lehman, J. A., Staples, J. E., & Fischer, M. (2014). West Nile virus and other arboviral diseases—United States, 2013. *MMWR. Morbidity and Mortality Weekly Report, 63*(24), 521–526. PMID: 24941331

Montgomery, J. M., Hossain, M. J., Gurley, E., Carroll, D. S., Croisier, A., Bertherat, E., Asgari, N., Formenty, P., Keeler, N., Comer, J., Bell, M. R., Akram, K., Molla, A. R., Zaman, K., Islam, M. R., Wagoner, K., Mills, J. N., Rollin, P. E., Ksiazek, T. G., & Breiman, R. F. (2008). Risk factors for Nipah virus encephalitis in Bangladesh. *Emerging Infectious Diseases, 14*(10), 1526–1532. DOI: 10.3201/eid1410.060507 PMID: 18826814

Moseman, E. A., Blanchard, A. C., Nayak, D., & McGavern, D. B. (2020). T cell engagement of cross-presenting microglia protects the brain from a nasal virus infection. *Science Immunology, 5*(48), Article eabb1817. DOI: 10.1126/sciimmunol.abb1817

Nonyong, P., Ekalaksananan, T., Phanthanawiboon, S., Aromseree, S., Phadungsombat, J., Nakayama, E. E., Shioda, T., Sawaswong, V., Payungporn, S., Thaewnongiew, K., Overgaard, H. J., Bangs, M. J., Alexander, N., & Pientong, C. (2021). Dengue virus in humans and mosquitoes and their molecular characteristics in northeastern Thailand 2016-2018. *PLoS One, 16*(9), e0257460. Advance online publication. DOI: 10.1371/journal.pone.0257460 PMID: 34520486

Olson, J. K., Girvin, A. M., & Miller, S. D. (2001). Direct activation of innate and antigen-presenting functions of microglia following infection with Theiler's virus. *Journal of Virology, 75*(20), 9780–9789. DOI: 10.1128/JVI.75.20.9780-9789.2001 PMID: 11559811

Pellett, P. E., Mitra, S., & Holland, T. C. (2014). Basics of virology. In *Handbook of Clinical Neurology* (Vol. 123, pp. 45–66). Elsevier. DOI: 10.1016/B978-0-444-53488-0.00002-X

Pérez-Vélez, C. M., Anderson, M. S., Robinson, C. C., McFarland, E. J., Nix, W. A., Pallansch, M. A., Oberste, M. S., & Glodé, M. P. (2007). Outbreak of neurologic enterovirus type 71 disease: A diagnostic challenge. *Clinical Infectious Diseases, 45*(8), 950–957. DOI: 10.1086/521895 PMID: 17879907

Principi, N., & Esposito, S. (2015). Enterovirus D-68: An emerging cause of infection. *Expert Review of Respiratory Medicine, 9*(6), 711–719. DOI: 10.1586/17476348.2015.1109451 PMID: 26535922

Rizzo, C., Napoli, C., Venturi, G., Pupella, S., Lombardini, L., Calistri, P., Monaco, F., Cagarelli, R., Angelini, P., Bellini, R., Tamba, M., Piatti, A., Russo, F., Palù, G., Chiari, M., Lavazza, A., & Bella, A. (2016). West Nile virus transmission: Results from the integrated surveillance system in Italy, 2008 to 2015. *Eurosurveillance*, *21*(37), 30340. Advance online publication. DOI: 10.2807/1560-7917.ES.2016.21.37.30340 PMID: 27684046

Robertson, S. J., Mitzel, D. N., Taylor, R. T., Best, S. M., & Bloom, M. E. (2009). Tick-borne flaviviruses: Dissecting host immune responses and virus countermeasures. *Immunologic Research*, *43*(1–3), 172–186. DOI: 10.1007/s12026-008-8065-6 PMID: 18841330

Rotbart, H. A. (2000). Viral meningitis. *Seminars in Neurology*, *20*(3), 277–292. DOI: 10.1055/s-2000-9427 PMID: 11051293

Rubin, S., Eckhaus, M., Rennick, L. J., Bamford, C. G. G., & Duprex, W. P. (2015). Molecular biology, pathogenesis and pathology of mumps virus. *The Journal of Pathology*, *235*(2), 242–252. DOI: 10.1002/path.4445 PMID: 25229387

Sheybani, F., Haddad, M., & Shirazinia, M. (2023). Epidemiology and etiology of community-acquired CNS infections in Iran: A narrative review. *Future Neurology*, *18*(4), FNL73. Advance online publication. DOI: 10.2217/fnl-2023-0017

Thong, W. Y., Han, A., Wang, S. J., Lin, J., Isa, M. S., Koay, E. S., & Tay, S. K. (2017). Enterovirus infections in Singaporean children: An assessment of neurological manifestations and clinical outcomes. *Singapore Medical Journal*, *58*(4), 189–195. DOI: 10.11622/smedj.2016099 PMID: 27245861

Travassos da Rosa, J. F. S., Travassos da Rosa, A. P. A., Vasconcelos, P. F. C., Pinheiro, F. P., Rodrigues, S. G., Travassos da Rosa, E. S., & Dias, L. B. (1998). Arboviruses isolated in the Evandro Chagas Institute, including some described for the first time in the Brazilian Amazon region, their known hosts, and their pathology for man. In Travassos da Rosa, J. F. S., Travassos da Rosa, A. P. A., & Vasconcelos, P. F. C. (Eds.), *An overview of arbovirology in Brazil and neighbouring countries* (pp. 19–31). Instituto Evandro Chagas.

Tumani, H., Huss, A., & Bachhuber, F. (2017). The cerebrospinal fluid and barriers - Anatomic and physiologic considerations. In *Handbook of Clinical Neurology* (Vol. 146, pp. 21–32). Elsevier., DOI: 10.1016/B978-0-12-804279-3.00002-2

Van der Linden, L., Wolthers, K. C., & van Kuppeveld, F. J. M. (2015). Replication and inhibitors of enteroviruses and parechoviruses. *Viruses*, *7*(8), 4529–4562. DOI: 10.3390/v7082832 PMID: 26266417

Vergnano, S., Kadambari, S., Whalley, K., Menson, E. N., Martinez-Alier, N., Cooper, M., Sanchez, E., Heath, P. T., & Lyall, H. (2015). Characteristics and outcomes of human parechovirus infection in infants (2008-2012). *European Journal of Pediatrics*, *174*(7), 919–924. DOI: 10.1007/s00431-014-2483-3 PMID: 25573462

APPENDIX

Table 1. Summary of neurotropic viruses, neuropathology and presentation

	Neurotropic viruses	Portal of entry in host	Entry in CNS	Mechanisms of neuropathology	Clinical presentation
A	**Entero virus**	Gastrointestinal tract	• BBB • Infected immune cells • Via nerves (motoneurons)	• Induction of oxidative stress and activation of apoptosis signalling pathway • Alteration of autophagy and impairment of Mitophagy	Aseptic meningitis, encephalitis, AFM, cognitive impairments in motor skills, problem-solving abilities, socialization, communication, neuronal development delay, ADHD, and epilepsy.
B	**JE**	Vector borne	Via olfactory bulb or the choroid plexus	• Induction of oxidative stress and activation of apoptosis signalling pathway • Alteration of autophagy and impairment of Mitophagy • Dysregulation of Neuroinflammation • Dysregulation of Neurotransmitter • Protein misfold & aggregate	Encephalitis
C	**Dengue**	Vector borne	• Hematogenous spread • BBB • Through Dendritic cells and lymphatics	• Induction of oxidative stress and activation of apoptosis signalling pathway • Protein misfold & aggregate	encephalopathy, encephalitis, and other CNS implications to peripheral neuromuscular issues
D	**Zika**	Vector borne	• Hematogenous spread • BBB • Through Dendritic cells and lymphatics	• Induction of oxidative stress and activation of apoptosis signalling pathway • Disrupts neuronal metabolism	encephalopathy, encephalitis, meningitis, myelitis, and seizures
E	**WNV**	Vector borne	Via olfactory bulb or the choroid plexus	• Induction of oxidative stress and activation of apoptosis signalling pathway • Protein misfold & aggregate	Encephalitis
F	**Mumps**	• Respiratory tract • Direct contact	• Via olfactory bulb or the choroid plexus • Through infected lymphocytes	• Disrupts neuronal metabolism	Meningitis, Encephalitis

continued on following page

Table 1. Continued

	Neurotropic viruses	Portal of entry in host	Entry in CNS	Mechanisms of neuropathology	Clinical presentation
G	**Measles**	Respiratory tract	Passive transport through infected lymphocytes	• Disrupts neuronal metabolism	acute disseminated encephalomyelitis (ADEM), measles inclusion body encephalitis (MIBE), and subacute sclerosing panencephalitis (SSPE)
H	**Nipah & Hendra**	Direct contact	• BBB • Via olfactory bulb	• Disrupts neuronal metabolism	aseptic meningitis, diffuse encephalitis, and focal brainstem involvement
I	**HSV**	• Oral mucosa/skin • Genitourinary tract	• BBB • Via olfactory bulb and Trigeminal nerve	• Induction of oxidative stress and activation of apoptosis signalling pathway • Alzheimer's disease pathological hallmark	Aseptic meningitis, acute encephalitis, and cognitive impairment.
J	**VZV**	• Respiratory tract • Direct contact	Via infected T Cells	• Alzheimer's disease pathological hallmark	segmental motor weakness, myelitis, cranial nerve syndromes, Guillain–Barre syndrome, meningoencephalitis, and zoster sine herpete
K	**EBV**	• Epithelial cells of oropharynx • Epithelial cells of cervix	BBB	• Dysregulation of Neuroinflammation	Aseptic meningitis, encephalitis, transverse myelitis, cerebellitis, ataxia, Guillian–Barré syndrome, Alzheimer's Disease, and Parkinson's disease.
L	**CMV**	• Direct contact • Transfusion/organ transplant • Transplacental	BBB	• Dysregulation of Neuroinflammation	Aseptic meningitis, polyradiculopathy, myelitis, ventriculitis, dementia, cranial nerve involvement, microcephaly, periventricular calcifications, convulsions, spastic tetraplegia, and hydrocephalus suppress the development of neural stem cells.

continued on following page

Table 1. Continued

	Neurotropic viruses	Portal of entry in host	Entry in CNS	Mechanisms of neuropathology	Clinical presentation
M	**SARS CoV 2**	Respiratory tract	• BBB • Via Cranial nerves	• Disrupts neuronal metabolism • Protein misfold & aggregate	Encephalitis, encephalopathy, seizures, epilepsy, and Alzheimer's Disease.
N	**Influenza**	Respiratory tract	• BBB • Via Cranial nerves	• Induction of oxidative stress and activation of apoptosis signalling pathway	febrile seizures, encephalopathy, encephalitis, Reye's-like syndrome, acute disseminated encephalomyelitis, and acute necrotizing encephalitis (ANE)
O	**Adeno virus**	Respiratory tract	• BBB Via olfactory bulb	• Induction of oxidative stress and activation of apoptosis signalling pathway	Aseptic meningitis convulsions, encephalitis, and acute disseminated encephalomyelitis.

Chapter 6
Parasitic and Fungal Infections of the CNS:
Insights Into Pathogens, Diagnosis, Treatment, and Future Prospects

Sonam Yadav
https://orcid.org/0000-0002-6440-4675
Indian Pharmacopoeia Commission, Ministry of Health and Family Welfare, Government of India, Ghaziabad, India

Tabish Qidwai
Shri Ramswaroop Memorial University, Lucknow, India

ABSTRACT

Central nervous system (CNS) infections involve the brain, spinal cord, optic nerves, and their protective membranes. These infections are medical emergencies with high morbidity, mortality, and potential long-term complications that significantly affect quality of life. Parasitic infections are common in regions with poor sanitation but can also occur in non-endemic areas due to international travel and immunosuppression from Human Immunodeficiency Virus (HIV) or post-transplant medications. Fungal and parasitic CNS infections present with diverse clinical symptoms and are often associated with high mortality in resource-limited settings. Survivors frequently suffer from neurological complications such as motor and sensory deficits, cognitive impairment, and seizures. Diagnosis can be challenging due to the complexity of parasite life cycles, geographic variations, and overlapping clinical features. This chapter reviews major parasitic and fungal pathogens affecting the CNS, highlighting their pathogenesis, diagnostic approaches, treatment strategies, recent developments, and key aspects of prevention and control.

DOI: 10.4018/979-8-3693-4070-7.ch006

INTRODUCTION

Numerous pathogens, including various bacteria, viruses, fungi, and parasites, have the capacity to infect the human central nervous system (CNS). Their primary targets of infection are the brain and spinal cord, and they can spread via the blood-brain barrier (BBB) or the blood-cerebrospinal fluid barrier (BCSFB) through a variety of molecular pathways (Güémez and García, 2021). Globally, parasitic infections that impact the CNS continue to be a significant cause of illness and mortality. Millions of children and adults in low- and middle-income countries suffer from the neurological, cognitive, and mental health issues caused by these parasitic infections; however, owing to increased international travel and immunosuppression caused by Human Immunodeficiency Virus (HIV) infection or post-transplantation therapy, sporadic cases also occur in nonendemic areas (Snydman et al., 2006). An organism that feeds on the host while living on or inside another organism of a different species (spp.) is called a parasite. Many parasites spp. live in typical vertebrates, and parasites may not necessarily cause harm to their host. Many parasites spp. have the ability to infiltrate the human neurological system, and in certain situations, this infiltration can result in a substantial burden of morbidity and mortality (Garcia, 2021).

The prevalence of invasive fungal diseases has increased, making them a global issue. To promote worldwide awareness and response to fungal infections, the World Health Organization (WHO) created the first list of fungal priority pathogens in 2022. Our understanding of fungal infections and their diversity has improved owing to the development of advanced genetic and molecular techniques, but our capacity to precisely diagnose and calculate the actual burden of these illnesses is still hampered by a lack of readily available, high-quality diagnostic techniques. The increase in the number of immunocompromised people is one of the major contributing factors to the increased incidence of fungal infections, along with a number of other factors. Life expectancy has increased and improved for those with autoimmune illnesses, HIV, solid or stem cell transplants, cancer, and intrusive devices with advancements in medical therapies. However, these developments have also made these people more vulnerable to serious fungal infections. The role of fungi in CNS illnesses is becoming more widely acknowledged. High death rates are a result of their propensity to affect the most susceptible people, diagnostic difficulties, and a lack of effective treatments (Lino et al., 2024).

Particularly in low- and middle-income nations, parasitic diseases that affect the CNS pose serious risks. Various unicellular and multicellular organisms, including worms and protozoa, are the causative agents. In some situations, certain parasitic agents are extremely feared, such as cerebral malaria in tourists returning from endemic areas with fever and any neurological symptoms, or cerebral toxoplasmosis in HIV-positive patients. Patients with nonspecific symptoms, such as meningitis, encephalitis, ventriculitis, myelitis, or brain abscess, with fever and headaches as the main complaints, may be suspected of having parasitic infections of the CNS. The location and size of the lesions determine the clinical presentation, but different parasites can cause the same symptoms, making diagnosis difficult. Despite being endemic in tropical nations, several CNS parasitic infections are currently spreading throughout the world as a result of international migration and travel (Coyle, 2021).

Commonly opportunistic, fungal infections of the CNS arise from hematogenous dissemination in immunocompromised hosts. Immunocompetent people, however, are increasingly being mentioned as potential hosts for these infections. Fungal infections frequently result from the direct inoculation of fungal spores, such as during surgery or trauma. Crucially, the pathophysiology of CNS lesions is influenced by fungal morphology. The main causes of meningitis (dimorphic fungi) or meningoencephalitis (Cryptococcus and Candida spp.) are fungi that grow as budding yeasts in vivo. *Candida albicans* (*C. albicans*) and other yeast-to-hyphae transition-exhibiting spp. can be more invasive, resulting in brain abscesses and necrosis. Filamentous fungi, which produce large hyphae, are prone to macrovascular invasion, which can result in cerebral abscesses, aneurysms, and hemorrhagic stroke. Candidiasis is the most prevalent nosocomial infection, whereas cryptococcal meningoencephalitis is the most common fungal infection of the CNS. Additionally, cerebral phaeohyphomycoses primarily affect individuals with intact immune systems, AND aspergillosis and mucormycosis are relatively uncommon but extremely harmful in immunocompromised patients (Le Govic et al., 2022).

This book chapter aims to provide an overview of parasitic and fungal pathogens, such as Candida spp., Toxoplasma spp., Paragonimus spp., Plasmodium spp., Histoplasma spp., and Blastomyces spp. and so on, that can cause CNS infections and may soon emerge as emerging pathogens. There has also been a discussion of the pathogenesis, diagnosis, treatment, and prospects for the future. Figure 5.1 shows a graphical representation of parasitic and fungal infections of the CNS.

Figure 1. Graphical representation of Parasites and Fungi infecting the CNS

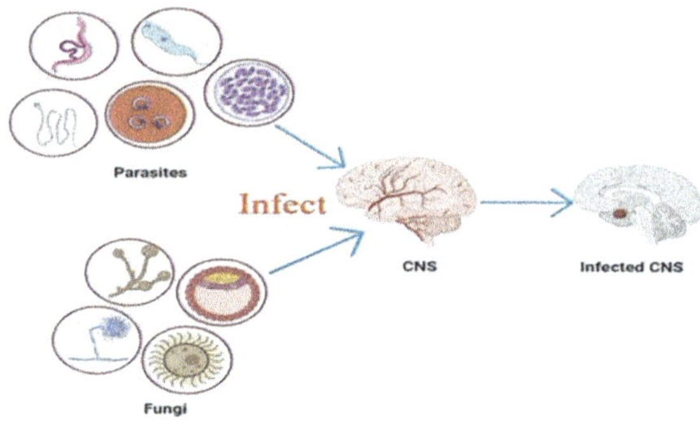

PARASITIC DISEASES OF THE CNS

Cysticercosis

The larvae of the cestode *Taenia solium* (*T. solium*) is caused by the prevalent debilitating disease known as human cysticercosis. According to antiquated conservative estimate, up to 50 million people worldwide may have cysticercosis. In Sub-Saharan Africa, India, Asia, and Central and South America, it is especially prevalent in rural or peri-urban settings. The adult life stage of the cestode *T. solium* is exclusively found in humans (Sylvia Van Belle et al., 2021). Cysticercosis frequently affects muscle tissue, the eye, and the CNS. The brain parenchyma, ventricles (20–25%), or subarachnoid space (2%–3%) are frequently affected. The parenchymal type of this parasite is primarily observed in the corticomedullary junction. One patient may have lesions in multiple phases of the disease at the same time, and multiple anatomic sites are frequently involved (Razek et al., 2011). When humans accidentally become intermediate hosts after ingesting the eggs in an infected host's feces, cysticercosis results. After being exposed to gastric acid, the eggs transform into L1s, move across the intestinal epithelium, and settle in a variety of tissues, with a strong preference for the CNS. This leads to a condition known as neurocysticercosis (NCC). Recurrent seizures are the primary sign of human cysticercosis (Sylvia Van Belle et al., 2021).

Seizures are the most prevalent symptom, occurring in approximately 70% of cases and varying in intensity and type. Frequent headaches are caused by inflammation or elevated pressure. Depending on where the cysticerci are located, neurological deficiencies may present as weakness, sensory abnormalities, visual disturbances, aphasia, or cranial nerve palsies. Possible symptoms include depression, psychosis, personality changes, memory problems, and cognitive impairment. Hydrocephalus, which is characterized by headaches, vomiting, papilledema, and altered mental status, can result from cysticerci obstructing the flow of cerebrospinal fluid. A diagnosis can be difficult because symptoms can overlap with other neurological conditions and the presentation varies from person to person (Garcia et al., 2014, Zammarchi et al., 2017).

Toxoplasmosis

The intracellular parasitic protist *Toxoplasma gondii* (*T. gondii*) is the cause of toxoplasmosis, a common human illness that can develop into more severe forms in immunocompromised people or during pregnancy (Sanchez et al., 2023). In the majority of hosts, *T. gondii* causes a latent infection that lasts a lifetime in tissues such as cardiac muscle, skeletal muscle, or the CNS, which consists of the brain, spinal cord, and retina. The main ways in which humans contract *T. gondii* are through vertical transmission or contaminated food or water. *T. gondii* is globally widespread, with seroprevalence rates varying significantly, ranging from under 10% to over 60%. *T. gondii* spreads throughout the host during an acute infection as a tachyzoite, the parasite's fast-replicating form that the host immune system targets. As the infection worsens, *T. gondii* changes into a slowly replicating bradyzoite, which encysts, and enters the chronic stage of infection. Tachyzoites and bradyzoites undergo a variety of changes, some of which are believed to allow bradyzoites to evade immune recognition and cause chronic infection. The brain is the primary organ involved in persistence and encystment in both humans and rodents (Mendez and Koshy, 2017).

There is some disagreement about Toxoplasma neurotropism or whether its affinity for the CNS is greater than or different from that of other organs, although Toxoplasma clearly causes pathology in the CNS and is frequently portrayed as a neurotropic parasite. Although *T. gondii* spreads widely during acute infection, the mouse CNS actually has significantly lower parasite loads than other organs do. As a result, Toxoplasma is hardly a pathogen that is primarily neurotropic and has a greater affinity for the CNS than for other organs. Nevertheless, the parasite circumvents BBB restriction to create infection, which appears to be typical for infections in humans and rodents (Schlüter and Barragan, 2019). Immunocompromised people are susceptible to CNS toxoplasmosis, which necessitates prompt diagnosis and treatment to avoid serious neurological consequences. In addition to serological testing and cerebrospinal fluid (CSF) analysis for antibody and deoxyribonucleic acid (DNA) detection, the diagnosis includes neuroimaging, which reveals distinctive ring-enhancing lesions on magnetic resonance imaging (MRI) (Q. Liu et al., 2015).

Echinococcosis

Human echinococcosis is caused by infection of the larval stages of the taeniid cestodes belonging to the genus Echinococcus. *Echinococcus granulosus* (*E. granulosus*), which causes cystic echinococcosis; *Echinococcus multilocularis* (*E. multilocularis*), which causes alveolar echinococcosis; and *Echinococcus vogeli (E. vogeli)* and *Echinococcus oligarthrus* (*E. oligarthrus*), which cause polycystic echinococcosis, are the four spp. that are of public health concern out of the six that have been identified (Moro and Schantz, 2009). The majority of human infections are caused by *E. granulosus* and *E. multilocularis*, two of the four spp. Slowly growing solitary brain cysts are a common feature of CNS disease. The patient may continue to have no symptoms, depending on the size and location of the cyst. However, as the size of the CNS lesion increases, symptoms such as headache, nausea, vomiting, seizures, hemiparesis, dysarthria, and cranial nerve palsies may develop as a result of the lesion's local effects or as a result of elevated intracranial pressure (ICP) (Archibald and Quisling, 2013).

Through the oral route, *E. granulosus* infects humans by releasing oncospheres from ingested eggs that pass through the intestinal wall and enter different organs, mainly the liver and lungs. Oncospheres rarely may enter the bloodstream and travel to the CNS, where they may cause cysts to form in the spine or surrounding tissues. In an effort to contain the infection, the host immune system frequently produces fibrous encapsulation in response to the growing cysts (Jacquier and Piroth, 2018, Imperato et al., 2016). Although their potential for zoonotic transmission is unknown, two new spp. have recently been identified: *Echinococcus felidis* (*E. felidis*) in African lions and *Echinococcus shiquicus* (*E. shiquicus*) in small mammals from the Tibetan Plateau. These illnesses can be considered emerging or re-emerging diseases, according to numerous studies, and they are becoming a greater public health concern (Moro and Schantz, 2009).

Schistosomiasis

Bilharziasis, another name for schistosomiasis, is a parasitic disease that can infect both people and animals. Schistosoma trematode worms are the cause, and they can infect humans with both acute and chronic illnesses (Ekloh et al., 2024). Humans are the definitive hosts of five major schistosome spp.: In Africa and the Middle East, *Schistosomiasis haematobium* (*S. haematobium*) is found; in Africa, the Middle East, South America, and the Caribbean, *Schistosomiasis mansoni* (*S. mansoni*) is found; in Japan, China, Indonesia, and the Philippines, *Schistosomiasis japonicum* (*S. japonicum*) is found; in Southeast Asia, *Schistosomiasis mekongi* (*S. mekongi*) is found; and in West and Central Africa, *Schistosomiasis intercalatum*

(*S. intercalatum*) is found (Hughes and Biggs, 2002). Schistosomiasis transmission is influenced primarily by specific environmental factors that impact intermediate hosts. The proximity of people to bodies of water (dams, irrigation projects) and specific socioeconomic factors (poverty, migration, climate change) are the primary causes of schistosomiasis transmission (Ekloh et al., 2024).

The life cycles of all human schistosomes are comparable. There are distinct sexes in the parasite. The male worm's gynecophoric channel is occupied by the longer, thinner female worm. The freshwater snail serves as the intermediate host for the asexual cycle, whereas humans are the primary host for the sexual cycle. Schistosome spp. can be spread only by specific snail spp. that are members of the genus Biomphalaria (*S. mansoni*), Bulinus (*S. haematobium*), or Oncomelania (*S. japonicum*). Each of the many eggs the female produces contains a miracidium larva. Proteolytic enzymes secreted by ciliated miracidium larva aid in the migration of eggs to the intestine or bladder. Either urine or faeces are used to expel the eggs. Each egg releases a miracidium larva when it comes into contact with water. With the aid of cilia, the miracidium swims and locates a freshwater snail, which serves as its intermediate host. It then enters the snail and develops asexually into secondary larvae known as cercaria. When snails are stimulated by light, hundreds of these cercarial larvae are released. With the embryonic characteristics of an adult worm, cercarial larvae have a large head and a bifurcated tail. When these larvae come into contact with human skin, they whirl around in the water and pierce the dermis. They lose their tail as they pierce the human skin and move through the bloodstream to the heart, lungs, liver, and portal vein, where they develop over the course of several weeks. The cycle restarts when the adult worm's mate and move upstream to the mesenteric veins, their ultimate destination (Sah et al., 2015).

Paragonimiasis

The discovery of adult flatworms in the lungs of Lutra spp. in Brazil in 1850 was the first documented sight of Paragonimus. The most common spp. in China is *Paragonimus westermani (P. westermani)*, which is also the most widely distributed. Researchers have named eggs, metacercariae, and adults with larger triple chromosome *Paragonimus* and smaller double chromosome Paragonimus separately during the time when morphology observation was the main identification method (Zhou et al., 2021). Aquatic snails are the first intermediate host in the life cycle of Paragonimus *spp.* parasites, followed by freshwater decapod crustaceans as the second intermediate host and humans and other mammals as the definitive host. Eating raw or pickled freshwater crabs or crayfish that contain infectious forms known as metacercariae can infect humans. The consumption of untreated river or stream water is also thought to be a potential source of infection (Liu et al., 2024).

Cerebral Malaria (CM)

CM is caused by *Plasmodium falciparum* (*P. falciparum*). Clinical signs of CM, a severe form of malaria, include fever, coma, parasitemia, and other symptoms. The mortality rate for CM is approximately 25–35%, with nearly 90% of deaths resulting from malarial complications (Shaikh et al., 2024). When a person infected with *P. falciparum* is profoundly unconscious and has no other explanation for their coma, it is clinically diagnosed. It affects people who have not developed a specific immunity to *P. falciparum*, and children in sub-Saharan Africa bear the majority of the burden. Systemic endothelial activation, patchy endothelial damage, low platelet counts, decreased anticoagulant levels, and the production of procoagulant microparticles and activated thrombin are linked to *P. falciparum* infection. The adherence of *P. falciparum*-infected erythrocytes (PfIE) in cerebral vessels is a noticeable pathological characteristic (Moxon et al., 2009).

The pathophysiology of CM has been linked in part to disruptions in the brain's microcirculation. Plasmodium falciparum erythrocyte membrane protein 1 (PfEMP1), a particular cell-surface ligand expressed by infected red blood cells (iRBCs), binds to the brain endothelium to cause *P. falciparum*-infected RBCs (PfRBCs) to adhere to it through a process called sequestration. Since there is currently no evidence that PfRBCs enter the brain parenchyma, it is likely that iRBCs remain in the vascular space after being sequestered. Numerous downstream vascular effects, such as increased vasoconstriction, decreased cerebral blood flow, vascular obstruction, and disruption of BBB integrity, are caused by PfRBC sequestration (Shikani et al., 2012).

Chagas Disease

The flagellate parasite that causes Chagas disease, *Trypanosoma cruzi* (*T. cruzi*), is a protozoan that is highly significant in Latin America (Buscaglia, 2003). The presence of the parasite in the CNS during the acute phase or as a result of reactivation during chronic disease is one of the complications of Chagas disease. Immunocompromised patients are more likely to experience this reactivation. The mortality rate for CNS Chagas disease varies according to the stage of the disease; it is approximately 10% during acute illness and 79–100% during reactivation. Confusion, headache, hypertonia, convulsions, meningismus, focal neurological deficits, fever, and altered mental status are typical clinical signs and symptoms observed in patients with cerebral Chagas (Shelton and Gonzalez, 2023).

Evasion from both peripheral and intra-CNS immune responses is necessary for successful spread from a point of entry to the CNS, either by breaching or rupturing the BCSFB or BBB. Tight junctions, which are especially noticeable in the BBB, allow macromolecules and hydrophilic molecules to selectively pass through the

BBB and BCSFB. Furthermore, compared with parenchymal vessels, leptomeningeal vessels and CNS areas that contain BCSFB (such as the choroid plexus and brain circumventricular organs) are more permeable. Furthermore, the meninges have a more robust immune response than the brain parenchyma. Additionally, astrocyte-released cytokines and chemokines, which trigger the expression of brain endothelial cell (BEC) adhesion molecules in response to infection, facilitate the increased passage of circulating immune cells, such as monocytes, T cells, and macrophages, through BECs when activated (Useche et al., 2022). Depending on the type and stage of infection, trypanosomiasis has a different pathophysiology in the CNS. *Trypanosoma brucei (T. brucei)* spp., the parasites that cause human african trypanosomiasis (HAT), go through a complicated life cycle in the tsetse fly vector, where they proliferate and mature into epimastigotes in the salivary glands. During a tsetse fly bite, these forms are injected into the human bloodstream, where they quickly divide via binary fission and differentiate into trypomastigotes (Papagni et al., 2023). Table 5.1 summarizes the parasitic diseases affecting the CNS.

Table 1. Major Parasitic Diseases and their Epidemiological Characteristics

Parasitic Diseases	Cysticercosis	Toxoplasmosis	Echinococcosis	Schistosomiasis	Paragonimiasis	Malaria	Chagas disease
Causative organism	*T. solium*	*T. gondii*	*E. granulosus, E. multilocularis*	*S. japonicum, mansoni, haematobium*	*P. westermani*	*P. falciparum*	*T. cruzi*
Vector/ intermediate host	Pigs, humans	Cats, intermediate hosts in nature (birds & rodents)	Sheep, goats, cattle, pigs, yaks or other farm animals. Small mammals (rodents and lagomorphs)	Fresh water snail	Fresh water snails, crustacean-eating mammals	Vector borne, Anopheles mosquito	Triatomine bug
Mode of transmission	Fecal–oral, ingestion of eggs from human feces	Ingestion of oocysts (cat feces) or tissue cysts, blood transfusion.	Ingestion of contaminated soil, water or food, contact with infected animals	Penetration of skin by cercariae in freshwater	Fecal–oral, raw, undercooked freshwater crustaceans	Insect bite	Insect bite
Endemic regions	Rural areas with poor sanitation, and Latin America, Africa and Asia.	Worldwide, greatest burden in SubSaharan Africa.	Middle East, Europe, Pacific, Latin America; North America	Tropical and subtropical areas of SubSaharan Africa, Latin America and Asia.	East and Southeast Asia, West and Central Africa, Central and South America.	Tropics from Sub-Saharan Africa, Latin America, Asia and Oceania.	Latin America.

PATHOGENESIS OF PARASITIC INFECTIONS OF THE CNS

Hematogenic spread is the main way that infectious organisms enter the CNS. Viruses typically enter the bloodstream after first colonizing the body's mucosal surfaces, where they often multiply at extra neural sites before passing through the blood-brain barrier (BBB) and entering the CNS. Depending on the virus, CNS entry may occur via the choroid plexus, through infection of cerebral microvascular endothelial cells, direct passage through cerebral capillary endothelial cells, or via infected leukocytes via a "Trojan horse" mechanism. Additionally, some viruses may reach the CNS directly through peripheral nerves or the olfactory nerve. The mode of CNS entry significantly influences the pattern of viral spread within the central nervous system.

Similarly, bacterial infections of the CNS typically begin with mucosal colonization in the nasopharynx, facilitated by bacterial surface traits that promote adhesion and persistence. After gaining access to the bloodstream, bacteria must resist host defenses, which they achieve primarily through polysaccharide capsules that inhibit complement-mediated lysis and neutrophil phagocytosis. Sustained bacteraemia is believed to contribute to the penetration of bacteria into the subarachnoid space. Once there, local immune responses are insufficient to contain the infection. As a result, a vigorous inflammatory response is triggered, contributing significantly to the morbidity and mortality associated with bacterial meningitis. This inflammatory cascade increases BBB permeability, leading to cerebral edema—which may be vasogenic, cytotoxic, or interstitial in nature elevates intracranial pressure and potentially fatal brain herniation. In addition, the resulting reduction in cerebral blood flow causes relative anoxia and subsequent neuronal damage.

Infections may also reach the CNS via septic emboli originating from distant sites (such as an infected heart valve) or by contiguous spread from adjacent structures in cases of otitis, sinusitis, mastoiditis, or septic phlebitis. Furthermore, in certain viral and mycoplasmal infections—as well as postvaccination—an immune response may be triggered not only against the infectious agent but also against myelin basic protein. This autoimmune process may lead to peripheral nerve dysfunction through demyelination of peripheral nerves and nerve roots or acute disseminated encephalomyelitis (ADEM) when CNS myelin is affected (Marko Pokorn, 2004).

FUNGAL DISEASES OF THE CNS

Neurocandidiasis

In addition to being a beneficial fungus for human skin and mucous membranes, *C. albicans* causes both systemic and local infections. Systemic candidiasis is a bloodstream infection that affects the CNS. Preterm and full-term babies are more likely than children or adults to have this pathogen moving to the CNS. CNS fungal invasion is present in 50% of neonatal patients with systemic candidiasis and is linked to a 70% mortality rate. Meningitis, meningoencephalitis, brain abscess, and ventriculitis are the clinical manifestations of neurocandidiasis. During necropsy, brain abscesses have been discovered in the cerebral cortex, basal ganglia, cerebellum, and other brain regions. They are characterized by fungal invasion into the brain parenchyma encircled by inflammatory cells (Flores-Maldonado et al., 2023).

Since the hyphal-expressed protein Amyotrophic lateral sclerosis-3 (Als3) has been demonstrated to mediate brain infection by this fungus and to attach to brain endothelial cells that constitute the BBB, it was previously believed that hyphae are necessary for *C. albicans* to penetrate the CNS by invading and disrupting the BBB. (Fu et al., 2023). Particularly vulnerable to candidiasis are immunocompromised individuals, those with neutropenia, diabetes, acquired immune deficiency syndrome (AIDS), or significant wounds (burns and surgeries), preterm newborns, transplant recipients, and those who have undergone catheterization. Lung, pulmonary, and digestive tract infections can be caused by disseminated candidiasis. Fungemia is a hallmark of the disseminated type that can occur in patients with a markedly compromised immune system. CNS involvement is typically observed in people who have undergone neurological surgery or who develop disseminated candidiasis. The development of a biofilm, which shields yeast cells from microglial activity (phagocytosis, cytokines), is a distinctive trait of *Candida* spp. Undiagnosed neuroinfection is thought to affect 6% of individuals with disseminated candidiasis (Góralska et al., 2018).

Histoplasmosis

CNS histoplasmosis can result from an infection with *Histoplasma capsulatum* (*H. capsulatum*), especially in areas where the disease is endemic. This infection highlights the substantial influence of fungal pathogens on brain health by causing neuroinflammation and cognitive impairment (Nanda et al., 2024). The clinical appearance may be entirely asymptomatic (for example, incidental mediastinal lymphadenopathy on a computed tomography (CT) scan during cancer staging) or it may spread through lymphatics and blood to cause severe disseminated disease. The number of fungal spores mostly determines symptoms, whereas the host's immunological status determines how much organ involvement occurs. Immunocompetent patients account for 70% of asymptomatic cases on average (Khalaf et al., 2022).

A systemic illness is caused by *H. capsulatum* when bird or guano feces are inhaled. Round, oval, 1–5 mm fungus that seems basophilic by hematoxylin and eosin (H&E) stains and has a translucent halo that stains when impregnated with Grocott silver Global occurrence A reservoir is a soil that has a large amount of nitrogen. AIDS patients and cancer patients have CNS diseases and other widespread diseases. When many infections do not cause any symptoms if left untreated, histoplasmosis is lethal (Deigendesch et al., 2017).

Blastomycosis

The thermally dimorphic fungus Blastomyces grows as a mold in the environment and transforms into yeast inside the organism. It consists of several spp. that typically live in soils close to waterways and have varying geographic distributions. *Blastomyces dermatitidis* (*B. dermatitidis*) is by far the most prevalent infection. Eighty-two cases of CNS blastomycosis were discovered in case reports and retrospective studies. The majority either failed to identify the spp. of Blastomyces or were caused by *B. dermatidis*. Meningitis, meningoencephalitis, ventriculitis, intracranial, epidural, and spinal cord mass lesions, or a combination of these can be symptoms of CNS blastomycosis. Even though CNS involvement is uncommon, the propensity of Blastomyces spp. for hematogenous dissemination makes them a plausible cause of CNS disease, especially considering their growing geographic range. Except for *Blastomyces helices (B. helices)*, which typically affect immunocompromised hosts, blastomycosis typically affects immunocompetent people (Lino et al., 2024).

The majority of the knowledge regarding the clinical, therapeutic, and diagnostic aspects of blastomycosis has been derived from *B. dermatidis* infections. The lungs are the main organs impacted by infection, which usually occurs via inhalation of conidia. Approximately 25 to 50% of *B. dermatidis* infections can spread outside the lungs, generally to the skin, bones, or genitourinary system. Except for *B. helicus*, which typically affects immunocompromised hosts, blastomycosis typically affects immunocompetent people (Schwartz and Kauffman, 2020).

Coccidioidomycosis

Valley fever, or coccidioidomycosis, is an ailment caused by the inhalation of airborne arthroconidia from the soil-dwelling fungus Coccidioides spp. Despite being regarded as an uncommon disease, environmental mycosis is becoming a greater public health concern because of an increase in cases and indications of its geographic spread (Williams and Chiller, 2022).

Californian *Coccidoides immitis (C. immitis)* infections and non-Californian *Coccidoides posadasii (C. posadasii)* infections mostly attack the lungs and only rarely move to the CNS. The fungus creates spherules that range in size from 20 to 100 mm. occurs in South America, Mexico, and the southwestern United States (US). Dry, sandy soil makes up the reservoir. Inhalation is the method of transmission. In the US, there are 150,000 new infections annually; in Mexico, the frequency ranges from 10% to 40%. occurs in people who are immunocompetent and infrequently in those who are immunocompromised. Periodic acid-Schiff (PAS) and Grocott stains emphasize immature forms, although mature spherules may exhibit little to no PAS-positivity (Deigendesch et al., 2017).

Paracoccidioidomycosis (PCM)

In Latin America, where an estimated 10 million people are affected, PCM is one of the most common endemic mycoses. It is contracted by inhaling fungal infection propagules while engaging in activities in rural locations, and it primarily affects male patients who are in their productive years. A small and unknown percentage of infected people may develop the disease throughout the course of their lives, while the majority of them remain asymptomatic. Since the public systems of most endemic countries do not report people with PCM, the incidence rate is unknown (Haran et al., 2024).

Conidia and/or mycelial pieces found in the soil might cause infection when inhaled. According to previous studies, the female hormone estrogen prevents infection from developing by preventing the change from a mycelial to a yeast-like form. There are two different types of this disease: the acute or juvenile form, which affects children of both sexes and can progress quickly, and the chronic or adult form, which affects men and has a longer latency period. The following ideas underpin the development of the illness and the spread of the fungus in PCM: However, specific immunity against *Paracoccidioides brasiliensis* (*P. brasiliensis*) antigens are lacking and can be influenced by other antigens. PCM is a mycosis that affects healthy people (thus, it occurs without the use of immunosuppressive medications or illnesses) (Lauana Aparecida Santos et al., 2020).

Sporotrichosis

People who live in tropical and subtropical areas are particularly susceptible to sporotrichosis, a mycosis caused by fungus that are found around the world and are members of the Sporothrix genus. As a sapronotic infection, this dimorphic fungus can infect humans through soil and plants, which is why they are called "rose gardener's disease." In Southeast Brazil in particular, zoonotic transmission occurs, especially by cats. Sporotrichosis usually manifests as cutaneous or cutaneous-lymphatic, and more than 95% of cases take this form (Bonifaz and Tirado-Sánchez, 2017). The majority of CNS sporotrichosis case series exclusively include people who have underlying immunosuppression, primarily HIV infection.

CNS sporotrichosis may appear as a secondary cause of broad dispersion or as a single, isolated case of chronic meningitis. Although it is uncommon, isolated CNS involvement usually occurs in immunocompetent patients. Since CNS invasion frequently occurs via hematogenous dissemination, the majority of individuals with CNS involvement also have concurrent cutaneous disease. Lumbar puncture was performed on 53 individuals with disseminated sporotrichosis during a 1999–2020 investigation conducted at a Brazilian reference facility. Seventeen patients (32%) received a meningitis diagnosis. Every patient had a concurrent skin illness. HIV infection was the most common comorbidity among the 17 meningitis patients (88%), followed by prolonged steroid usage (6%) and drinking (6%) (Lima et al., 2022).

Cryptococcus

The fungus most frequently linked to CNS illnesses is Cryptococcus spp. With a global distribution, *Cryptococcus neoformans* (*C. neoformans*) is frequently discovered in soil that has been tainted by bird droppings. Both *C. neoformans* var neoformans and *C. neoformans* var gattii are types of bacteria. The ecology, natural distribution, epidemiology, presentation, clinical course, and treatment of these two spp. are different. While *C. neoformans* var gattii is more frequently found in Southeast Asia, Africa, Australia, and some regions of southern California, *C. neoformans* var neoformans is widespread globally and causes the majority of infections in individuals in the U.S.

Inhalation causes the first infection with Cryptococcus spp., which results in pneumonitis, which is typically asymptomatic even in patients with compromised immune systems. Patients with symptoms typically have fever, cough, and a range of radiographic abnormalities on their chest, including lobar infiltrates and nodular, pleural-based lesions. Even in immunocompromised patients, the first pneumonia usually goes away on its own. Many organs in the body become seeded as a result of pneumonitis dissemination, with the CNS being especially susceptible (Archibald and Quisling, 2013). The most prevalent opportunistic invasive infection in people with HIV is cerebral cryptococcosis. The polysaccharide moieties in the Cryptococcus cell wall, such as melanin, glucuronoxylomannan and glucuronoxylomannogalactan, decrease the activity of oxidative bursts and normal macrophages, respectively (Pathakumari et al., 2020).

Meningitis, which affects up to 40% of patients and is thought to be an indicator disease in the development of fulminant AIDS, is one of the most prevalent types of CNS cryptococcosis. Currently, patients with AIDS who have cryptococcal meningitis have a high mortality rate (between 15% and 39%). Globally, there were approximately 223,100 cases of cryptococcal meningitis among HIV/AIDS patients in 2014: 162,500 in sub-Saharan Africa, 43,200 in the Asia-Pacific region, 5300 in Latin America, 4400 in Europe, 3300 in North Africa and the Middle East, 3000 in North America, and 1400 in the Caribbean. Globally, the incidence of cryptococcal meningitis is 181,100 individuals annually, with sub-Saharan Africa accounting for 75.04% of these deaths (Rajasingham et al., 2017). Following arrest in the brain capillaries, *C. neoformans* transmigrates across the BBB into the brain parenchyma. Research has demonstrated that *C. neoformans* can be directly transcytosed through the endothelium of the brain via in vitro methods. Interactions between cryptococcal hyaluronic acids and endothelium-expressed cell surface adhesion receptor (CD44) induce transcytosis (Shi and Mody, 2016). Table 5.2 summarizes the fungal diseases of the CNS.

Table 2. Major Fungal Diseases and their Epidemiological Characteristics

Fungal Diseases	Neurocandidiasis	Histoplasmosis	Blastomycosis	Coccidioidomycosis	PCM	Sporotrichosis	Cryptococcus
Causative organism	*C. albicans*	*H. capsulatum*	*B. dermatitidis*	*C. immitis*	*P. brasiliensis*	*S.schenckii*	*C. neoformans, C. neoformans gattii*
Vector/ intermediate host	Endogenously, contagion	Sail, chicken, bird, and bat excreta.	Soil, decaying wood, dogs, inhalation	Contaminated soil, rodents, inhalation	Vegetation, soil inhalation	Soil and plant inhalation	Soil, wood, bird excreta, juices, milk.
Mode of transmission	Oroesophageal region, vagina	Lungs, reticuloendothelial system	lungs	lungs	lungs	Musculoskeletal tissue, mucosa, viscera.	lungs
Endemic regions	Worldwide	Worldwide; Central & eastern US	North America, Africa	Southwest US, Mexico, South America	South and Central America	Central and South America, US, Japan.	Worldwide; frequent in Europe.

PATHOGENESIS OF FUNGAL INFECTIONS OF THE CNS

Fungi thrive in environments that are rich in water and organic material. Fungal enzymes break down organic matter proteins, carbohydrates, and other macromolecules into smaller molecules that they may readily consume to sustain their life processes. Certain fungi, particularly in immunocompromised individuals, can become opportunistic pathogens and invade various organs, including the central nervous system (CNS), leading to distinct clinical syndromes depending on the fungal species involved.

The CNS is typically thought of as an immunologically favorable location. In addition to the brain's unique, comparatively impermeable blood-brain barrier (BBB), the subarachnoid areas around it have strong meningeal barriers. These highly vascularized tissues provide effective defenses against fungal diseases. In healthy individuals, activated T-lymphocytes are typically allowed to cross the BBB for immunological monitoring. However, common (opportunistic or pathogenic) fungi can readily overcome these anatomical and functional barriers to create clinical symptoms in immunocompromised situations.

For example, *C. neoformans* is one of the most common fungal pathogens affecting the CNS. It causes cryptococcal meningitis, a life-threatening condition predominantly observed in individuals with advanced HIV/AIDS or other immunosuppressive conditions. Aspergillus species can lead to cerebral aspergillosis, often presenting as brain abscesses, especially in neutropenic patients. Candida species, although more commonly associated with systemic candidiasis, may also cause Candida meningitis or encephalitis, particularly in neonates or those undergoing neurosurgical procedures. Histoplasma capsulatum and Coccidioides immitis can also disseminate to the CNS, where they can cause chronic meningitis or granulomatous lesions, especially in endemic regions. Additionally, Mucorales species (causing mucormycosis) may invade the CNS via the paranasal sinuses, particularly in patients with uncontrolled diabetes mellitus or haematological malignancies.

Like bacterial infections, fungal infections in the CNS can cause humoral and cellular reactions that may help the host eradicate the infection. The immunopathogenesis of CNS fungal infections may be partially explained by the relative expression of cytokines and chemokines that enhance and repress the immune system, as well as the activation of resident brain cells by fungi. Major histocompatibility complex (MHC) class I and class II molecules are expressed by activated resident brain cells, including microglia, astrocytes, and endothelial cells, which function as antigen-presenting cells. They also generate cytokines, chemokines, and compounds with antifungal properties such as nitric oxide (NO), and express complement receptors. They also have the ability to phagocytose. As antigen-presenting cells, microglia promote T-cell growth and cytokine release, which in turn encourages these cells to consume and more efficiently eliminate invasive fungus. As an essential part of the innate immune system, the complement (C) system is crucial for the host's defense against infections. It also has a strong propensity to start inflammation, which, if left unchecked, can cause pathological alterations and severe tissue damage. It is widely acknowledged that the C system plays a crucial role in mediating fungal cytolysis. Additionally, activated microglial cell expression of C-receptors plays a crucial role in mediating phagocytosis.

It is unclear how human CNS fungal infections are immunopathogenic. Understanding the pathophysiology, pathogenicity, and immunological response of the host defense against the majority of fungal diseases can be improved by investigating their genetic sequences. Our knowledge of CNS mycoses will improve with more research in these fields (Raman Sharma, 2010).

DIAGNOSIS AND TREATMENT

Treatment options for CNS parasitic infections are varied and include both medicinal and surgical interventions. Pharmacotherapy to eradicate the parasite and supplementary care to avoid or treat complications resulting from parasite invasion are common components of medical treatment (e.g., anticonvulsants for patients presenting with seizures). Similarly, surgical intervention may be required to treat parasite-related complications (e.g., hydrocephalus) or for the direct removal of parasitic lesions, such as CNS cysts.

According to recent clinical guidelines, such as those of the Infectious Diseases Society of America (IDSA) and the WHO, early and accurate identification of microbial pathogens is essential to guide timely clinical response. The conventional methods used in clinical microbiology laboratories include direct microscopic examination, culture techniques, and antigen/antibody detection assays.

For fungal identification, techniques utilizing optical brighteners (e.g., Calcofluor or Blankophor) offer high sensitivity and specificity. For neuroinfection diagnostics, biopsy material stained with H&E, as well as PAS or Gomori methenamine silver (GMS), remains essential. Guidelines also recommend confirmatory culture and serological testing of both blood and CSF whenever possible. Czapek-Dox and Sabouraud media are commonly employed, although their effectiveness varies by the etiological agent. For example, in *Candida* spp. infections, peripheral blood cultures are often the most effective diagnostic method.

Serological testing, including enzyme-linked immunosorbent assay (ELISA), enzyme immunoassay (EIA), and indirect hemagglutination, remains foundational. Notably, immunofluorescence techniques have significantly advanced and are recommended for their improved specificity and sensitivity (Góralska et al., 2018).

For most fungal and parasitic CNS infections, the current WHO and Centers for Disease Control and Prevention (CDC) guidelines recommend targeted antifungal and antiparasitic agents. However, treatment must be tailored—some antiparasitic medications may provoke harmful inflammatory responses or be ineffective if the parasite is already dead (e.g., calcified neurocysticercosis). Surgical approaches, such as echinococcosis, may be combined with perioperative antihelminthic therapy, as supported by consensus recommendations (Carpio et al., 2016).

As of the most recent updates, five major classes of antifungal agents recommended for clinical use: azoles, polyenes, echinocandins, allylamines, and pyrimidine analogs. The azole class, especially triazoles (fluconazole, voriconazole), is highlighted in the IDSA guidelines for its broad spectrum of activity against CNS fungal infections and good CSF penetration. Despite their widespread use, concerns remain regarding hepatotoxicity, drug interactions, and emerging resistance, particularly in Candida species.

The most recent antifungal class, echinocandins (e.g., caspofungin, anidulafungin and micafungin), has shown promise, especially in combination therapy for invasive candidiasis and aspergillosis, and is endorsed for certain high-risk cases. According to IDSA 2023 guidelines, echinocandins are also recommended for empiric treatment in immunocompromised patients and intensive care unit (ICU) settings.

Prophylactic antifungal therapy is now a standard recommendation for immunocompromised individuals (e.g., HIV/AIDS patients, transplant recipients, long-term ICU patients) using oral azoles, especially fluconazole. The guidelines emphasize initiating empirical amphotericin B when a fungal infection is suspected, with targeted therapy adjusted on the basis of diagnostic confirmation.

The recommended treatments include the following:

- **Aspergillosis:** Amphotericin B, voriconazole, posaconazole, caspofungin
- **Mucormycosis:** Amphotericin B
- **Candidiasis:** Triazole or Echinocandins
- **Cryptococcosis:** Amphotericin B + flucytosine, followed by fluconazole for maintenance therapy in AIDS patients (Raman Sharma, 2010).

Recent diagnostic advances have also improved clinical outcomes. Nucleic acid amplification techniques (e.g., PCR, RT-PCR) are now widely used in laboratories because of their high sensitivity and specificity. These are endorsed in the latest European Society of Clinical Microbiology and Infectious Diseases (ESCMID) and IDSA diagnostic protocols for rapid detection of CNS pathogens. RT-PCR, in particular, has proven useful not only for diagnosis but also for monitoring treatment efficacy in RNA-virus-related neuroinfections.

Recent studies also highlight that early RT-PCR for the diagnosis of viral CNS infections can significantly reduce hospital stays, avoid unnecessary antibiotic use, and limit the need for additional laboratory tests (He et al., 2016). Table 5.3 represents the methodologies for diagnosing parasitic and fungal infections of the CNS.

Table 3. Methodologies for Diagnosing Parasitic and Fungal Infections of the CNS

S. No.	Methodologies	Diagnosis
1.	**Culture method**	Identification at species level.
2.	**Microscopy**	Visualization of parasites and fungal structures; Analysis of shape, tracking of motion, and classification of microorganisms.
3.	**Histopathology**	Detection of tissues invasion by fungi; Detection of the host response or tissue necrosis.
4.	**Chromogenic media**	Detection in polymicrobial samples; Detection and identification at the species level.
5.	**Fluorescence in situ hybridization (FISH)**	Accurate identification of *Candida* spp. Infections.
6.	**Matrix-Assisted Laser Desorption Ionization-Time of Flight (MALDI-TOF) - Mass spectrometry**	Identification of the pathogen at the genus, spp. and strain levels.
7.	**Serological methods (1,3 β-D-glucan, galactomannan)**	Detection of relevant fungal pathogens.
8.	**Neuroimaging (CT scan and MRI)**	Monitor the progression of the infection.
9.	**PCR-based methods**	Allows species identification and intraspecies differentiation.
10.	**Pan-omics molecular assays**	Technology for pathogen detection and discovery.

Emerging Molecular Diagnostics in CNS Infections

Recent advances in molecular diagnostics have revolutionized the detection and management of CNS infections. These techniques offer superior sensitivity, specificity, and rapid turnaround times, greatly improving clinical decision-making and patient outcomes.

Next-Generation Sequencing (NGS)

NGS allows for unbiased, broad-spectrum pathogen detection from clinical samples and is especially useful in cases with atypical presentations or unknown etiologies. It enables:

- Simultaneous detection of bacteria, viruses, fungi, and parasites
- Identification of novel or rare pathogens
- Genomic characterization for antimicrobial resistance and strain typing

Utility: Particularly valuable in immunocompromised patients or when conventional tests are inconclusive.

MALDI-TOF mass spectrometry

MALDI-TOF is now widely used for the rapid identification of cultured organisms:

- Detecting pathogens on the basis of their unique protein fingerprints
- Delivers results within minutes once cultures are available
- Reducing the need for extensive biochemical tests

Utility: Especially beneficial for fungal species and fastidious bacteria in CNS infections.

Pan-Omics Approaches

These integrated platforms include genomics, transcriptomics, proteomics, and metabolomics to provide a holistic understanding of infection:

- Help in host-pathogen interaction analysis
- Identification of biomarkers for early detection and treatment monitoring
- Support precision medicine strategies

Utility: This method is still largely research-based but shows promise for individualized CNS infection profiling.

Table 5.4 complements these diagnostic advances by summarizing the current first-line therapeutic options for major CNS parasitic and fungal infections, aiding in rapid clinical decision-making once a diagnosis is established. Figure 5.2 illustrates the chemical structures of the drug regimens for CNS parasitic infection and Figure 5.3 represents the chemical structures of the drug regimens for CNS fungal infection.

Table 4. First-Line Therapies for Common CNS Parasitic and Fungal Infections

First-Line Therapy for Parasitic Infections of the CNS		
S. No.	**Parasitic Infections**	**First-Line Therapy**
1.	NCC	Albendazole with corticosteroids
2.	Toxoplasmosis	Sulfadiazine + pyrimethamine + leucovorin
3.	Echinococcosis	Albendazole pre/post-surgery
4.	Schistosomiasis	Praziquantel

continued on following page

Table 4. Continued

First-Line Therapy for Parasitic Infections of the CNS		
S. No.	**Parasitic Infections**	**First-Line Therapy**
5.	Paragonimiasis	Praziquantel
6.	CM	IV artesunate
7.	Chagas Disease	Benznidazole or Nifurtimox
First-Line Therapy for Fungal Infections of the CNS		
S. No.	**Fungal Infections**	**First-Line Therapy**
1.	Candidiasis	Liposomal Amphotericin B or Echinocandins
2.	Histoplasmosis	Liposomal Amphotericin B (initial) → Itraconazole (maintenance)
3.	Blastomycosis	Liposomal Amphotericin B (initial) → Itraconazole (maintenance)
4.	Coccidioidomycosis	High-dose Fluconazole
5.	PCM	Itraconazole
6.	Sporotrichosis	Amphotericin B
7.	Cryptococcus	Amphotericin B + Flucytosine

Figure 2. Chemical Structures of the Drug Regimens for CNS Parasitic Infection

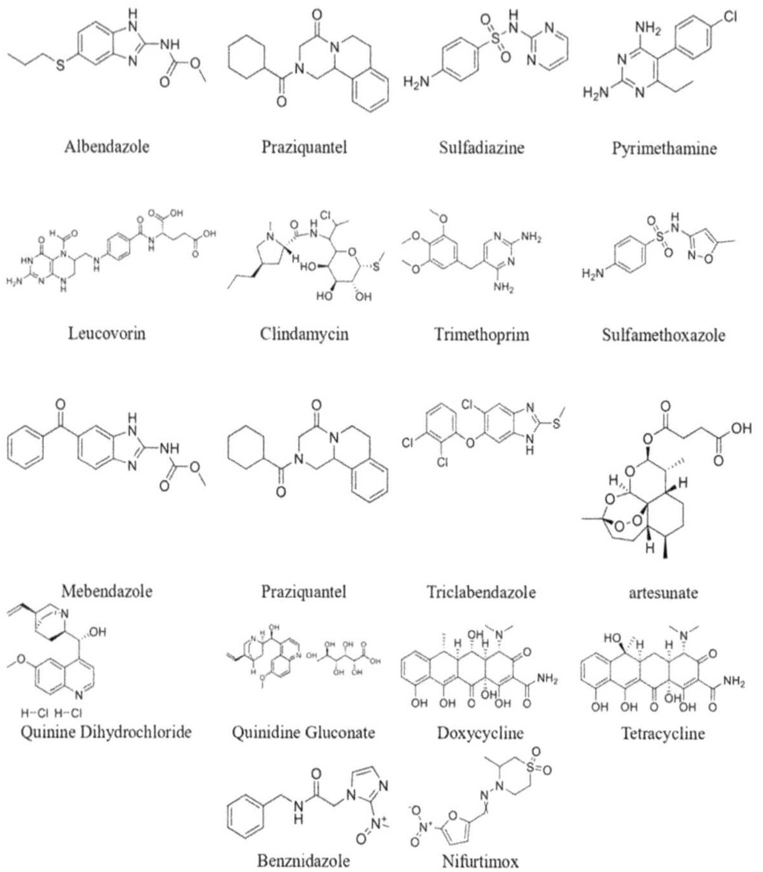

Figure 3. Chemical Structures of the Drug Regimens for CNS Fungal Infection

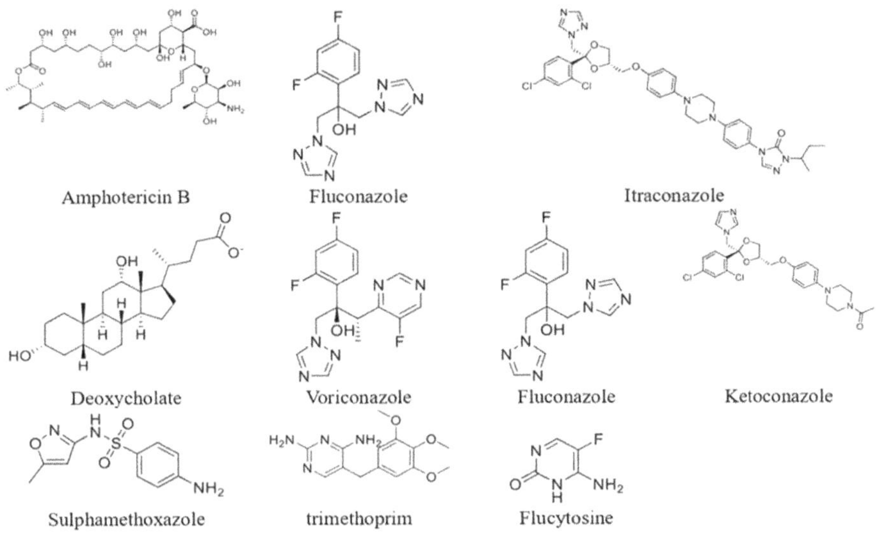

FUTURE PROSPECTS

Despite the progress made by WHO programs, there are still many obstacles to overcome in the prevention and control of neglected illnesses, which calls for ongoing attention and persistent work. Accurately estimating the disease burden among marginalized and neglected groups, who frequently lack access to healthcare and suffer a disproportionate number of chronic illnesses, is a crucial problem. Addressing these issues calls for consistent attention and a coordinated global effort. The following priority actions are advised to make significant progress:

- **Enhance Data on Marginalized Populations:** Accurately estimating the disease burden among underserved populations, which are frequently left out of regular healthcare systems, is crucial. To properly collect these data, inclusive health surveillance systems and targeted research must be implemented.
- **Advance Diagnostic Tools and Accessibility:** Especially in environments with limited resources, immediate investment is required in quick, accurate, and reasonably priced diagnostic techniques. Better illness management and early detection might be possible with this approach (Carpio et al., 2016).

- **Ensuring Equitable Access to Treatment:** To guarantee the prompt delivery of efficient treatments and interventions to populations at risk, supply chains and procurement processes must be strengthened.
- **Encouraging Innovation in Prevention and Treatment:** The creation of innovative medications and vaccines should be given top priority. Promoting integrated vector management can assist in effectively using pooled resources to combat a variety of vector-borne illnesses.
- **Protect high-risk groups:** National and regional health programs should incorporate early interventions for vulnerable groups, especially children and people living with HIV.
- **Strengthening Surveillance and Monitoring:** To follow disease trends, evaluate the effectiveness of interventions, and direct resource allocation, reliable, real-time monitoring technologies are essential.
- **Establish Mycology Centers of Excellence:** These establishments, which are modeled after the National Institutes of Health's (NIH) Cancer Centers, foster multidisciplinary research on fungal diseases by bringing together specialists in the fields of human, plant, and wildlife health to promote advancements in fungal biology and ecology.
- **Expand Public Education and Outreach:** National campaigns should promote preventative measures and increase knowledge of fungal infections, particularly in parks and schools. To slow the spread of pathogens, public awareness is essential.
- **Boost Academia-Industry Collaboration:** Research on neglected diseases and mycology can benefit from cross-sector collaborations, targeted support for graduate and postdoctoral researchers, and increased innovation (Case et al., 2022).
- **Leverage Genomic and Transcriptomic Technologies:** Pathogen virulence, genetic variation, and host interactions should be studied via state-of-the-art sequencing technologies (e.g., PacBio, Oxford Nanopore, and Illumina). Targeted interventions and insights into the mechanisms of antifungal resistance can be obtained by combining genomes, transcriptomics, and bioinformatics (Ball et al., 2020).
- **Adoptive Methodologies in Field Research:** To improve data dependability, future research must follow established methods, such as well-matched case-control designs, and make use of cutting-edge diagnostics including PCR, electroimmunotransfer blot (EITB), Ag ELISA, and neuroimaging (Carpio et al., 2016).
- **Maintaining and Standardizing Genomic Databases:** Investing in unified fungal genome databases with uniform taxonomy and annotation would ex-

pedite research, make data exchange easier, and allow multiomics data to be integrated for scientific discoveries (Case et al., 2022).

CONCLUSION

This chapter provides a comprehensive review of the pathogenesis, diagnostic methods, current treatment strategies, and future outlook for common parasitic and fungal infections affecting the CNS. With high rates of morbidity and mortality, infectious diseases—particularly parasitic and fungal CNS infections—continue to pose a serious threat to global health. In some areas, the effects of these illnesses are especially severe, making public health issues worse. Parasites that primarily infect humans can sometimes migrate to unusual locations, such as the brain or spinal cord, complicating both their identification and treatment. The necessity for better management techniques is highlighted by infection persistence. New therapeutic alternatives are desperately needed, even if the evidence base for current medicines has been strengthened. Given the present medications' subpar efficacy and toxicity, this is particularly important. Therefore, lowering the burden of these diseases requires strengthening preventative and control measures.

Antifungal medications such as amphotericin B, fluconazole, itraconazole, and voriconazole are frequently suggested for the efficient treatment of fungal CNS infections. These medications are essential for treating the serious consequences of fungal infections on the CNS. On the other hand, combination medicines are frequently used to treat parasitic infections. Depending on the particular parasite, regimens using sulfadiazine or pyrimethamine with leucovorin are frequently employed, in addition to additional medications such as mebendazole, praziquantel, and benznidazole.

Although fungal and parasite infections of the CNS are uncommon, they have significant effects. A comprehensive strategy is needed because of the difficulties in detecting these illnesses, the lack of public awareness, and the shifting dynamics of population health, including zoonotic threats. To solve these problems, the veterinary, medicinal, and environmental sectors must work together. Reducing the impact of these illnesses on public health requires updating health policy, improving public knowledge, and fortifying surveillance systems.

Furthermore, more studies on parasitic and fungal pathogens are desperately needed. The development of improved antifungal and antiparasitic drugs, new diagnostic techniques, and possible vaccinations will enhance the results and reduce the risk of parasitic and fungal CNS infections. To improve the public health response overall and guarantee that future treatment and preventative techniques that are more effective, it is imperative that these research initiatives be advanced.

To achieve substantial progress in the fight against parasite and fungal diseases of the CNS, an integrated strategy involving prevention and treatment as well as continuous research is ultimately needed.

LIST OF ABBREVIATIONS

Acquired Immune Deficiency Syndrome (AIDS)
Amyotrophic lateral sclerosis-3 (Als3)
Blastomyces dermatitidis (*B. dermatitidis*)
Blastomyces helices (*B. helices*)
blood-brain barrier (BBB)
blood-cerebrospinal fluid barrier (BCSFB)
brain endothelial cells (BEC)
Candida albicans (*C. albicans*)
central nervous system (CNS)
Centers for Disease Control and Prevention (CDC)
Cerebral malaria (CM)
cerebrospinal fluid (CSF)
Coccidoides immitis (*C. immitis*)
Coccidoides posadasii (*C. posadasii*)
complement (C)
computed tomography (CT)
Cryptococcus neoformans (*C. neoformans*)
deoxyribonucleic acid (DNA)
Echinococcus felidis (*E. felidis*)
Echinococcus granulosus (*E. granulosus*)
Echinococcus multilocularis (*E. multilocularis*)
Echinococcus shiquicus (*E. shiquicus*)
Echinococcus oligarthrus (*E. oligarthrus*)
Echinococcus vogeli (*E. vogeli*)
Electroimmunotransfer Blot (EITB)
Enzyme Immunoassay (EIA)
Enzyme-linked immunosorbent assay (ELISA)
European Society of Clinical Microbiology and Infectious Diseases (ESCMID)
Fluorescence *in situ* hybridization (FISH)
Gomori methenamine silver (GMS)
hematoxylin and eosin (H&E)
Histoplasma capsulatum (*H. capsulatum*)
Human African trypanosomiasis (HAT)

Human Immunodeficiency Virus (HIV)
Infectious Diseases Society of America (IDSA)
infected red blood cells (iRBCs)
intensive care unit (ICU)
intracranial pressure (ICP)
Magnetic resonance imaging (MRI)
Major Histocompatibility Complex (MHC)
Matrix-Assisted Laser Desorption Ionization-Time of Flight (MALDI-TOF)
National Institutes of Health (NIH)
neurocysticercosis (NCC)
nitric oxide (NO)
paracoccidioidomycosis (PCM)
Paracoccidioides brasiliensis (*P. brasiliensis*)
Paragonimus westermani (*P. westermani*)
Periodic acid-Schiff (PAS)
Plasmodium falciparum (*P. falciparum*)
P. falciparum-infected erythrocytes (PfIE)
Plasmodium falciparum erythrocyte membrane protein 1 (PfEMP1)
P. falciparum-infected RBCs (PfRBCs)
polymerase chain reaction (PCR)
Reverse transcriptase (RT)
Ribonucleic acid (RNA)
Schistosomiasis haematobium (*S. haematobium*)
Schistosomiasis intercalatum (*S. intercalatum*)
Schistosomiasis japonicum (*S. japonicum*)
Schistosomiasis mansoni (*S. mansoni*)
Schistosomiasis mekongi (*S. mekongi*)
species (spp.)
Taenia solium (*T. solium*)
Toxoplasma gondii (*T. gondii*)
Trypanosoma brucei (*T. brucei*)
Trypanosoma cruzi (*T. cruzi*)
United States (US)
World Health Organization (WHO)

REFERENCES

Archibald, L. K., & Quisling, R. G. (2013). Central Nervous System Infections. *Textbook of Neurointensive Care*, 427–517. DOI: 10.1007/978-1-4471-5226-2_22

Ball, B., Langille, M., & Geddes-McAlister, J. (2020). Fun(gi)omics: Advanced and Diverse Technologies to Explore Emerging Fungal Pathogens and Define Mechanisms of Antifungal Resistance. *mBio*, *11*(5), e01020-20. Advance online publication. DOI: 10.1128/mBio.01020-20 PMID: 33024032

Bonifaz, A., & Tirado-Sánchez, A. (2017). Cutaneous Disseminated and Extracutaneous Sporotrichosis: Current Status of a Complex Disease. *Journal of Fungi (Basel, Switzerland)*, *3*(1), 6. DOI: 10.3390/jof3010006 PMID: 29371525

Buscaglia, C., & Di Noia, J. M. (2003). Trypanosoma cruzi clonal diversity and the epidemiology of Chagas' disease. *Microbes and Infection*, *5*(5), 419–427. DOI: 10.1016/S1286-4579(03)00050-9 PMID: 12737998

Carpio, A., Romo, M. L., Parkhouse, R. M. E., Short, B., & Dua, T. (2016). Parasitic diseases of the central nervous system: Lessons for clinicians and policy makers. *Expert Review of Neurotherapeutics*, *16*(4), 401–414. DOI: 10.1586/14737175.2016.1155454 PMID: 26894629

Case, N. T., Berman, J., Blehert, D. S., Cramer, R. A., Cuomo, C., Currie, C. R., Ene, I. V., Fisher, M. C., Fritz-Laylin, L. K., Gerstein, A. C., Glass, N. L., Gow, N. A. R., Gurr, S. J., Hittinger, C. T., Hohl, T. M., Iliev, I. D., James, T. Y., Jin, H., Klein, B. S., & Kronstad, J. W. (2022). The future of fungi: threats and opportunities. *G3 Genes|Genomes|Genetics, 12*(11). DOI: 10.1093/g3journal/jkac224

Coyle, C. M. (2021). The returned traveler with neurologic manifestations: Could my patient have a parasite? *Current Opinion in Infectious Diseases*, *34*(3), 245–254. DOI: 10.1097/QCO.0000000000000732 PMID: 33769967

Deigendesch, N., Costa Nunez, J., & Stenzel, W. (2017). Parasitic and fungal infections. *Handbook of Clinical Neurology*, *145*, 245–262. DOI: 10.1016/B978-0-12-802395-2.00018-3 PMID: 28987173

Dorovini-Zis, K., Schmidt, K., Huynh, H., Fu, W., Whitten, R. O., Milner, D., Kamiza, S., Molyneux, M., & Taylor, T. E. (2011). The Neuropathology of Fatal Cerebral Malaria in Malawian Children. *American Journal of Pathology*, *178*(5), 2146–2158. DOI: 10.1016/j.ajpath.2011.01.016 PMID: 21514429

Ekloh, W., Asafu-Adjaye, A., & Nii, C. (2024). A comprehensive exploration of schistosomiasis: Global impact, molecular characterization, drug discovery, artificial intelligence and future prospects. *Heliyon*, *10*(12), e33070–e33070. DOI: 10.1016/j.heliyon.2024.e33070 PMID: 38988508

Flores-Maldonado, O., González, G. M., Enríquez-Bañuelos, J. F., Andrade, Á., Treviño-Rangel, R., & Becerril-García, M. A. (2023). Candida albicans causes brain regional invasion and necrosis, and activation of microglia during lethal neonatal neurocandidiasis. *Microbes and Infection*, *25*(6), 105119. DOI: 10.1016/j.micinf.2023.105119 PMID: 36758890

Fu, Y., Phan, Q. T., Luo, G., Solis, N. V., Liu, Y., Cormack, B. P., Edwards, J. E.Jr, Ibrahim, A. S., & Filler, S. G. (2013). Investigation of the Function of Candida albicans Als3 by Heterologous Expression in Candida glabrata. *Infection and Immunity*, *81*(7), 2528–2535. DOI: 10.1128/IAI.00013-13 PMID: 23630968

Garcia, H. H. (2021). Parasitic Infections of the Nervous System. *Continuum (Minneapolis, Minn.)*, *27*(4), 943–962. DOI: 10.1212/CON.0000000000000986 PMID: 34623099

Garcia, H. H., Nash, T. E., & Del Brutto, O. H. (2014). Clinical symptoms, diagnosis, and treatment of neurocysticercosis. *Lancet Neurology*, *13*(12), 1202–1215. DOI: 10.1016/S1474-4422(14)70094-8 PMID: 25453460

Góralska, K., Blaszkowska, J., & Dzikowiec, M. (2018). Neuroinfections caused by fungi. *Infection*, *46*(4), 443–459. DOI: 10.1007/s15010-018-1152-2 PMID: 29785613

Güémez, A., & García, E. (2021). Primary Amoebic Meningoencephalitis by Naegleria fowleri: Pathogenesis and Treatments. *Biomolecules*, *11*(9), 1320. DOI: 10.3390/biom11091320 PMID: 34572533

Haran, H., Santos, I. C., Batista, R. L., & Silva-Vergara, M. L. (2024). Congestive heart failure associated with itraconazole in a patient with paracoccidioidomycosis. *The Brazilian Journal of Infectious Diseases : an Official Publication of the Brazilian Society of Infectious Diseases*, *28*(5), 103868–103868. DOI: 10.1016/j.bjid.2024.103868 PMID: 39276794

He, T., Kaplan, S., Kamboj, M., & Tang, Y.-W. (2016). Laboratory Diagnosis of Central Nervous System Infection. *Current Infectious Disease Reports*, *18*(11), 35. Advance online publication. DOI: 10.1007/s11908-016-0545-6 PMID: 27686677

Hughes, A. J., & Biggs, B. A. (2002). Parasitic worms of the central nervous system: An Australian perspective. *Internal Medicine Journal*, *32*(11), 541–553. DOI: 10.1046/j.1445-5994.2002.00265.x PMID: 12412938

Imperato, A., Consales, A., Ravegnani, M., Castagnola, E., Bandettini, R., & Rossi, A. (2016). Primary Hydatid Cyst of the Brain in a Child: A Case Report. *Polish Journal of Radiology / Polish Medical Society of Radiology*, *81*, 578–582. DOI: 10.12659/PJR.898619 PMID: 27994696

Jacquier, M., & Piroth, L. (2018). Vertebral Hydatidosis. *The New England Journal of Medicine*, *379*(2). Advance online publication. DOI: 10.1056/NEJMicm1714206 PMID: 29996078

Khalaf, S. A., Patel, P., Caruso, C. R., Parrett, T., & Bran, A. (2022). CNS Histoplasmosis as a Gliosarcoma mimicker: The diagnostic dilemma of solitary brain lesions. *IDCases*, *27*, e01364. DOI: 10.1016/j.idcr.2021.e01364 PMID: 35024338

Le Govic, Y., Demey, B., Cassereau, J., Bahn, Y.-S., & Papon, N. (2022). Pathogens infecting the central nervous system. *PLoS Pathogens*, *18*(2), e1010234. DOI: 10.1371/journal.ppat.1010234 PMID: 35202445

Lima, M. A., Freitas, D. F. S., Oliveira, R. V. C., Fichman, V., Varon, A. G., Freitas, A. D., Lamas, C. C., Andrade, H. B., Veloso, V. G., Almeida-Paes, R., Almeida-Silva, F., Zancopé-Oliveira, R. M., de Macedo, P. M., Valle, A. C. F., Silva, M. T. T., Araújo, A. Q. C., & Gutierrez-Galhardo, M. C. (2022). Meningeal Sporotrichosis Due to Sporothrix brasiliensis: A 21-Year Cohort Study from a Brazilian Reference Center. *Journal of Fungi (Basel, Switzerland)*, *9*(1), 17. DOI: 10.3390/jof9010017 PMID: 36675837

Lino, R., Guimarães, A. R., Sousa, E., Azevedo, M., & Santos, L. (2024). Emerging Fungal Infections of the Central Nervous System in the Past Decade: A Literature Review. *Infectious Disease Reports*, *16*(5), 952–976. DOI: 10.3390/idr16050076 PMID: 39452161

Liu, K., Sun, Y.-C., Pan, R.-T., Xu, A.-L., Xue, H., Tian, N., Zheng, J.-X., Shi, F.-Y., Lu, Y., & Li, L.-H. (2024). Infection and biogeographical characteristics of Paragonimus westermani and P. skrjabini in humans and animal hosts in China: A systematic review and meta-analysis. *PLoS Neglected Tropical Diseases*, *18*(8), e0012366–e0012366. DOI: 10.1371/journal.pntd.0012366 PMID: 39102441

Liu, Q., Wang, Z.-D., Huang, S.-Y., & Zhu, X.-Q. (2015). Diagnosis of toxoplasmosis and typing of Toxoplasma gondii. *Parasites & Vectors*, *8*(1), 292. Advance online publication. DOI: 10.1186/s13071-015-0902-6 PMID: 26017718

Mazumder, R., & Lee, J. K. (2022). Epileptogenesis in Common Parasitic Infections. *Current Neurology and Neuroscience Reports*, *22*(4), 285–291. DOI: 10.1007/s11910-022-01187-6 PMID: 35332514

Mendez, O. A., & Koshy, A. A. (2017). Toxoplasma gondii: Entry, association, and physiological influence on the central nervous system. *PLoS Pathogens*, *13*(7), e1006351. DOI: 10.1371/journal.ppat.1006351 PMID: 28727854

Moro, P., & Schantz, P. M. (2009). Echinococcosis: A review. *International Journal of Infectious Diseases*, *13*(2), 125–133. DOI: 10.1016/j.ijid.2008.03.037 PMID: 18938096

Moxon, C. A., Heyderman, R. S., & Wassmer, S. C. (2009). Dysregulation of coagulation in cerebral malaria. *Molecular and Biochemical Parasitology*, *166*(2), 99–108. DOI: 10.1016/j.molbiopara.2009.03.006 PMID: 19450727

Nanda, E. (2024). The brain pathobiome in Alzheimer's disease. *Neurotherapeutics; the Journal of the American Society for Experimental NeuroTherapeutics*, *21*(6), e00475–e00475. DOI: 10.1016/j.neurot.2024.e00475 PMID: 39510900

Papagni, R., Novara, R., Minardi, M. L., Frallonardo, L., Panico, G. G., Pallara, E., Cotugno, S., Ascoli Bartoli, T., Guido, G., De Vita, E., Ricciardi, A., Totaro, V., Camporeale, M., Segala, F. V., Bavaro, D. F., Patti, G., Brindicci, G., Pellegrino, C., Mariani, M. F., & Nicastri, E. (2023). Human African Trypanosomiasis (sleeping sickness): Current knowledge and future challenges. *Frontiers in Tropical Diseases*, *4*, 1087003. Advance online publication. DOI: 10.3389/fitd.2023.1087003

Pathakumari, B., Liang, G., & Liu, W. (2020). Immune defence to invasive fungal infections: A comprehensive review. *Biomedicine and Pharmacotherapy*, *130*, 110550. DOI: 10.1016/j.biopha.2020.110550 PMID: 32739740

Pokorn, M. (2004). Pathogenesis and Classification of Central Nervous System Infection. *PubMed*, *15*(3), 68–71. PMID: 29988854

Rajasingham, R., Smith, R. M., Park, B. J., Jarvis, J. N., Govender, N. P., Chiller, T. M., Denning, D. W., Loyse, A., & Boulware, D. R. (2017). Global burden of disease of HIV-associated cryptococcal meningitis: An updated analysis. *The Lancet. Infectious Diseases*, *17*(8), 873–881. DOI: 10.1016/S1473-3099(17)30243-8 PMID: 28483415

Raman Sharma, R. (2010). Fungal infections of the nervous system: Current perspective and controversies in management. *International Journal of Surgery*, *8*(8), 591–601. DOI: 10.1016/j.ijsu.2010.07.293 PMID: 20673817

Razek, A. A. K. A., Watcharakorn, A., & Castillo, M. (2011). Parasitic Diseases of the Central Nervous System. *Neuroimaging Clinics of North America*, *21*(4), 815–841. DOI: 10.1016/j.nic.2011.07.005 PMID: 22032501

Reddy, G., Kiran, K., Padmavathi, A. R., & Nancharaiah, Y. V. (2022). Fungal infections: Pathogenesis, antifungals and alternate treatment approaches. *Current Research in Microbial Sciences, 3*, 100137. DOI: 10.1016/j.crmicr.2022.100137 PMID: 35909631

Sah, V. K., Wang, L., Min, X., Rizal, R., Feng, Z., Ke, Z., Deng, M., Li, L., & Li, H. (2015). Human schistosomiasis: A diagnostic imaging focused review of a neglected disease. *Radiology of Infectious Diseases (Beijing, China), 2*(3), 150–157. DOI: 10.1016/j.jrid.2015.11.007

Sanchez, S. G., Bassot, E., & Cerutti, A., Hoa Mai Nguyen, Amel Aïda, Blanchard, N., & Sébastien Besteiro. (2023). The apicoplast is important for the viability and persistence of *Toxoplasma gondii* bradyzoites. *Proceedings of the National Academy of Sciences of the United States of America, 120*(34). DOI: 10.1073/pnas.2309043120

Santos, L. A., Grisolia, J. C., Malaquias, L. C. C., Paula, F. B. A., Dias, A. L. T., & Burger, E. (2020). Medication association and immunomodulation: An approach in fungal diseases and in particular in the treatment of paracoccidioidomycosis. *Acta Tropica, 206*, 105412–105412. DOI: 10.1016/j.actatropica.2020.105412 PMID: 32135141

Schlüter, D., & Barragan, A. (2019). Advances and Challenges in Understanding Cerebral Toxoplasmosis. *Frontiers in Immunology, 10*, 242. Advance online publication. DOI: 10.3389/fimmu.2019.00242 PMID: 30873157

Schwartz, I. S., & Kauffman, C. A. (2020). Blastomycosis. *Seminars in Respiratory and Critical Care Medicine, 41*(1), 31–41. DOI: 10.1055/s-0039-3400281

Shaikh, M. S., Baig, M. S., Ali, S. S., Ahmad, A., Shaikh, M. M., Mahaparale, P. R., & Faiyazuddin, M. (2024). Review on cerebral malaria—Pathogenesis and role of EphA2 receptor in maintaining blood brain barrier integrity. *Health Sciences Review (Oxford, England), 11*, 100175. DOI: 10.1016/j.hsr.2024.100175

Shelton, W. J., & Gonzalez, J. M. (2023). Outcomes of patients in Chagas disease of the central nervous system: A systematic review. *Parasitology*, 1–9. DOI: 10.1017/S0031182023001117 PMID: 37987164

Shi, M., & Mody, C. H. (2016). Fungal Infection in the Brain: What We Learned from Intravital Imaging. *Frontiers in Immunology, 7*. Advance online publication. DOI: 10.3389/fimmu.2016.00292 PMID: 27532000

Shikani, H. J., Freeman, B. D., Lisanti, M. P., Weiss, L. M., Tanowitz, H. B., & Desruisseaux, M. S. (2012). Cerebral Malaria. *American Journal of Pathology, 181*(5), 1484–1492. DOI: 10.1016/j.ajpath.2012.08.010 PMID: 23021981

Snydman, D. R., Walker, M., Kublin, J. G., & Zunt, J. R. (2006). Parasitic Central Nervous System Infections in Immunocompromised Hosts: Malaria, Microsporidiosis, Leishmaniasis, and African Trypanosomiasis. *Clinical Infectious Diseases*, *42*(1), 115–125. DOI: 10.1086/498510 PMID: 16323101

Useche, Y., Pérez, A. R., de Meis, J., Bonomo, A., & Savino, W. (2022). Central nervous system commitment in Chagas disease. *Frontiers in Immunology*, *13*, 975106. Advance online publication. DOI: 10.3389/fimmu.2022.975106 PMID: 36439149

Van Belle, S., de Lange, A., Tomes, H., Lucas, R., Naidoo, V., & Raimondo, J. V. (2021). Peripheral Taenia infection increases immunoglobulins in the central nervous system. *International Journal for Parasitology*, *51*(8), 685–692. DOI: 10.1016/j.ijpara.2020.12.008 PMID: 33753094

Williams, S. L., & Chiller, T. (2022). Update on the Epidemiology, Diagnosis, and Treatment of Coccidioidomycosis. *Journal of Fungi (Basel, Switzerland)*, *8*(7), 666. DOI: 10.3390/jof8070666 PMID: 35887423

Zammarchi, L., Bonati, M., Strohmeyer, M., Albonico, M., Requena-Méndez, A., Bisoffi, Z., Nicoletti, A., García, H. H., & Bartoloni, A. (2017). Screening, diagnosis and management of human cysticercosis and*Taenia solium*taeniasis: Technical recommendations by the COHEMI project study group. *Tropical Medicine & International Health*, *22*(7), 881–894. DOI: 10.1111/tmi.12887 PMID: 28449318

Zhou, X.-J., Yang, Q., Tan, Q.-H., Zhang, L.-Y., Shi, L.-B., & Zou, J.-X. (2021). Paragonimus and its hosts in China: An update. *Acta Tropica*, *223*, 106094–106094. DOI: 10.1016/j.actatropica.2021.106094 PMID: 34389330

Chapter 7
Current Trends in Biomarkers and Diagnosis of Prevalent Neurological Infectious Diseases

Kavita Verma
https://orcid.org/0009-0004-3518-7546
Dr. Rammanohar Lohia Avadh University, Ayodhya, India

Priyanka
Dr. Rammanohar Lohia Avadh University, Ayodhya, India

Sarika Singh
CSIR-Central Drug Research Institute, Lucknow, India

Neelam Yadav
https://orcid.org/0000-0002-2245-7824
Dr. Rammanohar Lohia Avadh University, Ayodhya, India

ABSTRACT

Infections of the central nervous system (CNS) are linked to high rates of morbidity and death and account for a significant portion of the global illness burden. To reduce the likelihood of unfavorable results, prompt diagnosis and the start of the right treatment are essential. Nevertheless, there are insufficient instruments available to reliably identify infections, gauge the degree of injuries, and forecast results. The identification of biomarkers for structural neurological damage may be a useful tool

DOI: 10.4018/979-8-3693-4070-7.ch007

in tackling these obstacles. Authors provide an overview of the experimental and clinical studies on neurological damage biomarkers in a variety of CNS infectious diseases in this chapter. According to the research findings, the biomarkers S100B and neuron-specific enlose (NSE), among others, may be able to provide light on the pathogenesis of central nervous system infections as well as the severity, progression, and treatment response of injuries in both adults and children. Scientists are still in the early stages of researching the usefulness of biomarkers in CNS illnesses.

INTRODUCTION

Disorders known as neurodegenerative diseases (NDDs) impact the peripheral and central nervous systems. Along with other risk factors contributing to Alzheimer's disease (AD) sporadic occurrences, infection may be involved in late-onset AD. Over the last three decades, the onset of AD has been related to infectious microorganisms like viruses, bacteria, fungi, and protozoa (Long & Holtzman, 2019; Rahman, Bajgai, Fadriquela, Sharma, Trinh Thi et al, 2021). The most intricate biological organ on the planet is the human brain. However, humans are not unbeatable and can suffer from a wide range of illnesses, some of which are related to brain disorders (Perrachione & Perrachione, 2008). As a result of accumulated tau and A pathologies, neurodegeneration occurs just before the clinical presentation of AD, which is the development of cognitive impairment. This is succeeded by a brain cellular malfunction (Long & Holtzman, 2019). NDDs can arise from a variety of factors, including injury to the nervous system, ischemia, endoplasmic reticulum (ER) cellular and oxidative stress, inflammation, aberrant autoimmune-mediated neuronal demise, protein accumulation in neural tissue, and viral or prion infections (Dugger & Dickson, 2017). Furthermore, misfolded protein build up in the central nervous system (CNS) like insoluble clumps (or inclusions) and progressive neuronal loss inside the afflicted areas are the most common characteristics of neurodegeneration, which encompasses a wide range of clinically and pathologically diverse illnesses (Akter, Rahman, Behl et al, 2021; Peng et al., 2020; Rahman, Akter, & Kamal, 2021). Weakness and cognitive decline are symptoms of amyotrophic lateral sclerosis (ALS); symptoms of Parkinson's disease (PD) include reduced motor ability and attention issues; and among the signs of Alzheimer's disease (AD) are memory loss and personality abnormalities (Akter, Chowdhury, & Rahman, 2021; Bhattacharya et al., 2021; Rahman, Bajgai, Fadriquela, Sharma, Trinh Thi et al, 2021).

One of the most difficult and complicated subjects in modern neuro medicine is the study and creation of therapeutic approaches for NDDs. At the same time, any possible risks or development expenses are outweighed by the social and economic advantages of at least partially resolving these challenges. Despite being identified more than a century ago, prevalent neurodegenerative conditions, such as Parkinson's and Alzheimer's are still incurable. Although the pathophysiology of these disorders has been greatly advanced, the precise processes and causes of neurodegeneration are still unclear (Fahn, 2018; Knopman et al., 2021).

In addition to guiding clinical diagnosis, biomarkers can be used to assess treatment response, estimate illness risk or prognosis, and determine disease stage (Kobeissi & Zanotti-Cavazzoni, 2010). During clinical trials, biomarkers can be employed to identify a particular diagnostic subgroup (stratification or enrichment of patients), ensure appropriate target engagement for therapy, identify therapeutic side effects on the course of the illness and evaluate clinical effectiveness and/or safety (Hansson, 2021). One major development in the field of neurology research has been the development of biomarkers based on blood. The detection of analytes in a variety of biofluids at incredibly low concentrations has been made possible by recent technological advancements, despite early scepticism regarding peripheral markers because of the physical limitations brought about by the blood-brain barrier (BBB) (Hampel et al., 2018).

Over the past twenty years, some genes have shown multiple mutations generating familial variations of important neurodegenerative illnesses. This has sparked a new wave of investigation into the etiology of neurodegeneration and its underlying mechanisms enabling neuronal protection (Rahman, Bajgai, Fadriquela, Sharma, Trinh et al, 2021; Sierksma et al., 2020). Numerous potential neurodegenerative pathways have been proposed based on transgenic disease models and toxicological data. Similar traits and processes, such as the build-up of intrinsically disordered proteins as aggregates, oxidative stress and mitochondrial dysfunction and neuroinflammation have been utilized to design therapeutic approaches that target the prevention or deceleration of disease progression as opposed to treating its symptoms (Schneider et al., 2020).

A diminished blood-brain barrier (BBB) is one of the consequences of viral and bacterial infections. This can occur either directly or indirectly through a central nervous system infection, and it causes broad cerebral dysfunction following the inflammatory reaction throughout the system (Al-Obaidi & Desa, 2018). Alzheimer's patients with increases in TNF-α, a measure of systemic inflammation, have been found to have more cognitive impairment. Recent discoveries from preclinical and clinical studies indicate that microglia are activated following central nervous system infestation by bacteria, fungi, viruses, and parasites. Microglia, a hallmark of brain inflammation, possess several attributes for neuroinflammation, such as immunosuppression, cytotoxicity, regeneration and repair, due to their capacity to acquire different activation states or phenotypes. According to recent studies, infection with bacteria belonging to the Enterobacteriaceae family speeds up the development of AD in a model of Drosophila by boosting hemocyte migration of the immune system to the brain (Wu et al., 2017).

However, diagnosis is challenging since many NDDs share similar symptoms and traits. In order to identify characteristics that might aid in diagnosis, several research have been conducted to look at the clinical features, in addition to the molecular mechanisms that result in these disorders. In light of this, the present chapter is focus on and provide an overview of neurological illnesses and associated biomarkers.

NEURODEGENERATION, INFLAMMATION AND TUMORIGENESIS

The pathogenic role and fundamental molecular mechanisms behind neurodegeneration are unclear, despite the fact that they include complex genetic, environmental, and endogenous factors associated with aging (Jellinger, 2009). These days, NDDs are classified according to the main substances discovered in their protein deposits as well as their established genetic pathways. Because of the severe structural defects in proteins that underlie these ailments, they are known as "protein misfolding" diseases or proteinopathies (Golde & Miller, 2009). Inflammatory cells and mediators can start a variety of basic pathways underpinning neurodegeneration at different points in the neurodegenerative cascade.

Apoptosis: Caspases regulate apoptosis, a specific kind of programmed cell death (Karthika et al., 2021). The formation of membrane-encased apoptotic bodies, which are quickly phagocytosed by near bycells or macrophages, is its defining feature. While a number of neurodegenerative diseases have been shown to have apoptotic pathways in animal models, human tissues show less evidence of these mechanisms. Human striatal brain tissue exhibited cytochrome c release and activation of caspase 1,-3,-8, and -9 in models of Huntington's disease (HD). Similar findings have been reported for caspase activation and neuronal death in HIV-associated neurodegeneration and amyotrophic lateral sclerosis (ALS) (Ghavami et al., 2014).

Necroptosis is a type of programmed cell death in which the integrity of the plasma membrane is lost without caspase activation. The two primary effector proteins in necroptosis are mixed-lineage kinase domain-like and receptor-interacting serine/threonine protein kinase 1 (RIPK1) (MLKL). As demonstrated in models of ALS in mice, astrocytes emit TNF-α, FasL-, and TRAIL, which can activate RIPK1 and MLKL and promote necroptosis (Re et al., 2014). Pathological specimens from individuals with ALS showed evidence of RIPK1-caused axonal degeneration (Ito et al., 2016).

Autophagy, which is often referred to as programmed cell death of type II, is characterized by the accumulation of autophagic vacuoles when a cell dies, which may include potentially hazardous elements including damaged organelles or proteins. Over autophagy can trigger self-destruction and cellular death. Damaged neurons in individuals with AD, HD and PD were revealed to have autophagosomes. Autophagy can also be triggered by a wide range of additional factors, including oxidative stress, hypoxia, mitochondrial toxins and starvation (Vives-Bauza et al., 2010).

The proximal neuronal cell body experiences retrograde degeneration can be caused by axonal injury or transection. This degenerative modification inside the cellular system includes neuronal perikaryon chromatolysis and apoptosis. Due to the correlation between axonal damage and neuronal apoptosis, axotomy brought on by inflammation may trigger retrograde (secondary) death of the cell bodies of neurons (Chitnis & Weiner, 2017).

The term “astrogliopathy” encompasses a wide range of conditions related to astrocyte malfunction. ARTAG (Aging-related tau astrogliopathy) is the term used to describe the aberrant accumulation of improperly tau protein that is phosphorylated in astrocytes observed in Alzheimer's disease (AD), frontal temporal lobe dementia (FTLD), and corticobasal degeneration (Kovacs et al., 2017). Neuromyelitis optica (NMO), which mimics multiple sclerosis, is characterized by myelitis and optic neuritis.NMO is associated with antibodies against aquaporin-4 (AQP4), a protein that interacts with astrocyte water channels. One of NMO's pathological characteristics is perivascular immunoglobulin deposition, complement activation, and a marked decrease of immunoreactivity for glial fibrillary acidic protein (GFAP) and the astrocytic proteins AQP4 (Lucchinetti et al., 2014).

The body's immune cells initiate inflammatory cascades to shield tissue from trauma or invading infections, which is how inflammation starts. Successful inflammatory responses eradicate germs, start wound healing and angiogenesis, and finally go down. Acute neuroinflammatory responses are necessary and beneficial for the neuronal environment because they help remove pathogens and repair the brain. Continuous gliosis and apoptosis may ensue from unchecked inflammatory cytokine production when major hazards to the neuronal microenvironment for instance protein aggregates, especially as neurofibrillary tangles and Lewy bodies, form in the brain and maintain inflammation for a prolonged period of time. Because of prolonged activation, chronic inflammation is linked to almost all neurological disorders, including ALS, PD, and AD (Jung et al., 2019).

In contrast, inflammation has been linked to several disorders, defying this protective homeostatic system. Its effect on neurological illnesses has led to the hypothesis that it contributes significantly to the course of disease in recent years. To communicate with astrocytes and neurons, microglia in the CNS (central nervous system) adopt phagocytic morphologies and release pro-inflammatory cytokines. Until the brain environment is no longer in danger, this can lead to synaptic phagocytosis, neurodegeneration, decreased neuronal function, production of inflammatory cytokines, microglial activation, along with additional microglial activation. Additionally, during the inflammatory process known as astrogliosis, astrocytes are stimulated. A persistent low-grade inflammatory state is typically the outcome of dysregulated cytokine expression in older individuals, which is defined as increased production of pro-inflammatory cytokines and a decline in the availability of anti-inflammatory cytokines. This kind of auto-inflammatory disease that develops with aging is known as "inflammatory aging" (Franceschi et al., 2018).

Research indicates that neurogenesis—the development of new neurons—and tumor-induced neuronal sprouting, or axonogenesis towards the tumour micro-environment—may play significant roles in the initiation and progression of cancer, in addition to blood and lymphatic vessels. Pre-neoplastic lesions have been seen to exhibit neurogenesis and axonogenesis, suggesting that these processes may be involved in the early stages of the pre-malignant phase of cancer (Mauffrey et al., 2019).

INFLAMMATION AND NEURODEGENERATION'S RELATIONSHIP

Because the neurological system in mammals is capable of directly sensing inflammatory stimuli, it may be used to identify a possible site of harm by inducing pain and modifying the immune system's response to infection. Evidence suggests that central muscarinic signalling influences obesity-related inflammation and inflammatory colitis, and experimental sepsis, despite ongoing research on afferent pathways and integration of immunological information in the brain (Ji et al., 2014).

The immune system is always scanning the body for signs of harm, including chemicals generated by the body itself and potential pathogens. Under normal circumstances, inflammation is a well-regulated, constantly-adjusting response. Innate immunity is essential for halting more incursions by inducing inflammation once pathogens have passed past the epidermal and mucosal barriers. Following the removal of the infection's source, tissue healing and functional recovery depend on the inflammatory response. If the damage is gone, the specific systems that cause and control inflammation will respond less strongly. Sepsis and multiple organ failure can be brought on by infections with highly pathogenic bacteria or by large pathogen loads (Deutschman & Tracey, 2014).

The autoimmune disease Systemic lupus erythematosus (SLE) is relapsing-remitting that affects several organs, including the central nervous system. Lack of immunity against self-antigens and aberrant B- and T-cell reactions are immunological characteristics. Tissue accumulation of immunoglobulin complexes might result in systemic inflammation. One might detect anti-nuclear antibodies in individuals with different autoimmune disorders, but they are present in up to 98% of patients. Unknown medical illness neuropsychiatric SLE (NPSLE) presents with a range of clinical symptoms. A research found that between 12% and 95% of individuals suffer from neurological and behavioural issues. An SLE clinical presentation that is more severe is predicted when there is CNS involvement (Mak et al., 2012). Because neuropsychiatric symptoms can show in an extensive variety of sensory, motor, cognitive, and behavioural domains, diagnosis can be difficult (Jeltsch-David & Muller, 2014).

INFECTIONS AND NEUROINFLAMMATION

According to certain theories, viruses can replicate in CCR5+ T cells and macrophages in the CNS. HIV proteins Tat and gp120, for example, have been shown to induce neuronal dysfunction through miRNA disruption and neuronal death through an increase in CXCR4-PKC (Chang et al., 2011). Significantly, similar to HIV infection, further assaults propagated by viruses are linked to elevated levels of lipopolysaccharide (LPS) concentrations, increased cytokine secretion, increased cholesterol, APOE4, insulin resistance and insufficient testosterone, these factors lead to CNS inflammation. Furthermore, due to chronic stress, age-related enhancement of the provoking reaction seems to be the primary initiating mechanism for tissue injury linked to a variety of age-related diseases (Brew et al., 2009). BBB endothelial cells, which possess the molecular tools necessary to identify bacterial and viral antigens, can cause local inflammation. Pattern recognition receptors (PRRs) are the initial line of protection against the invasion of microbes because they are able to recognize antigenically a wide range of conserved molecular determinants referred to as pathogen-associated molecular patterns (PAMPs). The state of NDDs can be impacted by peripheral elements like the gut flora. Severe NDDs are associated with abnormalities in the normal composition of the flora, which interfere with brain development and plasticity and lead to behavioral problems (El Aidy et al., 2014).

SIGNIFICANCE OF BIOMARKERS IN NEUROPATHOLOGY

Biomarkers are quantifiable, objective indications of either disease or usual functioning. They offer data on pathogen activity and dynamic processes that support prognostication, diagnosis and assessment of therapy safety and effectiveness. Additionally, they may serve as stand-in indicators for clinical or scientific outcomes, such as the efficacy of cutting-edge therapies. Numerous biological fluids, including blood and urine, are readily collected for research, and their measurement is user-independent (Berger, 2006). An expanding number of acute and chronic CNS disorders are being studied for biomarkers associated with CNS pathologies (Kuhle & Petzold, 2011).The cerebral extracellular fluid (CEF) contains a collection of breakdown products and damaged cells due to CNS infection, trauma, hypoxia, inflammation, or degeneration. Additionally, the blood-brain barrier (BBB) is more permeable. These products diffuse into the CSF along concentration gradients and enter the circulation through a leaky blood-brain barrier, making them quantifiable markers of brain damage. Sequential sampling offers information on the progression of the damage, cell specificity suggests the kind and may be the location of the injury, and the extent to which certain concentrations of biomarkers are elevated indicates the severity of the injury (Lamers et al., 2003).

High brain sensitivity and specificity are desirable qualities in biomarkers for brain damage. Their release ought to correspond with the time profile of that injury and be linked to permanent brain damage. Since the brain is a multicellular, highly complex and varied organ, brain diseases differ in shape and severity. Although it's not always available, CSF reflects changes in the brain more accurately than serum does. Because the BBB limits the size and quantity of the biomarker that can filter the circulation, serum levels may depend on both the level of BBB disruption—which frequently happens in brain injury—and the degree of cell damage (Berger, 2006). The separation in length between the afflicted area and the compartment of CSF, the regional variations in brain biomarker protein levels, and the degradation of biomarkers by proteinases inside the CSF or parenchyma may all alter biomarker concentrations even in the presence of CSF variability (Lamers et al., 1995). Furthermore, biomarker analysis is limited to quantitative measurements and is not able to capture the qualitative and quantitative aspects of brain activity (Sandler et al., 2010). Using a panel of biomarkers as opposed to individual ones and combining them with clinical and radiological techniques is one method to get around some of these restrictions (Berger, 2006).

Biomarkers of CNS damage show potential as diagnostic and prognostic indicators in studies of traumatic brain injury (TBI) (Berger et al., 2007; Sandler et al., 2010), subarachnoid haemorrhage (Wiesmann et al., 1997), dementia, cardiac arrest (Böttiger et al., 2001), Alzheimer's disease, stroke and several other diseases. Less study has been done on their involvement in CNS infections. But two important biomarkers that show promise have come to light from the researches that are now available: S100B and NSE (Neuron-Specific Enolase). We mainly discuss these proteins in this chapter, but we also provide a brief summary of research on additional putative biomarkers.

LIMITATIONS OF BIOMARKERS

Some methodological errors can occur while analyzing biomarkers. The method used to get the samples affects how suitable they are; for instance, blood samples that have been hemolyzed may contain biomarkers that have been liberated from erythrocytes (Lima et al., 2004). It is important to utilize tubes that are appropriate for the biomarker of interest since the collecting tube can affect biomarker concentrations (Teunissen et al., 2011). In order to prevent antigen degradation, samples should ideally be kept at 70 °C as soon as feasible; however, this depends on the stability of the biomarker. Long-term storage and repeatedly freezing and thawing can also cause biomarker degradation (Butterfield et al., 2011). The immunoassay is now the main technique used to test for biomarkers. It has a strong sensitivity, is easy to use and affordable, and is available in a variety of commercial kits. By making use of the great specificity and affinities with which antibodies attach to their antigens, this method guarantees that in a sample, only the target antigen will bind, even in the presence of several other analytes and at extremely low concentrations. Antibodies specific to the target biomarker are coated on immunoassay plates. When experimental samples are put on the plate, the antibody and biomarker bond together; the amount of binding indicates how much of the biomarker is present. An auxiliary reaction is used to evaluate the binding event since the interaction between the antigen and antibody is not linked to a measurable physical or chemical change. In this reaction, one of the immunoreactants is labelled with a material that can be readily detected by spectrophotometry (Warsinke et al., 2000). Several widely utilized choices include enzymes (RIAs and ELISAs), fluorophores (immune fluorometric assays), and chemiluminescent chemicals (chemiluminescence immunoassay). Platforms vary depending on the label and antibody that are utilised to identify the antibody-antigen interaction. There is also a growing availability of label-free electrochemical immunoassays that detect antibody-antigen binding by using variations in charge densities or conductivities (Warsinke et al., 2000). Standardized operating and testing protocols are necessary since various assays have varied upper and lower detection limits. As a result, it is difficult to compare reference values and the outcome associated with pathology across testing platforms. Large-scale multi-center trials would make it possible to gather enough data for research with adequate power to set standards, reference values, and suitable cut-off values that are particular to a given illness. A significant portion of biomarker research is still restricted to specialized labs or projects; yet, the creation of quick, easy-to-use, low-tech tests that may be employed whenever needed at the clinic and hospital levels is necessary for the full biomarker translation from bench to bedside (Berger, 2006).

S100B

S100B is a member of the S100 family, which is a broader group of small acidic proteins with a molecular weight of 10–12 kDa with subunits A and B (Infante et al., 2003). These proteins control a variety of intracellular functions, including as transcription, differentiation, and cell division. The action of S100 proteins is dependent on their extracellular concentration; the trophic effects occur at nanomolar doses, while for concentrations of micromolar, they may induce apoptosis and harm to cells. Subunit B is produced by Schwann cells, oligodendrocytes, and astrocytes and is present in the CNS in the greatest numbers (Infante et al., 2003). It contributes to the growth and maintenance of cells, intracellular signal transduction, and cell-to-cell communication (Steiner et al., 2007). There are several S100B assays that can identify S100 AB and BB, however, there is still no consensus on the S100B reference range as of yet. Therefore, reference intervals for the population are needed for laboratories doing S100B tests, and patient studies need to have a control group that is typical of the community. S100B leaks into the CSF and enters the bloodstream as a result of brain damage through CSF circulation or a brief rupture of the BBB (Hampel et al., 2018). The kidneys break down S100 B, which is then eliminated in the urine. Following an acute injury, concentrations typically return to baseline within 24 hours; hence, prolonged elevations in S100 B might indicate continuing or secondary cellular damage (Raabe & Seifert, 2000). By triggering apoptosis, releasing proinflammatory cytokines and nitric oxide from astrocyte cells, and promoting oxidative stress, S100B may have a neurotoxic impact at higher doses (Steiner et al., 2007). Consequently, elevated amounts may both worsen and reflect tissue injury. Blood, urine, and CSF are just a few of the biological substances in which this protein is easily measured. It is a good option for routine monitoring in the lab and batch analysis in research as it does not deteriorate after freezing and is stable over a broad temperature range of 48 hours or more following collection (70 °C at room temperature) (Gazzolo et al., 2004).

There is an increase in S100B in a number of CNS disorders, such as stroke (Bertsch et al., 2001), subarachnoid haemorrhage (Wiesmann et al., 1997), Alzheimer's disease (Ghavami et al., 2014), dementia (Infante et al., 2003), and traumatic brain injury (Berger et al., 2007; Sandler et al., 2010). Skin, adipocytes, skeletal muscle, melanocytes and white and brown fat are examples of extracranial sources of S100B (Mazzini et al., 2009). Clinical reports of melanomas or lengthy bone injuries indicate elevated blood concentrations (Lamers et al., 2003).

Due to various developmental phases, S100B concentrations change from the fetal stage until old age (Tiu et al., 2000). Differential levels of S100B in cord blood and amniotic fluid correspond to different phases of fetal development, suggesting that elevated S100B within a healthy range may reflect its neurotrophic function in brain development (Gazzolo et al., 2001). Consequently, S100B's role in glial cell maturation, synaptic development, and general brain morphogenesis—all of which are more prevalent in the early stages of infancy—is most likely what accounts for the age-related variations in S100B concentrations (Portela et al., 2002).

Nonetheless, the age-related pattern of variability in the currently available studies is challenging to understand. Serum samples were obtained by Portela et al. (2002) from 3 distinct age categories of healthy donors: infants (4–16 years old), adults (18–70 years old), and adults. While no sex-based differences were discovered, there was a clear adverse relationship with S100B, with infants exhibiting the greatest amounts. By the age of twenty, the baseline concentrations appeared to be settled. In a comprehensive investigation comprising 1004 children between the ages of 0 and 15, Gazzolo et al. (2003) likewise found a relationship between age and S100B concentrations in blood. The periods with the greatest values were the first year of life and the years between seven and thirteen. The largest development and maturation spikes are thought to coincide with two eras: infancy and the early phases of adolescence, according to the authors' premise. There were also observed sex-based differences in S100B peaks, which might be another illustration of how the development process varies between the sexes. Serum S100B concentrations decreased with age, according to Bouvier et al. (2011). The results of their study on a kid cohort only demonstrated that the greatest S100B concentrations were observed before the age of two. This finding might be explained by the blood-brain barrier's permeability, accelerated turnover of proteins in neuronal cells, reduced synthesis of S100B in the kidneys, and dynamic CNS development in babies younger than two years old. Conversely, Spinella et al. (2004) found a significant correlation between CSF S100B and age after studying 107 pediatric patients whose ages ranged from 3 days to 17.8 years. Age was shown to have a significant positive correlation with S100B, but it only accounted for 4% of the variance. These results were verified in research done on adults, by Nygaard et al. (1997), who found that age increased the level of S100B in the CSF and that age explained 30% of the variability in women and 43% in men. Men had considerably greater overall S100B concentrations than women. S100B was not detected in the serum samples used in the investigation. Unlike the previously cited studies, Wiesmann et al. (1998) found no significant differences related to sex or age.

Because age appears to have the most impact early in life, the results across studies may seem inconsistent, depending on if children are included in the research or not. The heterogeneity of the normal cohorts chosen in order to create reference intervals is troublesome since, in addition, a significant percentage of the inter individual variance cannot be explained, and sample numbers per age group are often insufficient to adequately correct for this variability. Selecting "normal" samples is a subjective procedure as well. For invasive procedures such as lumbar punctures, for instance, study subjects with symptoms suggestive of a neurological illness may be selected, although, in other studies, subjects in perfect health have been selected. Consequently, the characteristics of the study populations are crucial factors to take into account to make when establishing reference values, contrasting controls and cases, or evaluating the function of S100B or any other biomarker conditions of sickness.

CNS INFECTION RESEARCH STUDIES

Experimental Studies

Bertsch et al. (2001) evaluated serum S100B in a CNS Candida albicans-infected animal model. They discovered that compared to control mice, concentrations in infected animals were considerably higher. They peaked one day after infection and then began to fall. S100B's kinetics seem to mimic the infectious process, in which pathogen entrance into the central nervous system triggers an instantaneous inflammatory response, cell lysis, and disruption of the blood-brain barrier. Tissue damage stops and S100B concentrations return to normal after the infection is controlled. Garnier et al. (2009) discovered that fetal lambs in utero exposed to infection experienced white matter impairment in a sheep model. The function of S100B as a marker of hypoxia distress in foetal sheep is revealed by an additional experimental paradigm. Elevated levels of plasma S100B have been linked to signs of metabolic acidosis, peripheral blood flow redistribution, and currently utilized markers of neonatal hypoxia (Giussani et al., 2005).

Clinical Studies in Adults

Adult patients with a range of neurological diseases, such as multiple sclerosis, hydrocephalus, meningitis, dementia, acute cerebral infarction, diseases of the motor neurons, and lymphatic leukemia, had their CSF analyzed by Infante et al. (2003). The groups who experienced meningitis, dementia, and acute cerebral infarction showed a considerable rise in S100B levels, with dementia being linked with the highest values. According to the authors, S100B in acute limiting damage may be reaching its peak early and quickly escape the system; in such a scenario when the sampling was conducted in relation to the injury's commencement is critical for correct evaluation. Long-term elevations in S100B most likely indicate persistent damage or glial cell activation by inflammation. Adults with cerebral infections had greater blood S100B levels than those with extracerebral infections. Patients with bacterial meningitis reported greater quantities than those with viral meningitis, while patients with viral encephalitis showed the greatest concentrations. These results are consistent with the known cellular damage linked to these illnesses. Nevertheless, despite radiological and clinical abnormalities, several of those patients with meningitis and encephalitis did not show elevated levels, indicating that S100B may occasionally give false-negative outcomes when employed as a marker of brain damage. Given that S100B is a protein generated from the brain; this result could be explained by the fact that the researchers used blood samples rather than CSF. Furthermore, sampling for one of these patients with encephalitis was done a few days after for the patients whose concentrations were higher; as S100B has been known to peak earlier in the course of the disease, the peak could have gone unnoticed (Infante et al., 2003; Lins et al., 2005). Additionally, the authors speculate that S100B could provide false-positive results since it was elevated in several instances with extracranial infections and no signs of cerebral involvement. Although the precise extracranial causes of these elevations in S100B remain unknown, in majority of these cases S100B was only slightly elevated and did not approach the high level associated with encephalitis. CNS infections were often the main cause of elevated S100B.

Clinical Studies in Children

After looking at reference values in newborns, Spinella et al. (2004) discovered that children with confirmed meningitis had considerably higher quantities of CSF S100B when comparing them to healthy children. In a study by Hamed et al. (2009), 40 children with bacterial meningitis had their S100B concentrations as well as indicators of oxidative stress and antioxidative activity measured. Serum and CSF samples both showed elevated S100B levels. These researchers argued that increased intrathecal synthesis of S100B and indicators of oxidative activity indicate brain damage resulting from bacterial meningitis, and that the quantities of these markers correlate with the degree of the injury. Increases in CSF S100B were seen in a study of 56 babies who had bacterial meningitis; the children who also had encephalitis had the highest levels.

Neuron-Specific Enolase

The dimer protein Enolase is made up of the α, β, and γ subunits, and is a glycolytic enzyme. The stable, cell-specific isoenzyme of enolase is called NSE (γ-enolase). NSE is mostly found in neurons as well as neuroendocrine cells, but it is also present in lymphocytes and smooth muscle, erythrocytes, and the liver; in the latter, it is often present in low quantities (10ng/mg) and is commonly in the hybrid (αδ) enolase type (Lamers et al., 2003). NSE is only found in the cytoplasm of neurons in the brain.

NSE shows signs of enzymatic activity and is a good indicator of the overall neuron function. Serum concentration reference intervals span from 5 to 15 ng/mL. NSE readily diffuses into the extracellular space and CSF with damage to neuronal membranes (Lima et al., 2004). Consequently, a number of cerebral pathologies, such as amyotrophic lateral sclerosis, cervical spondylosis, spinocerebellar degeneration, encephalitis, cerebral infarction, Parkinson's disease, polyradiculoneuritis, and traumatic brain injury, have been linked to elevated NSE concentrations in the CSF and serum (Berger et al., 2005). Additionally, NSE is elevated in pediatric neuroblastoma and small-cell lung cancer (Lamers et al., 2003).

The goal of Van Engelen et al. (1992) was to define reference values for MBP (myelin basic protein), S100B, and NSE. A total of 79 control patients, aged 1 to 60, had their CSF samples taken.Their results indicate a considerable rise with age, with a 1% annual median rise across all 3 indicators. This observation may be explained by a concurrent decrease in CSF bulk flow and/or a rise in cell and loss of myelin with ageing. Nygaard et al. (1998) examined the levels of CSF and blood NSE in healthy people between the ages of 20 and 90.

Age and sex did not differ in the serum, but there was a positive, significant correlation with age in the CSF, with greater levels in men. The rise in NSE with age, according to the authors, might be caused by a decrease in CSF bulk flow, an increase in NSE half-life, or increasing NSE concentrations in the face of steady cell turnover. Similar pathways might underlie sexual reliance. Furthermore, no relationship between the NSE concentrations in the two bodily fluids was found in this investigation. The correlation with age is not a constant finding, though. Rodriguez Nunez et al. (1999) investigated 37 children who have NSE in their CSF ranging in age from one month to thirteen years in a pediatric investigation. Their results did not point to a relationship with age. In a study of 108 adults alone, Casmiro et al. (NSE Study Group et al., 2005) examined serum and CSF levels and discovered a strong correlation with age; however, the majority of the patients in their sample were over 60. There were no connections between CSF NSE and serum, nor were there any correlations between sex and NSE concentrations.

Together with the findings of Nygaard et al. (1998), these results imply that serum cannot replace CSF and that the existence of CNS damage is not always ruled out by serum NSE within the reference period, albeit further testing in a patient sample with CNS illness is needed to confirm this. The same restrictions and cautious interpretation apply to research on NSE reference intervals as they do to S100B.

Studies in CNS Infections

The concentrations of NSE in CNS infection experimental models have not been studied, as far as the authors know. However, as ischemia is a significant predictor of poor outcomes in CNS infections, an investigation of NSE in a model of ischemia rats is pertinent. Hardemark et al. (1988) sampled CSF in the middle cerebral artery both before and after closure over a few days in order to link NSE concentrations with the size and progression of infarcts in rats. After occlusion, NSE peaked between 24 and 72 hours later, and it took six days for it to return to baseline. The area under the NSE concentration curve and NSE concentrations were substantially linked with infarct size. These results imply that the size and progression of infarcts are reflected in the sequential examination of CSF NSE. The dynamic aspect of the ischemia process, which can last for many days and varies between individuals, is reflected in the temporal change of NSE. Therefore, it is crucial to take into account when sampling should be done as the damage develops.

The relationship between NSE concentrations and the degree of neurological damage was investigated by Lima et al. (2004). 51 individuals, of which 11 have meningitis, 7 with encephalic traumas, 25 individuals with neurocysticercosis and 8 control healthy individuals—had blood and CSF samples taken. Age or sex disparities were not discovered. NSE was exclusively elevated in CSF and in the group with encephalic injury. It is important to note that none of the meningitis group had neurological impairments; therefore it is questionable how much neurological damage was sustained. In contrast to controls, Song et al. (2012) assessed NSE in the serum and CSF of adult individuals with aseptic meningitis (n = 28) and tuberculous meningitis (TBM) (n = 15).The ratio of CSF to serum NSE was considerably greater in the TBM group, despite the fact that serum and CSF NSE concentrations did not differ significantly among the three groups. This ratio's potential use as a marker for diagnosis was demonstrated by the substantial correlation it showed between it and the TBM diagnosis in both univariate and multivariate analyses. This study's tiny sample size gives an incomplete picture of meningitis-related NSE concentrations.

There is a paucity of literature on biomarkers for pediatric brain damage, with the majority of the studies focusing on traumatic brain injury (Berger et al., 2005; Sandler et al., 2010). In order to determine the value of CSF indicators of cell hypoxia and NSE in the differential diagnosis of meningitis, Rodriguez-Nunez et al. (2003) looked at these markers. NSE concentrations in cases of bacterial meningitis and tuberculosis meningitis were not significantly more than those in the controls, nor did they differ based on sex or between meningitis groups, according to their examination of 160 children in control and 100 children with meningitis caused by bacteria, viruses, or tuberculosis. The only group with a significantly elevated NSE was the viral meningitis group; however, this was explained by the fact that nine patients with mumps aetiology had the highest total NSE concentrations. This study had two limitations: first, the TBM group was extremely small, consisting of just 0.9% of the cases of meningitis; second, the CSF samples were taken at an extremely early stage of the disease (1–16 hours following the beginning of symptoms). It is possible that the samples were obtained before hypoxia was strong enough to trigger cell death and raise NSE, as experimental studies in animal models revealed that NSE tended to rise beyond 24 hours postinjury (Hårdemark et al., 1988). The CSF and serum NSE concentrations of 20 children who are comatose with Reye syndrome, acute encephalopathy, and acute encephalitis were shown to be considerably higher in these individuals than in the controls NSE was linked to neurological impairment and was greater at first, then increased with time in individuals with more severe brain injury and worse prognoses. Their results confirm the variation in NSE concentrations amongst patients and at different phases of the illness. The authors of this study discovered a strong association between serum and CSF NSE, in contrast to previous research.

Combining Biomarkers

For individuals suffering from both bacterial and viral meningitis, Lins et al. (Giussani et al., 2005) sequentially linked CSF and serum tests of S100B and NSE. Serum and CSF S100B levels were considerably higher in individuals with bacterial meningitis alone, according to results from 32 adult patients. Elevated levels of S100B were linked to increased CSF/serum albumin ratios and lesions on computed tomography or MRI. S100B declined in the majority of patients following the initial samples, with the exception of a patient with TBM, whose biomarker concentrations in blood and CSF increased and peaked on day 27. This study did not show a substantial rise in NSE. Among those patients who have a variety of neurological diseases, such as meningitis, encephalitis, cerebral infarction, sclerosis, Parkinson's disease, among other conditions, looked at CSF S100B and NSE. Although not necessarily at the same time, NSE and S100B levels were raised in a number of these circumstances, indicating that the sort of tissue injury—glial vs neuronal—may be reflected in their presence. Before NSE concentrations normalizing, S100B concentrations did so sooner, and concentrations were greatest in cases of encephalitis and cerebral infarction.

Other Potential Biomarkers

While the majority of research in the literature focuses on S100B and NSE, additional biomarkers are also being studied. Van Engelen et al. (1992) investigated CSF concentrations of S100B, NSE, and MBP (myelin basic protein), a marker of the degradation of myelin, in a case series of three individuals suffering from cerebral infective illness. All three biomarker concentrations were found to be elevated, and their relative values were found to correspond with the kind of damage; MBP concentrations were greater than S100B and NSE concentrations in individuals with demyelinating diseases. Children who had acute encephalopathy or encephalitis were studied by Tsukahara et al. (2013) for CSF S100B, GFAP (glial fibrillary acidic protein), a marker of glial damage, and tau protein, a microtubule-associated protein present in neuronal axons. S100B exhibited the strongest predictive accuracy in terms of outcome, and concentrations of CSF biomarkers were only elevated in individuals who had bad outcomes. While the tau protein exhibited 85% specificity and 70% sensitivity, GFAP had a weak sensitivity of 40% but a very high specificity of 100%. The optimal predictive value for the result was achieved by combining multiple markers. Grahn et al. (2013) evaluated CSF S100B, GFAP, and neurofilament protein light chain (NFL), a putative marker of neuronal damage, in a cohort of patients with CNS infections caused by the varicella zoster virus. The NFL and GFAP had the largest and longest increases, respectively, whereas the concentrations of S100B were within the reference ranges. This implies that astrogliosis may have been a part of the damage while the cell membrane of an astrocyte was still intact and that NFL elevation may have been caused by a chronic or subsequent lesion. Research on biomarkers for adult encephalitis is summarized in a review conducted by Bonneh Barkay and colleagues (Bonneh-Barkay & Hayasaka, 2011); soluble Fas (an apoptotic marker) and CSF NSE, S100B, GFAP, NFL, and other proinflammatory cytokines were found in HSV encephalitis. In cases of influenza-associated encephalitis, the interleukin-6 cytokines and tumor necrosis factor-along with their metabolites, showed potential. Research was done on CSF S100B and NFL in cases of West Nile virus encephalitis. Studies on HIV encephalitis have looked at CSF HIV-1 RNA, immune-stimulating agents such as neopterin, and inflammatory markers. Proteomics, metabolomics, transcriptomics, and genomics advances provide avenues for examining different molecular features of the host-pathogen relationship in CNS infections. Among these are metabolic or molecular signatures unique to a pathogen, changes in patterns of gene expression in hosts caused by the pathogen, genetic predisposition to infections, genetic variation between individuals as a response to being exposed to pathogens, and the relationship between patterns of gene expression and the course of a disease. Therefore, these technologies have the capacity to find biomarkers that might lead to an accurate diagnosis of the disease. and the pathogen causing it, enable early selection of the most appropriate course of treatment, identify patients who are more likely to experience a poor prognosis and severe disease, and enable treatment that is customized to the unique characteristics of both the host and the pathogen. However, this subject is still in its infancy, especially when it comes to CNS infections (Brand et al., 2010). Pneumococcal meningitis patients'

CSF protein composition was examined using 2-dimensional gel electrophoresis by Goonetilleke et al. (2010) in the realm of proteomics. Increases in a number of proteins were linked to cellular damage, inflammation, and metabolic disruption in non-survivors; these findings may offer new insights into potential biomarkers and therapeutic targets. 18 proteins with differential expression were discovered by Kataria et al. (2011) in a proteomics investigation conducted on the CSF of TBM patients. GFAP, a sign of tissue damage, antithrombin-III, an indicator of the role that coagulation pathways play, and arachidonate 5-lipoxygenase, which weakens the host's immunological responses and contributes to the pathophysiology of tuberculosis, were among the upregulated proteins of human origin. Human proteins that were down regulated included transthyretin, which helps to lessen inflammation, brain edema, and neuronal death, and apolipoprotein E and A-1, which are significant for their anti-inflammatory qualities as well as for neural development and repair, immunological control, and neural growth. Mycobacterial proteins found in the CSF may serve as diagnostic markers for meningitis patients, enabling prompt identification of the etiological agent. High-throughput technology called metabolomics makes it possible to analyze all of the metabolites that are present in biological samples comprehensively and objectively. Because it offers insight into the cumulative impacts of the infected organism's metabolites, inflammatory cells, and brain cellular responses to pathogens and medicines, it is increasingly being exploited in drug development, therapeutics, and disease diagnostics (Zhang et al., 2012). Coen et al. (2005) improved the accuracy of regular CSF cell counts and chemical assays and showed that metabolomics of the CSF may be used to quickly detect meningitis and ventriculitis in patients. Subramanian et al. (2005) created an expert system that uses a special mix of clinical characteristics and metabolic fingerprints to help with the differential diagnosis of meningitis.

FUTURE WORK

It is necessary to do more thorough research using larger panels of markers. In addition to being helpful in monitoring damage to different tissue types, a combination of neurological indicators may also lessen the impact of extracranial sources. Combining indicators for inflammation and tissue damage has shown to have significant predictive value in traumatic brain injury and may also be helpful in cases of central nervous system infections. There isn't much research on CNS infections that look at biomarkers and outcomes. Finding the strength of the relationships with biomarkers in viral damage is crucial since these are the current methods available. Numerous studies have established strong connections between biomarker levels and clinical and radiological outcomes in traumatic brain injury (TBI) (Berger et al., 2007; Townend & Ingebrigtsen, 2006).

CONFLICT OF INTEREST

The authors declare no conflicts of interest exist.

REFERENCES

Akter, R., Chowdhury, M. A. R., & Rahman, M. H. (2021). Flavonoids and polyphenolic compounds as potential talented agents for the treatment of Alzheimer's disease and their antioxidant activities. *Current Pharmaceutical Design*, *27*(3), 345–356. DOI: 10.2174/1381612826666200515120047

Akter, R., Rahman, M. H., Behl, T., Chowdhury, M. A. R., Manirujjaman, M., Bulbul, I. J., Elshenaw, S. E., Tit, D. M., & Bungau, S. (2021). Prospective role of polyphenolic compounds in the treatment of neurodegenerative diseases. *CNS & Neurological Disorders - Drug Targets*, *20*(5), 430–450. DOI: 10.2174/18715273 20666210218084449

Al-Obaidi, M. M. J., & Desa, M. N. M. (2018). Mechanisms of blood brain barrier disruption by different types of bacteria, and bacterial–host interactions facilitate the bacterial pathogen invading the brain. *Cellular and Molecular Neurobiology*, *38*(7), 1349–1368. DOI: 10.1007/s10571-018-0619-z

Berger, R. P. (2006). The use of serum biomarkers to predict outcome after traumatic brain injury in adults and children. *The Journal of Head Trauma Rehabilitation*, *21*(4), 315–333. DOI: 10.1097/00001199-200607000-00010

Berger, R. P., Adelson, P. D., Pierce, M. C., Dulani, T., Cassidy, L. D., & Kochanek, P. M. (2005). Serum neuron-specific enolase, S100B, and myelin basic protein concentrations after inflicted and noninflicted traumatic brain injury in children. *Journal of Neurosurgery. Pediatrics*, *103*(1), 61–68. DOI: 10.3171/ped.2005.103.1.0061

Berger, R. P., Beers, S. R., Richichi, R., Wiesman, D., & Adelson, P. D. (2007). Serum biomarker concentrations and outcome after pediatric traumatic brain injury. *Journal of Neurotrauma*, *24*(12), 1793–1801. DOI: 10.1089/neu.2007.0368

Bertsch, T., Casarin, W., Kretschmar, M., Zimmer, W., Walter, S., Sommer, C., Muehlhauser, F., Ragoschke, A., Kuehl, S., Schmidt, R., & Pohlmann-Eden, B. (2001). Protein S-100B: A serum marker for ischemic and infectious injury of cerebral tissue. *Clinical Chemistry and Laboratory Medicine*, *39*(4), 319–323. DOI: 10.1515/CCLM.2001.050

Bhattacharya, T., Dey, P. S., Akter, R., Kabir, M. T., Rahman, M. H., & Rauf, A. (2021). Effect of natural leaf extracts as phytomedicine in curing geriatrics. *Experimental Gerontology*, *150*, 111352. Advance online publication. DOI: 10.1016/j.exger.2021.111352

Bonneh-Barkay, D., & Hayasaka, D. (2011). Biomarkers of encephalitis. In *Pathogenesis of encephalitis*. InTech. DOI: 10.5772/28567

Böttiger, B. W., Möbes, S., Glätzer, R., Bauer, H., Gries, A., Bärtsch, P., Motsch, J., & Martin, E. (2001). Astroglial protein S-100 is an early and sensitive marker of hypoxic brain damage and outcome after cardiac arrest in humans. *Circulation*, *103*(22), 2694–2698. DOI: 10.1161/01.CIR.103.22.2694

Bouvier, D., Castellani, C., Fournier, M., Dauphin, J. B., Ughetto, S., Breton, M., Labbé, A., Weinberg, A. M., & Sapin, V. (2011). Reference ranges for serum S100B protein during the first three years of life. *Clinical Biochemistry*, *44*(10-11), 927–929. DOI: 10.1016/j.clinbiochem.2011.04.012

Brand, H. K., Hermans, P. W. M., & de Groot, R. (2010). Host biomarkers and paediatric infectious diseases: From molecular profiles to clinical application. In *Hot topics in infection and immunity in children VI* (pp. 19–31). Springer.

Brew, B. J., Crowe, S. M., Landay, A., Cysique, L. A., & Guillemin, G. (2009). Neurodegeneration and ageing in the HAART era. *Journal of Neuroimmune Pharmacology*, *4*(2), 163–174. DOI: 10.1007/s11481-008-9143-3

Butterfield, L. H., Potter, D. M., & Kirkwood, J. M. (2011). Multiplex serum biomarker assessments: Technical and biostatistical issues. *Journal of Translational Medicine*, *9*, 173. Advance online publication. DOI: 10.1186/1479-5876-9-173

Casmiro, M., Maitan, S., De Pasquale, F., Cova, V., Scarpa, E., & Vignatelli, L.NSE Study Group. (2005). Cerebrospinal fluid and serum neuron-specific enolase concentrations in a normal population. *European Journal of Neurology*, *12*(5), 369–374. DOI: 10.1111/j.1468-1331.2004.00985.x

Chang, J. R., Mukerjee, R., Bagashev, A., Del Valle, L., Chabrashvili, T., Hawkins, B. J., He, J. J., & Sawaya, B. E. (2011). HIV-1 Tat protein promotes neuronal dysfunction through disruption of microRNAs. *The Journal of Biological Chemistry*, *286*(47), 41125–41134. DOI: 10.1074/jbc.M111.268466

Chitnis, T., & Weiner, H. L. (2017). CNS inflammation and neurodegeneration. *The Journal of Clinical Investigation*, *127*(10), 3577–3587. DOI: 10.1172/JCI90609

Coen, M., O'Sullivan, M., Bubb, W. A., Kuchel, P. W., & Sorrell, T. (2005). Proton nuclear magnetic resonance—Based metabonomics for rapid diagnosis of meningitis and ventriculitis. *Clinical Infectious Diseases*, *41*(11), 1582–1590. DOI: 10.1086/497832

Deutschman, C. S., & Tracey, K. J. (2014). Sepsis: Current dogma and new perspectives. *Immunity*, *40*(4), 463–475. DOI: 10.1016/j.immuni.2014.04.001

Dugger, B. N., & Dickson, D. W. (2017). Pathology of neurodegenerative diseases. *Cold Spring Harbor Perspectives in Biology*, *9*(7), a028035. Advance online publication. DOI: 10.1101/cshperspect.a028035

El Aidy, S., Dinan, T. G., & Cryan, J. F. (2014). Immune modulation of the brain-gut-microbe axis. *Frontiers in Microbiology*, *5*, 146. Advance online publication. DOI: 10.3389/fmicb.2014.00146

Fahn, S. (2018). The 200-year journey of Parkinson disease: Reflecting on the past and looking towards the future. *Parkinsonism & Related Disorders*, *46*(Suppl. 1), S1–S5. DOI: 10.1016/j.parkreldis.2017.07.020

Franceschi, C., Garagnani, P., Parini, P., Giuliani, C., & Santoro, A. (2018). Inflammaging: A new immune–metabolic viewpoint for age-related diseases. *Nature Reviews. Endocrinology*, *14*(10), 576–590. DOI: 10.1038/s41574-018-0059-4

Garnier, Y., Frigiola, A., Li Volti, G., Florio, P., Frulio, R., Berger, R., Alm, S., Von Duering, M. U., Coumans, A. B., Reis, F. M., Petraglia, F., & Huppertz, B. (2009). Increased maternal/fetal blood S100B levels following systemic endotoxin administration and periventricular white matter injury in preterm fetal sheep. *Reproductive Sciences (Thousand Oaks, Calif.)*, *16*(8), 758–766. DOI: 10.1177/1933719109335801

Gazzolo, D., Bruschettini, M., Corvino, V., Oliva, R., Sarli, R., Lituania, M., Bruschettini, P., & Michetti, F. (2001). S100B protein concentrations in amniotic fluid correlate with gestational age and with cerebral ultrasound scanning results in healthy fetuses. *Clinical Chemistry*, *47*(5), 954–956. DOI: 10.1093/clinchem/47.5.954

Gazzolo, D., Frulio, R., Bruschettini, P., Lituania, M., & Michetti, F. (2004). Effects of temperature on pre-analytical stability of S100B protein concentrations in urine of healthy full-term infants. *Clinica Chimica Acta*, *350*(1-2), 231–232. DOI: 10.1016/j.cccn.2004.08.001

Gazzolo, D., Michetti, F., Bruschettini, M., Marchese, N., Lituania, M., Mangraviti, S., Pedrazzi, E., & Bruschettini, P. (2003). Pediatric concentrations of S100B protein in blood: Age- and sex-related changes. *Clinical Chemistry*, *49*(6), 967–970. DOI: 10.1373/49.6.967

Ghavami, S., Shojaei, S., Yeganeh, B., Ande, S. R., Jangamreddy, J. R., Mehrpour, M., Christoffersson, J., Chaabane, W., Moghadam, A. R., Kashani, H. H., Hashemi, M., Owji, A. A., & Łos, M. J. (2014). Autophagy and apoptosis dysfunction in neurodegenerative disorders. *Progress in Neurobiology*, *112*, 24–49. DOI: 10.1016/j.pneurobio.2013.10.004

Giussani, D. A., Thakor, A. S., Frulio, R., & Gazzolo, D. (2005). Acute hypoxia increases S100β protein in association with blood flow redistribution away from peripheral circulations in fetal sheep. *Pediatric Research*, *58*(2), 179–184. DOI: 10.1203/01.PDR.0000169993.39867.5B

Golde, T. E., & Miller, V. M. (2009). Proteinopathy-induced neuronal senescence: A hypothesis for brain failure in Alzheimer's and other neurodegenerative diseases. *Alzheimer's Research & Therapy*, *1*(1), 5. Advance online publication. DOI: 10.1186/alzrt5

Goonetilleke, U. R., Scarborough, M., Ward, S. A., & Gordon, S. B. (2010). Proteomic analysis of cerebrospinal fluid in pneumococcal meningitis reveals potential biomarkers associated with survival. *The Journal of Infectious Diseases*, *202*(4), 542–550. DOI: 10.1086/654819

Grahn, A., Hagberg, L., Nilsson, S., Blennow, K., Zetterberg, H., & Studahl, M. (2013). Cerebrospinal fluid biomarkers in patients with varicella-zoster virus CNS infections. *Journal of Neurology*, *260*(7), 1813–1821. DOI: 10.1007/s00415-013-6883-5

Hamed, S. A., Hamed, E. A., & Zakary, M. M. (2009). Oxidative stress and S-100B protein in children with bacterial meningitis. *BMC Neurology*, *9*, 51. Advance online publication. DOI: 10.1186/1471-2377-9-51

Hampel, H., O'Bryant, S. E., Molinuevo, J. L., Zetterberg, H., Masters, C. L., Lista, S., Kiddle, S. J., Batrla, R., & Blennow, K. (2018). Blood-based biomarkers for Alzheimer disease: Mapping the road to the clinic. *Nature Reviews. Neurology*, *14*(11), 639–652. DOI: 10.1038/s41582-018-0079-7

Hansson, O. (2021). Biomarkers for neurodegenerative diseases. *Nature Medicine*, *27*(6), 954–963. DOI: 10.1038/s41591-021-01382-x

Hårdemark, H. G., Persson, L., Bolander, H. G., Hillered, L., Olsson, Y., & Påhlman, S. (1988). Neuron-specific enolase is a marker of cerebral ischemia and infarct size in rat cerebrospinal fluid. *Stroke*, *19*(9), 1140–1144. DOI: 10.1161/01.STR.19.9.1140

Infante, J. R., Martínez, A., Ochoa, J., Cañadillas, F., Torres-Avisbal, M., Vallejo, J. A., González, F. M., Pacheco, C., & Latre, J. M. (2003). Cerebrospinal fluid S-100 protein levels in neurological pathologies. *Journal of Physiology and Biochemistry, 59*(4), 255–261. DOI: 10.1007/BF03179892

Ito, Y., Ofengeim, D., Najafov, A., Das, S., Saberi, S., Li, Y., Hitomi, J., Zhu, H., Chen, H., Mayo, L., Geng, J., Elliott, J. L., & Yuan, J. (2016). RIPK1 mediates axonal degeneration by promoting inflammation and necroptosis in ALS. *Science, 353*(6299), 603–608. DOI: 10.1126/science.aaf6803

Jellinger, K. A. (2009). Recent advances in our understanding of neurodegeneration. *Journal of Neural Transmission (Vienna, Austria), 116*(9), 1111–1162. DOI: 10.1007/s00702-009-0240-y

Jeltsch-David, H., & Muller, S. (2014). Neuropsychiatric systemic lupus erythematosus: Pathogenesis and biomarkers. *Nature Reviews. Neurology, 10*(10), 579–596. DOI: 10.1038/nrneurol.2014.148

Ji, H., Rabbi, M. F., Labis, B., Pavlov, V. A., Tracey, K. J., & Ghia, J. E. (2014). Central cholinergic activation of a vagus nerve-to-spleen circuit alleviates experimental colitis. *Mucosal Immunology, 7*(2), 335–347. DOI: 10.1038/mi.2013.52

Jung, Y. J., Tweedie, D., Scerba, M. T., & Greig, N. H. (2019). Neuroinflammation as a factor of neurodegenerative disease: Thalidomide analogs as treatments. *Frontiers in Cell and Developmental Biology, 7*, 313. Advance online publication. DOI: 10.3389/fcell.2019.00313

Karthika, C., Hari, B., Rahman, M. H., Akter, R., Najda, A., Albadrani, G. M., Sayed, A. A., Akhtar, M. F., & Abdel-Daim, M. M. (2021). Multiple strategies with the synergistic approach for addressing colorectal cancer. *Biomedicine and Pharmacotherapy, 140*, 111704. Advance online publication. DOI: 10.1016/j.biopha.2021.111704

Kataria, J., Rukmangadachar, L. A., Hariprasad, G., Jithesh, O., Tripathi, M., & Srinivasan, A. (2011). Two dimensional difference gel electrophoresis analysis of cerebrospinal fluid in tuberculous meningitis patients. *Journal of Proteomics, 74*(10), 2194–2203. DOI: 10.1016/j.jprot.2011.06.020

Knopman, D. S., Amieva, H., Petersen, R. C., Chételat, G., Holtzman, D. M., Hyman, B. T., Nixon, R. A., & Jones, D. T. (2021). Alzheimer disease. *Nature Reviews. Disease Primers, 7*, 33. Advance online publication. DOI: 10.1038/s41572-021-00269-y

Kobeissi, Z. A., & Zanotti-Cavazzoni, S. L. (2010). Biomarkers of sepsis. *The Year Book of Critical Care Medicine, 227–228*. Advance online publication. DOI: 10.1016/S0733-8627(10)28015-5

Kovacs, G. G., Robinson, J. L., Xie, S. X., Lee, E. B., Grossman, M., Wolk, D. A., Irwin, D. J., Weintraub, D., Kim, C. F., Schuck, T., Yousef, A., Wagner, J. A., Trojanowski, J. Q., & Lee, V. M.-Y. (2017). Evaluating the patterns of aging-related tau astrogliopathy unravels novel insights into brain aging and neurodegenerative diseases. *Journal of Neuropathology and Experimental Neurology, 76*(4), 270–288. DOI: 10.1093/jnen/nlx007

Kuhle, J., & Petzold, A. (2011). What makes a prognostic biomarker in CNS diseases: Strategies for targeted biomarker discovery? Part 1: Acute and monophasic diseases. *Expert Opinion on Medical Diagnostics, 5*(4), 333–346. DOI: 10.1517/17530059.2011.586072

Lamers, K. J. B., van Engelen, B. G. M., Gabreels, F. J. M., Hommes, O. R., Borm, G. F., & Wevers, R. A. (1995). Cerebrospinal neuron-specific enolase, S-100 and myelin basic protein in neurological disorders. *Acta Neurologica Scandinavica, 92*(3), 247–251. DOI: 10.1111/j.1600-0404.1995.tb01694.x

Lamers, K. J. B., Vos, P., Verbeek, M. M., Rosmalen, F., van Geel, W. J. A., & van Engelen, B. G. (2003). Protein S-100B, neuron-specific enolase (NSE), myelin basic protein (MBP) and glial fibrillary acidic protein (GFAP) in cerebrospinal fluid (CSF) and blood of neurological patients. *Brain Research Bulletin, 61*(3), 261–264. DOI: 10.1016/S0361-9230(03)00033-X

Lima, J. E., Takayanagui, O. M., Garcia, L. V., & Leite, J. P. (2004). Use of neuron-specific enolase for assessing the severity and outcome of neurological disorders in patients. *Brazilian Journal of Medical and Biological Research = Revista Brasileira de Pesquisas Médicas e Biológicas, 37*(1), 19–26. DOI: 10.1590/S0100-879X2004000100003

Lins, H., Wallesch, C. W., & Wunderlich, M. T. (2005). Sequential analyses of neurobiochemical markers of cerebral damage in cerebrospinal fluid and serum in CNS infections. *Acta Neurologica Scandinavica, 112*(5), 303–308. DOI: 10.1111/j.1600-0404.2005.00491.x

Long, J. M., & Holtzman, D. M. (2019). Alzheimer disease: An update on pathobiology and treatment strategies. *Cell, 179*(2), 312–339. DOI: 10.1016/j.cell.2019.09.001

Lucchinetti, C. F., Guo, Y., Popescu, B. F., Fujihara, K., Itoyama, Y., & Misu, T. (2014). The pathology of an autoimmune astrocytopathy: Lessons learned from neuromyelitis optica. *Brain Pathology (Zurich, Switzerland)*, *24*(1), 83–97. DOI: 10.1111/bpa.12099

Mak, A., Cheung, M. W. L., Chiew, H. J., Liu, Y., & Ho, R. C. M. (2012). Global trend of survival and damage of systemic lupus erythematosus: Meta-analysis and meta-regression of observational studies from the 1950s to 2000s. *Seminars in Arthritis and Rheumatism*, *41*(6), 830–839. DOI: 10.1016/j.semarthrit.2011.11.002

Mauffrey, P., Tchitchek, N., Barroca, V., Bemelmans, A. P., Firlej, V., Allory, Y., Roméo, P. H., & Magnon, C. (2019). Progenitors from the central nervous system drive neurogenesis in cancer. *Nature*, *569*(7758), 672–678. DOI: 10.1038/s41586-019-1219-y

Mazzini, G. S., Souza, D. O., & Portela, L. V. (2009). The ischemic heart as an extracerebral source for S100B. *Resuscitation*, *80*(1), 144. DOI: 10.1016/j.resuscitation.2008.09.015

Nygaard, A., Langbakk, B., & Romner, B. (1998). Neuron-specific enolase concentrations in serum and cerebrospinal fluid in patients with no previous history of neurological disorder. *Scandinavian Journal of Clinical and Laboratory Investigation*, *58*(3), 183–186. DOI: 10.1080/00365519850186403

Nygaard, Ø., Langbakk, B., & Romner, B. (1997). Age- and sex-related changes of S-100 protein concentrations in cerebrospinal fluid and serum in patients with no previous history of neurological disorder. *Clinical Chemistry*, *43*(3), 541–543. DOI: 10.1093/clinchem/43.3.541

Peng, C., Trojanowski, J. Q., & Lee, V. M.-Y. (2020). Protein transmission in neurodegenerative disease. *Nature Reviews. Neurology*, *16*(4), 199–212. DOI: 10.1038/s41582-020-0313-2

Perrachione, T. K., & Perrachione, J. R. (2008). Brains and brands: Developing mutually informative research in neuroscience and marketing. *Journal of Consumer Behaviour*, *7*(4-5), 303–318. DOI: 10.1002/cb.257

Portela, L. V., Tort, A. B., Schaf, D. V., Ribeiro, L., Nora, D. B., Walz, R., Rotta, L. N., Silva, C. T., Busnello, J. V., Kapczinski, F., & Gonçalves, C. A. (2002). The serum S100B concentration is age dependent. *Clinical Chemistry*, *48*(6), 950–952. DOI: 10.1093/clinchem/48.6.950

Raabe, A., & Seifert, V. (2000). Protein S-100B as a serum marker of brain damage in severe head injury: Preliminary results. *Neurosurgical Review, 23*(3), 136–138. DOI: 10.1007/PL00011941

Rahman, M. H., Akter, R., & Kamal, M. A. (2021). Prospective function of different antioxidant containing natural products in the treatment of neurodegenerative diseases. *CNS & Neurological Disorders - Drug Targets, 20*(8), 694–703. DOI: 10.2174/1871527320666210218084449

Rahman, M. H., Bajgai, J., Fadriquela, A., Sharma, S., Trinh, T. T., Akter, R., Jeong, Y. J., Goh, S. H., Kim, C. S., & Lee, K. J. (2021). Therapeutic potential of natural products in treating neurodegenerative disorders and their future prospects and challenges. *Molecules (Basel, Switzerland), 26*(17), 5327. Advance online publication. DOI: 10.3390/molecules26175327

Rahman, M. H., Bajgai, J., Fadriquela, A., Sharma, S., Trinh Thi, T., Akter, R., Goh, S. H., Kim, C. S., & Lee, K. J. (2021). Redox effects of molecular hydrogen and its therapeutic efficacy in the treatment of neurodegenerative diseases. *Processes (Basel, Switzerland), 9*(2), 308. Advance online publication. DOI: 10.3390/pr9020308

Re, D. B., Le Verche, V., Yu, C., Amoroso, M. W., Politi, K. A., Phani, S., Ikiz, B., Hoffmann, L., Koolen, M., Nagata, T., Papadimitriou, D., Willey, J., Cleveland, D. W., Henderson, C. E., & Przedborski, S. (2014). Necroptosis drives motor neuron death in models of both sporadic and familial ALS. *Neuron, 81*(5), 1001–1008. DOI: 10.1016/j.neuron.2014.01.011

Rodríguez-Núñez, A., Cid, E., Eirís, J., Rodríguez-García, J., Camiña, F., Rodríguez-Segade, S., & Castro-Gago, M. (1999). Neuron-specific enolase levels in the cerebrospinal fluid of neurologically healthy children. *Brain & Development, 21*(1), 16–19. DOI: 10.1016/S0387-7604(98)00058-0

Rodríguez-Núñez, A., Cid, E., Rodríguez-García, J., Camiña, F., Rodríguez-Segade, S., & Castro-Gago, M. (2003). Neuron-specific enolase, nucleotides, nucleosides, purine bases, oxypurines and uric acid concentrations in cerebrospinal fluid of children with meningitis. *Brain & Development, 25*(2), 102–106. DOI: 10.1016/S0387-7604(02)00180-5

Sandler, S. J., Figaji, A. A., & Adelson, P. D. (2010). Clinical applications of biomarkers in pediatric traumatic brain injury. *Child's Nervous System, 26*(2), 205–213. DOI: 10.1007/s00381-009-0998-2

Schneider, A., Sari, A. T., Alhaddad, H., & Sari, Y. (2020). Overview of therapeutic drugs and methods for the treatment of Parkinson's disease. *CNS & Neurological Disorders - Drug Targets*, *19*(3), 195–206. DOI: 10.2174/1871527319666200402095644

Sierksma, A., Escott-Price, V., & De Strooper, B. (2020). Translating genetic risk of Alzheimer's disease into mechanistic insight and drug targets. *Science*, *370*(6512), 61–66. DOI: 10.1126/science.abb8575

Song, T. J., Choi, Y. C., Lee, K. Y., & Kim, W. J. (2012). Serum and cerebrospinal fluid neuron-specific enolase for diagnosis of tuberculous meningitis. *Yonsei Medical Journal*, *53*(6), 1068–1072. DOI: 10.3349/ymj.2012.53.6.1068

Spinella, P. C., Donoghue, A., Rajendra, A., Drott, H. R., Dominguez, T. E., & Helfaer, M. (2004). Cerebrospinal fluid levels of S-100β in children and its elevation in pediatric meningitis. *Pediatric Critical Care Medicine*, *5*(1), 53–57. DOI: 10.1097/01.PCC.0000102395.31510.4E

Steiner, J., Bernstein, H. G., Bielau, H., Berndt, A., Brisch, R., Mawrin, C., Keilhoff, G., & Bogerts, B. (2007). Evidence for a wide extra-astrocytic distribution of S100B in human brain. *BMC Neuroscience*, *8*, 2. Advance online publication. DOI: 10.1186/1471-2202-8-2

Subramanian, A., Gupta, A., Saxena, S., Gupta, A., Kumar, R., Nigam, A., Kumar, R., Mandal, S. K., & Roy, R. (2005). Proton MR CSF analysis and a new software as predictors for the differentiation of meningitis in children. *NMR in Biomedicine*, *18*(4), 213–225. DOI: 10.1002/nbm.942

Teunissen, C. E., Tumani, H., Bennett, J. L., Berven, F. S., Brundin, L., Comabella, M., Franciotta, D., Frederiksen, J. L., Fleming, J. O., Furlan, R., Hintzen, R. Q., Hughes, S. G., Jiménez Jiménez, F. J., Kroksveen, A. C., Kuhle, J., Magnussen, J. S., Petzold, A., Persson, L., Villoslada, P., & Zetterberg, H. (2011). Consensus guidelines for CSF and blood biobanking for CNS biomarker studies. *Multiple Sclerosis International*, *2011*, 246412. Advance online publication. DOI: 10.1155/2011/246412

Tiu, S. C., Chan, W. Y., Heizmann, C. W., Schäfer, B. W., Shu, S. Y., & Yew, D. T. (2000). Differential expression of S100B and S100A6 in the human fetal and aged cerebral cortex. *Brain Research. Developmental Brain Research*, *119*(2), 159–168. DOI: 10.1016/S0165-3806(99)00176-5

Townend, W., & Ingebrigtsen, T. (2006). Head injury outcome prediction: A role for protein S-100B? *Injury*, *37*(12), 1098–1108. DOI: 10.1016/j.injury.2006.07.014

Tsukahara, H., Fujii, Y., Matsubara, K., Yamada, M., Nagaoka, Y., Saito, Y., Yashiro, M., Tsuge, M., Goto, S., Kitamura, T., & Hata, A. (2013). Prognostic value of brain injury biomarkers in acute encephalitis/encephalopathy. *Pediatrics International, 55*(4), 461–464. DOI: 10.1111/ped.12074

Van Engelen, B. G. M., Lamers, K. J. B., Gabreels, F. J. M., Wevers, R. A., Van Geel, W. J. A., & Borm, G. F. (1992). Age-related changes of neuron-specific enolase, S-100 protein, and myelin basic protein concentrations in cerebrospinal fluid. *Clinical Chemistry, 38*(6), 813–816. DOI: 10.1093/clinchem/38.6.813

Vives-Bauza, C., de Vries, R. L. A., Tocilescu, M., & Przedborski, S. (2010). PINK1/Parkin direct mitochondria to autophagy. *Autophagy, 6*(2), 315–316. DOI: 10.4161/auto.6.2.11103

Warsinke, A., Benkert, A., & Scheller, F. W. (2000). Electrochemical immunoassays. *Fresenius' Journal of Analytical Chemistry, 366*(6-7), 622–634. DOI: 10.1007/s002160051559

Wiesmann, M., Missler, U., & Gottmann, D. (1998). Plasma S-100b protein concentration in healthy adults is age- and sex-independent. *Clinical Chemistry, 44*(5), 1056–1058. DOI: 10.1093/clinchem/44.5.1056

Wiesmann, M., Missler, U., Hagenström, H., & Gottmann, D. (1997). Plasma S-100 protein levels after aneurysmal subarachnoid haemorrhage. *Acta Neurochirurgica, 139*(12), 1155–1160. DOI: 10.1007/BF01408577

Wu, S. C., Cao, Z. S., Chang, K. M., & Juang, J. L. (2017). Intestinal microbial dysbiosis aggravates the progression of Alzheimer's disease in Drosophila. *Nature Communications, 8*, 24. Advance online publication. DOI: 10.1038/s41467-017-00040-9

Zhang, A., Sun, H., Wang, P., Han, Y., & Wang, X. (2012). Recent and potential developments of biofluid analyses in metabolomics. *Journal of Proteomics, 75*(4), 1079–1088. DOI: 10.1016/j.jprot.2011.10.027

Chapter 8
Role of Neurotransmitters in CNS Infections and Non-Drug Approaches in Modulating Their Functions

Abraham Olufemi Asuku
https://orcid.org/0000-0003-0071-0531
Bioresources Development Centre, National Biotechnology Research and Development Agency, Nigeria

Grace Ayobami Fajemidagba
https://orcid.org/0000-0002-9587-9307
Redeemers University, Ede, Nigeria

ABSTRACT

Neurotransmitters play a crucial role in regulating the central nervous system (CNS) and preserving homeostasis and appropriate neuronal function. This chapter sheds light on the problems caused by bacterial, fungal, and viral pathogens as it examines the complex link between neurotransmitters and CNS diseases. The authors explore the complex processes by which these diseases modify the production, release, and reception of neurotransmitters, highlighting the significant consequences for the general health of the nervous system. This chapter also looks into non-pharmacological methods as workable ways to change neurotransmitter levels in CNS diseases. The knowledge offered here serves as a basis for upcoming investigations and the treatment plans are meant to maintain brain function even in the face of infections and other challenges.

DOI: 10.4018/979-8-3693-4070-7.ch008

INTRODUCTION

Brief Overview of the Central Nervous System

The nervous system is a sophisticated neural network that coordinates and regulates all bodily functions. It is essentially separated into two distinct sections: the peripheral and central nervous systems. The peripheral nervous system comprises two parts: the somatic nervous system, which supplies skeletal muscle, and the autonomic nervous system, which controls involuntary visceral functions, while the central nervous system (CNS) is in charge of processing information from the peripheral nervous system.

Component of the CNS

The CNS includes the brain and spinal cord. The brain is the body's primary control center, responsible for sensation, reactions, cognition, memory, learning, sensation, communication, emotions, behavior, and physical movement. Aside from these, it regulates and coordinates a variety of physiological systems such as vision, breathing, body temperature, thirst, sleep, blood pressure, and appetite (Asuku et al., 2024a).

Conversely, the spinal cord is the caudal branch of the central nervous system, responsible for transmitting motor orders from the brain to the peripheral body and passing sensory information from the sensory organs to the brain. It is segmented and has 31 pairs of spinal neurons with both efferent and afferent components. The afferent nerves carry impulses from the muscles, skin, joints, and visceral organs, whereas the efferent nerves contain motor nerves, both somatic and autonomic, and innervate cardiac, skeletal, and smooth muscle, as well as secretory cells and glandular tissues.

Importance of Neurotransmitters in CNS Functions

The fundamental purpose of the CNS (central nervous system) is to analyze information from and provide information to the nerves in the peripheral nervous system via synapses, which connect one neuron to another. Neurotransmitters, which are endogenous chemical transmitters that amplify, transmit, and convert signals in cells, transmit nerve impulses from one neuron to another, or send signals between nerves and other cell types, play a crucial part in transferring information throughout the nervous system. Hundreds of these compounds have been identified, with many of them concentrated in various brain regions and the spinal cord, where they have a direct or indirect role in practically all physiological activities of the CNS

(Figure 1). They are the main regulators of neuronal development, differentiation, and survival, and they play critical roles in brain function as well as the maintenance of knowledge connections all through the nervous system that regulate multiple behavioral and physiological processes in the human body (Teleanu *et al.*, 2022).

They are divided into several systems, including cholinergic, glutamatergic, GABAergic, dopaminergic, serotonergic, histaminergic, and aminergic, each of which has a unique role in the modulation of central nervous system processes (Nimgampalle *et al.*, 2023). For example, the cholinergic system in the CNS, which uses the neurotransmitter acetylcholine, is crucial for sensory and motor processes such as purposeful movement control, awareness, cognitive behavior, learning, memory, sleep, attention, and arousal. The glutamatergic system, which secretes the neurotransmitter glutamate, is critical for long-term potentiation, learning, and recall. It also controls various muscular, sensory, and autonomic functions (Iovino *et al.,* 2020).

The GABAergic system regulates anxiety, alertness, muscular tension, recall, and epileptogenic activity, which comprises neurons that produce the inhibitory neurotransmitter gamma-aminobutyric acid to avoid or block nerve impulses and end a specific function. The dopaminergic system, which contains neurons that generate the endogenous catecholamine dopamine, regulates physiological and behavioral functions such as cognition, motivation, and motion. The serotonergic system, which is made up of neurons that release serotonin (5-hydroxytryptamine), plays a significant role in regulating wake and sleep states, motor activity, cognition, depression, and the circadian rhythm, secretion from the gastrointestinal tract and peristalsis, respiration, body temperature, vasoconstriction, behavior (e.g., feeding behavior, appetite, aggressive behavior, mood, depression), and neurological function (Niyonambaza *et al.*, 2019; Ou *et al.*, 2019). Histaminergic neurons release histamine, which modulates various physiological and behavioral activities including inflammation, allergies, wakefulness, cognition, arousal, hunger, and depression. The adrenergic system, which includes norepinephrine, has been shown to have major functions in arousal and concentration in the waking state, perceptual signal detection, mood regulation, memory, learning, attention, and depression. Others include neuropeptide Y, the most abundant peptide in the brain of mammals and one of the most widely expressed neurotransmitters in the nervous system, which has been shown to play a role in a variety of biological processes such as cortical excitability, response to stress, food intake, circadian rhythms, and cardiovascular function (Yi *et al.,* 2018). Glycine, the primary inhibitory neurotransmitter in the spinal cord, also functions as a neurotransmitter in the brainstem and medulla, where it co-agonists with glutamate for NMDA receptors. In early development, it plays a role in neuronal differentiation, proliferation, and connectivity, whereas in adults, it plays a part in voluntary control of movement, processing of sensory information, and auditory, cardiovascular, and respiratory functions (Niyonambaza *et al.*, 2019).

In general, neurotransmitters play an important role in conveying motor, sensory, and integrative neuronal signals, regulating a wide range of processes such as emotions, thinking, sleep patterns, movement, learning, and memory. Thus, the CNS controls smooth, skeletal, and cardiac muscles, secretions from the body, and organ functions via synaptic transmission (also known as neurotransmission); as a result, disruptions in neurotransmitter homeostasis result in dysregulation of central nervous system functions, which may lead to a variety of physical, psychotic, and neurodegenerative diseases (Teleanu *et al.*, 2022).

Figure 1. Neurotransmitter Systems and Their Functions

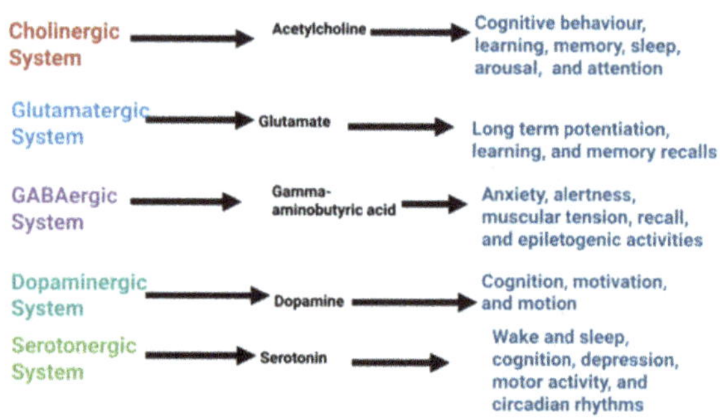

CNS INFECTIONS AND THE IMPACT ON NEUROTRANSMITTER REGULATION

CNS infections are defined as any infections that infiltrate the brain or spinal cord caused by a range of organisms such as bacteria, viruses, fungi, and protozoa. Common CNS diseases caused by these pathogens include meningitis, abscesses, and encephalitis. These diverse CNS infections advance quickly and inflict significant harm or even death if they are not addressed quickly and forcefully (Shinjyo & Kita, 2021).

Some infections are capable of communicating with receptors for neurotransmitters in the CNS. They impair neurons' biological activity, including metabolic pathways and neurotransmitter synthesis, resulting in alterations in neurotransmitter release, neurotransmitter levels, and neuronal communication within the CNS (Wongchitrat *et al.*, 2024).

ROLE OF NEUROTRANSMITTERS IN CNS INFECTIONS

Neurotransmitter Disruption in Viral Infections

Viral infections of the CNS can be chronic or acute in nature and are caused by a variety of viruses. These include meningitis, encephalitis, encephalomyelitis, and myelitis, as well as measles, Human immune virus-1 (HIV-1), and vacuolar myelopathy (Wongchitrat *et al.,* 2021). They affect neurotransmission systems, resulting in disruption of brain activity and contributing to virus-induced neuropathogenesis.

Mechanisms of Neurotransmitter Dysregulation During Infections

Mechanisms through which neurotransmitters get dysregulated by infection include:

1. Neurotoxicity: Certain viruses can cause neurotoxicity, resulting in neuronal death and malfunction. This can disrupt the circuits that control neurotransmitter release and uptake, causing neurotransmitter dysregulation. One example is neurotoxicity caused by glutamatergic system dysregulation, also known as glutamate-mediated excito-hyper-toxicity. It is a major mechanism of neuronal damage caused by viral infection. Study has indicated that viral proteins, such as HIV-1 proteins, stimulate the creation of a macromolecular complex including N-methyl-d-aspartic acid (NMDA) receptors, which promotes death in astrocytes and neurons. The compound increases glutamate levels, decreases NMDA receptors, activates TNF-α signaling, and causes redox imbalances in brain cells, leading to neuronal death. The glutamate-mediated excitotoxicity activation also elevates oxidative stress in the brain area involved in learning and memory deficits.
2. Viral infection also causes harm to neurotransmitter neuron-rich locations. Certain viruses directly infect neurons, glial cells, or neuron-rich parts of the brain, causing neuronal injury and dysfunction while altering neurotransmitter production, release, and uptake.
3. Changes in the equilibrium of other chemicals in the brain, such as chemokines and cytokines, are enzymes that can influence neurotransmitter signaling pathways: In some situations, viral infections can cause autoimmune reactions aimed at neurotransmitter receptors or neurotransmitter system components, resulting in abnormalities in neurotransmitter pathways (e.g. The encephalitis virus reduces muscarinic cholinergic signaling in several brain regions due to decreased expression levels of the cholinergic receptor muscarinic 2 and choline

acetyltransferase, resulting in a decrease overall muscarinic cholinergic binding (Wongchitrat *et al.,* 2024).

Neurotransmitter Alterations in Bacterial Infections

Impact of Bacterial Invasion on Neurotransmitter Synthesis

In addition to viral infections, bacterial infections also impact the CNS. Bacterial infections such as *Streptococcus agalactiae, Escherichia coli, Streptococcus pneumoniae, Mycobacterium tuberculosis,* and others infect the CNS (Govic *et al.,* 2022). Bacterial infections are broadly categorized into three types: meningitis, abscess, and encephalitis, based on the location and form of the inflammatory response caused by the infection.

Bacterial infections affect the body in a variety of ways, including their capacity to alter neurotransmitter production. Bacterial infection affects neurotransmitter release via the following mechanisms:

1. Activation of immune response: Pathogen invasion of the CNS triggers the immune response, resulting in the production of inflammatory chemicals such as cytokines, which activate responses of inflammation that regulate replication and/or coordinate elimination. These cytokines influence neurotransmitter generation and elimination in the brain. Pro-inflammatory cytokines, such as IL-1β, TNF-alpha, and IFN-α, can affect neurotransmitter production and functions. IL-1β influences the degeneration of dopaminergic neurons (Stojakovic *et al.,* 2017), TNF induces the death of dopaminergic neurons (Prajapati *et al.,* 2015), while IFN-α impacts serotonin, dopamine, and glutamate production; Indoleamine-2,3-dioxygenase (IDO), a neuroactive metabolite, is activated by IFN-α, causing a decrease in quinolinic acid (QA) and an increase in kynurenic acid (KA); the kynurenine pathway is activated, which decreases the formation of dopamine and serotonin (Hoyo-Becerra et al., 2014); quinolinic acid, which is produced by microglia, binds to NMDA receptors, causing glutaminergic system excitotoxicity; kynurenic acid, which is produced by astrocytes, causes a decrease in glutamatergic signaling (Hoyo-Becerra et al., 2014; Prajapati et al., 2015).
2. Neurotoxicity: Some bacteria create toxins that harm the CNS during infection, altering neurotransmitter-producing cells within the brain and hence influencing neurotransmitter synthesis, release, as well as function. Clostridial neurotoxins (Botulinum neurotoxin) are generated by Clostridium botulinum and interfere with the breakdown of acetylcholine, a neurotransmitter involved in muscular contraction.

3. Alteration of the gut microbiota: The gut microbiota is essential for the generation of neurotransmitters that include gamma-aminobutyric acid (GABA), serotonin, histamine, dopamine, glutamate, and norepinephrine (Leon & Dick, 2022). Following infection, the gut microbiota generates chemicals that trigger the "gut-brain axis" to affect neuronal circuits, autonomic function, and higher-order brain activity and conduct. Bacterial infections that disturb the balance of gut bacteria may influence neurotransmitter synthesis.

Fungal Infections and Neurotransmitter Imbalance

Fungal infections of the CNS are rather rare. While bacteria and viruses cause the bulk of CNS illnesses, fungi are becoming well-recognized as significant pathogens. Fungal pathogens that cause infections of the central nervous system include *Aspergillus spp., Cryptococcus neoformans, Histoplasma capsulatum, Coccidioides immitis, Candida spp., Zygomycetes, Histoplasma capsulatum, Aspergillus spp., Blastomyces dermatitidis, Penicillium spp, Candida spp., Paracoccidioides brasiliensis, Fusarium spp.,* and *Paracoccidioides brasiliensis,.* etc.(Gholami-Shabani *et al.,* 2018).

Fungus infection produces dangerous fungus metabolites known as mycotoxins. These mycotoxins have been discovered to directly disrupt various neurotransmitter systems, for example: Aflatoxin B1, a fungal mycotoxin causes a variety of responses in the CNS, which might impact the neurotransmitter levels of the infected host, such mycotoxins stimulate the generation of chemokines, cytokines, and antifungal chemicals such as nitric oxide (NO), which alters brain circuitry and may change neurotransmitter levels (Gholami-Shabani *et al.,* 2018). Also, mycotoxin-mediated astrocyte damage reduces neurotransmitter glutamate uptake and results in extracellular glutamate buildup, which causes excitotoxicity, functional impairment, and nerve cell death (Pei *et al.*, 2021). Mycotoxin signaling causes toxicological consequences comparable to those linked with brain disorders which include oxidative stress (Ehsanifar *et al.,* 2023), which may further impact neurotransmitter production, uptake, and function.

NON-DRUG APPROACHES FOR MODULATING NEUROTRANSMITTERS IN CNS INFECTIONS

Nutritional Interventions

Food consumption, diet adjustments, and dietary supplements are recognized as excellent alternative and complementary health choices and have been shown to have an important influence on the supply of antecedents for neurotransmitter production. Modulating neurotransmitter systems via pharmacological medications and non-drug techniques, such as dietary therapies, may help control CNS infection symptoms and perhaps improve outcomes.

Role of Specific Nutrients in Neurotransmitter Synthesis

There are several nutrients required for neurotransmitter production and regulation. Amino acids include tyrosine (Tyr) precursors, tryptophan (Trp) B-vitamins (especially folate, vitamin B12, and vitamin B6), vitamin C, leucine, valine, omega-3 fatty acids, isoleucine, phenylalanine, iron, vitamin D, and zinc.

Examples of Neurotransmitters and Particular Nutrients That Have a Role in Their Production

1. Dopamine: L-amino acid decarboxylase, commonly known as DOPA decarboxylase, catalyzes the synthesis of dopamine from its precursor, L-Dopa. L-Dopa is derived from an amino acid known as L-Tyrosine. The generation of dopamine is controlled by an amino acid called tyrosine, which is essential for its development. As a result, obtaining appropriate quantities of this essential amino acid is critical; it is present in all protein sources, including eggs, turkey, legumes (particularly soy), milk and other dairy products, and cattle. Some foods raise dopamine levels by giving L-DOPA. These foods include animal products such as poultry, meat, milk products, fish, eggs, chocolate, vegetables, and fruits like watermelon, apples, bananas, spinach, some beets, avocados, tomato, peas, sea vegetables, legumes, and peanuts, oregano, green vegetables, oats, rosemary, especially pumpkin seeds and sesame, turmeric, soy products, olive oil and some types of wheat. As a result, appropriate intake of these meals is critical for dopamine production (Hryhorczuk *et al.*, 2016; Gasmi *et al.*, 2023).
2. Acetylcholine: Acetylcholine is produced using the choline acetyltransferase enzyme and two chemical components, choline and acetyl-CoA. Acetyl CoA is obtained from food, whereas choline is obtained from food; hence, eating choline-rich foods such as green split peas, soybeans, turkey, salmon, mung beans, egg yolks, beef, liver, and lentils is beneficial (Gasmi *et al.*, 2023). Melatonin and vitamin C might also enhance cholinergic neurotransmission (Ayinla *et al.*, 2020)
3. Serotonin: The bioavailability of its precursor, the amino acid L-Tryptophan, is necessary for the synthesis of serotonin, and 5-Hydroxytryptophan converts it into serotonin through a metabolic process involving two enzymes, Tryptophan hydroxylase and amino acid decarboxylase (Jenkins et al., 2016). A variety of

dietary nutrients, such as oranges, kiwi, bacon, turkey, walnuts, bananas, chicory, cherries, coffee beans, cabbage, green grapes, brinjal, legumes, hickory peanuts, onion, hot peppers, green lettuce, papaya, pineapples, oats, green pears, potatoes, plums, green spinach, tomatoes, strawberries, and walnuts, increase serotonin levels (Ramakrishna *et al.,* 2011).

4. Gamma-Aminobutyric Acid (GABA): It is produced via the enzyme glutamic acid decarboxylase (GAD) from glutamate. It requires a cofactor called pyridoxal phosphate, which is derived through the consumption of dietary vitamin B6. Fruits like almonds, walnuts, and hazelnuts can help in GABA synthesis. They are high in glutamic acid and include important lipids that participate in the synthesis of GABA. Additional sources of glutamic acid include broad beans, lupins, and lentils. These meals also contain vitamin B and carbohydrates, which help GABA synthesis. Spinach, tomatoes, and parsley contain GABA precursors, as do eggs, salmon, and meat (Sarawagi *et al.*, 2021).
5. Glutamate: Another amino acid produced by the breakdown of glutamic acid by the glutaminase enzyme is glutamate, which is produced by the glutamine molecule. Foods high in protein naturally contain glutamic acid. Meat, seafood, soups, stews, and sauces are some examples of these foods. Likewise, glutamic acid salts like sodium, calcium, magnesium, and potassium, which can be added to some foods or sauces as flavor enhancers, cheeses, seaweeds, soy sauces, fish sauces, Solanum Lycopersicum L. (tomato), fermented beans, coffee powder, and spinach (Tennant, 2018; Valluzzi et al., 2019).
6. Histamine: Histamine comes naturally in some meals and is dispersed evenly throughout the body. Foods, like almonds, guava, brinjal, and salami, pepperoni, sausages, and hot dogs, cheese, canned meats, ketchup, beverages, kombucha, fish, milk products like kefir, yogurt, sour cream, cottage and ricotta cheese, buttermilk, sauerkraut, kimchi, seafood, pineapple, tamari, soya sauce, spinach, spoiled food, tea of any kind, coconut, vinegar, tomatoes, and yeast foodstuffs.

Dietary Strategies to Support Neurotransmitter Balance

Every neurotransmitter has a separately allocated substrate, thus it should be included in the diet in a general and equal amount to maintain neurotransmitter balance. Dietary routine can influence neurotransmitter physiology, for example, saturated fats excess found in butter, animal fats, and coconut oil may disrupt dopamine uptake in the brain, therefore a continuous high-fat diet intake can cause changes in dopamine reuptake, regardless of the degree or manifestation of the transporter that transports dopamine. As a result, it is critical to maintain a well-balanced, nutrient-dense diet (Gasmi *et al.,* 2023).

Lifestyle Modifications

1. Importance of Sleep and Its Impact on Neurotransmitters

Sleep is a reversible natural condition of rest for the brain and body with closed eyelids characterized by a loss of consciousness, diminished responsiveness to stimuli, and reduced bodily motions. While getting enough sleep improves mood and brain function while also preserving neurotransmitter balance and overall body health, several pieces of data suggest that sleep deprivation significantly alters neurotransmitter activity. The persistence or rise in wake-promoting neurotransmitter levels, which is usually accompanied by alterations in enzyme activity that facilitate neurotransmitter turnover, is one of the most consistently described effects of sleep deprivation (Longordo et al., 2009).

The influence of sleep deprivation on neurotransmitter patterns has been researched using various methodologies, and sleep deprivation has been shown to change neurotransmitter balance. Sleep deprivation seems to be associated with changes in neurotransmitter balance.

2. Exercise and Its Role in Promoting Neurotransmitter Homeostasis

Exercise is a type of physical activity that is designed and arranged to improve or sustain physical fitness and total bodily health. Exercise is broadly categorized into two types: dynamic exercise and static exercise; aerobic activity and anaerobic exercise; and light, moderate, and severe exercise. Dynamic exercise entails isotonic muscular contraction (i.e., consistent tension in the muscle as it changes length) and requires the body to move through a full range of motion, such as swimming, bicycling, walking, etc. Static exercise involves isometric muscular contraction (the contraction of skeletal muscle without a change in muscle length) without joint movement, such as moving a heavy item. Anaerobic exercise, also known as cardio exercise, consists of lower-intensity activities performed over a longer period with energy gained through utilizing nutrients in the presence of oxygen, such as medium to long-distance running/jogging, swimming, walking, cycling, and so on. Anaerobic exercise is defined as exertion for short periods (high-intensity activities that last from seconds to about 2 minutes), with the amount of energy needed for the workout being derived from burning glycogen that is kept in the muscles without oxygen. It is commonly used by athletes for developing strength, speed, and power and by bodybuilders for gaining muscle mass, such as pull-ups, push-ups, weightlifting, sprinting, and other forms of rapid bursts of strenuous exercise. Mild exercise is a basic type of exercise such as gentle walking. Moderate exercise does not need significant muscle action. Moderate exercise can be performed for a longer period and does not result in exhaustion at the end, e.g., fast walking and slow running, whereas severe exercise requires strenuous muscular activity with complete exhaustion at the end of the exercise as well as the severity is maintained only for a short period. Growing data suggests that exercise has a positive impact on humans. It achieves this through a variety of methods, including neurotransmitter regulation and its impacts on brain shape and function. Exercise has been shown in studies to affect neurotransmitter release and reuptake patterns. For example, acute aerobic exercise has been shown to affect neurotransmitter release and neuronal circuitry (Liu *et al.,* 2019).

Stress Management Techniques

Stress-Induced Neurotransmitter Imbalances

Stress is how the body responds to a change that necessitates a mental, physical, or emotional adaptation or response. It can stem scenario or thinking that causes frustration, anger, nervousness, or anxiety. It might be any actual or perceived threat to an organism's well-being (Asuku *et al.,* 2025).

Stress has been shown to change a variety of neurotransmitters, including the following:

1. Gamma-aminobutyric acid (GABA): Stress has been shown to change the composition of GABA neurotransmissions. Stress causes the amygdale and hypothalamus to release corticotrophin-releasing factor (CRF) and GABA. In contrast, stress inhibits vesicular glutamate transporter and its interaction with GABA-synthesizing enzyme glutamic acid decarboxylase (GAD65), resulting in lower GABA levels in the hippocampus (Bagosi *et al.*, 2012; Martisova *et al.*, 2012).
   2) Dopamine: Preclinical research indicates that dopamine responds unevenly to diverse stressful situations. Acute and manageable physical stress was shown to boost dopamine levels, however persistent and uncontrolled exposure to stress reduced dopamine release.
   3) Norepinephrine: Stress has been shown to enhance norepinephrine turnover in the locus ceruleus as well as the hippocampus.
   4) Serotonin: During psychological conflict in animals, hippocampal serotonin levels rise. Serotonin (5-hydroxytryptamine receptor 1A) receptors are reduced in several brain areas, like cortex and hippocampus after stress. Studies have shown that a considerable decrease in serotonin levels promotes stress response (Texel *et al.*, 2012).

NON-PHARMACOLOGICAL INTERVENTIONS FOR SUPPORTING CNS HEALTH

Physical Rehabilitation

Physical rehabilitation is a type of treatment that seeks to bring back function to those recuperating from an accident or surgery, and also to those who have a physical impairment or handicap. It entails avoiding, diagnosing, and treating crippling illnesses, disorders, and injuries using physical endeavors such as therapeutic exercise to manage and restore the body's natural functions, hence improving quality of life. It includes three main types of therapies: physical therapy, occupational therapy, and speech/language therapy. Physical therapy is concerned with improving the body's functionality, with its main emphasis on restoring the capacity to move, reducing pain, and improving gross motor abilities, whereas occupational therapy is concerned with improving the patient's capacity to perform activities of daily living that a person requires or wishes to perform daily. Despite these minor distinctions, both strive to promote a better standard of life with as much freedom as possible. For patients in the recovery phase after any sort of diagnosis, a mix of both therapies, including motor function, physiological awareness, and motivation, is frequently required for complete recovery.

Physical Therapy and Its Impact on Neurotransmitter Function

Physical therapy (PT) is the use of physical techniques to treat sickness or injury, including exercise, heat and cold treatments, massage, and stretching. There are many additional exercise-based alternatives. It can be conducted in hospitals, outpatient clinics, or even at home. Exercise, which is primarily used in this therapy, enhances neurogenesis, has anti-neuroinflammatory effects, and modulates neurotransmitter synthesis, release, and action, as well as neurotransmitter receptor modulation, implying that it plays an important role in the regulation of neurotransmitter functions.

Occupational Therapy in CNS Infection Recovery

Occupational therapy is the therapeutic application of everyday activities, or occupations, for the management of mental, physical, developmental, and emotional conditions that impair an individual's capacity to perform daily tasks. Occupational therapy and treatment, while similar to physical therapy, emphasize independence in performing daily activities. It has been discovered that approximately half of those diagnosed with infections of the CNS such as brain abscess and empyema present with neuro-musculoskeletal deficits, and one-third with mental deficits, necessitating the use of physical rehabilitation methods in addition to medical treatment (Gradidgei *et al.*, 2013).

Cognitive Interventions

Cognitive Rehabilitation and Its Influence on Neurotransmitter Systems

Restoring or strengthening previously learned behavioral patterns, as well as creating new forms of cognitive activity or compensatory responses to damaged neurological systems, are the goals of cognitive rehabilitation therapy (CRT), which is defined as methodical and functionally oriented therapeutic cognitive activities.

After discharge, individuals with CNS illnesses have reported a variety of impairments, including attention problems, memory and/or mental agility loss, decreased cognitive function speed, poor psychomotor performance, and difficulty falling asleep. These cognitive deficits can impact the patient's health-related quality of life, including their capacity to work and, therefore, CRT.

Alternative Therapies

Over the past few years, alternative and complementary medicine has grown in popularity throughout the world because it is seen as a natural source of therapy that is safe and efficient, with fewer negative consequences in sensitive and difficult conditions such as CNS disorders, as compared to synthetic drugs.

1. Acupuncture and Its Potential Impact on Neurotransmitter Release

Acupuncture is a classic form of therapy in Chinese medicine. It is effective in treating Alzheimer's disease, stroke, spinal cord injury, Parkinson's disease, depression, and other CNS problems. It can modulate brain activities by regulating central neurotransmitters since all acupuncture-influenced neurotransmitters are involved in practically all neural control, either directly or indirectly. Acupuncture research, particularly mechanistic investigations on acupuncture analgesia, has shown that acupuncture signal, either generated by manual acupuncture or electroacupuncture (Ea), astoundingly influences the release, synthesis, reuptake, and degradation of neurotransmitters which includes serotonin, noradrenalin, dopamine, and acetylcholine (ACh) either to enhance or reduce. Acupuncture increases the production of endogenous opioid peptides, dopamine, serotonin, and ACh, and inhibitory amino acids like GABA, glycine, taurine, and lactamine. It decreases the action of noradrenaline and excitatory amino acids like glutamate and aspartic acid.

2. Herbal Supplements and Their Role in Neurotransmitter Modulation

Natural medicine has long been utilized across the world to treat problems of the central nervous system. These herbal remedies are occasionally employed in place of conventional treatments for CNS disorders. They have been shown to play key roles in the medical management of a variety of neurological and pathophysiological problems, with no or little side effects. Many plant-based compounds have been shown to have positive benefits on the body's CNS. These herbs include *Desmodium adscendens, Cleome rutidosperma, Withania somnifera, Bacopa monnieri, Rauvolfia serpentina, Acorus calamus, and Emblica officinalis,* among others. These plants and their chemical contents are particularly beneficial in protecting humans from central nervous system (CNS) problems. The processes of action that they utilize include binding to CNS receptors with pharmacologic and therapeutic effects, normalizing hormones such as corticosterone, ameliorating depressive-like behaviors, anti-inflammatory effects, modifying neurotransmitter pathways such as acetylcholinesterase activity, stimulating γ-aminobutyric acid receptors, reducing reactive oxygen scavenging properties, and abrogating monoamine oxidase activity.

Plant Natural Compounds and Their Involvement in Neurotransmitter Regulation

The most prevalent class of natural chemicals are phenols. Phenolic compounds have been demonstrated to have a significant impact on a range of central nervous system functions and disorders through direct interaction with neurotransmitter systems, leading to sedative, anxiolytic, antipsychotic, cognitive enhancement, cholinergic upregulation, and antidepressant properties, in addition to their capacity to scavenge free radicals and reactive oxygen species and to chelate metals (Asuku et al., 2024b; Ayinla & Asuku, 2025).

Steroids or pentacyclic triterpenoids are examples of aglycones in the structurally diverse class of glycosidic compounds known as saponins. It has been demonstrated that saponins have a potent neuroprotective effect in preventing central nervous system disorders, including stroke, Parkinson's disease, Alzheimer's disease, and Huntington's disease. Terpenoids bind directly or allosterically to the GABAergic system, reducing issues including anxiety, insomnia, convulsions, pain, and cognitive deficits. They also inhibit cholinesterase via interacting with the octopaminergic and noradrenergic neurotransmitter systems.

CONCLUSION

To summarize, CNS infections may alter neurotransmitter levels, impacting the symptoms, course, and severity of the illness. Changes in serotonin, glutamate, or GABA levels, for example, impact mood and behavior, as well as cognitive function, which accounts for symptoms such as confusion, alterations in consciousness, mood disorders, or cognitive impairments encountered with CNS infections. During this illness, various neurotransmitters affect the body's reaction, including immunological response, brain barrier permeability, and neuroinflammatory processes, allowing it to modify, respond, and combat the infection.

Using non-drug approaches such as nutrients, exercises, and therapy for rehabilitation will provide a natural and likely safer approach to maintaining neurotransmitter balance than synthetic compounds, which easily change body composition and have negative consequences or additional restrictions or disadvantages after repeated use.

Future Directions for Research and Therapeutic Development

The link between CNS illnesses and neurotransmitters is complicated and varies based on the kind of infection, affected brain regions, and individual characteristics. More study is required to completely understand the processes by which the nervous system's illnesses affect neurotransmitter production, release, and absorption in the body. Understanding how neurotransmitters interact with CNS illnesses can lead to innovative therapeutic methods.

REFERENCES

Asuku, A. O., Adebayo, P. O., & Ogungbangbe, G. O. (2025). Stress and Gender Differences in Brain Development. In Moradikor, N., & Orish, C. (Eds.), *Stress and the Brain: Evidence from Molecular Mechanisms to Interventions and Therapies*. Elsevier. DOI: 10.1016/bs.pbr.2025.01.013

Asuku, A. O., Ayinla, M. T., & Ajibare, A. J. (2024a). Central Nervous System Regulation of Eating and Brain Functions. In Mohamed, W., & Kobeissy, F. (Eds.), *Nutrition and Psychiatric Disorders. Nutritional Neurosciences*. Springer. DOI: 10.1007/978-981-97-2681-3_4

Asuku, A. O., Ayinla, M. T., Ajibare, A. J., & Olajide, T. S. (2024b). Mercury chloride causes cognitive impairment, oxidative stress and neuroinflammation in male Wistar rats: The potential protective effect of 6-gingerol-rich fraction of Zingiber officinale via regulation of antioxidant defense system and reversal of pro-inflammatory markers increase. *Brain Research,* 148741: 1826. DOI: 10.1016/j.brainres.2023.148741

Ayinla, M. T., & Asuku, A. O. (2025). The neurotoxic effects of lead acetate and the abrogating actions of 6-gingerol-rich extract of ginger via modulation of antioxidant defence system, pro-inflammatory markers, and apoptotic cascade. *Naunyn-Schmiedeberg's Archives of Pharmacology*, *398*(7), 9341–9356. Advance online publication. DOI: 10.1007/s00210-025-03873-x PMID: 39937255

Ayinla, M. T., Asuku, A. O., Bayo-Olugbami, A., Ayeni, A. O., Abiola, A. A., & Owoyele, B. V. (2020). Melatonin and Vitamin C Modulate Cholinergic Neurotransmission and Oxidative stress in Scopolamine–induced Rat Model of Memory Impairment. *Journal of African Association of Physiological Sciences*, *8*(1), 20.

Bagosi, Z., Csabafi, K., Jászberényi, M., & Telegdy, G. (2012). The effects of corticotropin-releasing factor and the urocortin on hypothalamic gamma-aminobutyric acid release – The impacts on the hypothalamic-pituitary-adrenal axis. *Neurochemistry International*, *60*(4), 350–354. DOI: 10.1016/j.neuint.2012.01.007 PMID: 22306347

Ehsanifar, M., Reihane, R., Akram, G., & Joseph, P. (2023). Mold and Mycotoxin Exposure and Brain Disorders. *Journal of Integrative Neuroscience*, *22*(6), 137. DOI: 10.31083/j.jin2206137 PMID: 38176924

Gasmi, A., Aniqa, N., Alain, M., & Asma, G. (2022, December 26). Benahmed, Lyudmila, P., Sàdaf, N., Massimilian, P., Salvatore, C., & Geir, B. (2023). Neurotransmitters Regulation and Food Intake: The Role of Dietary Sources in Neurotransmission. *Molecules (Basel, Switzerland)*, *28*(1), 210. Advance online publication. DOI: 10.3390/molecules28010210 PMID: 36615404

Gholami-Shabani, M. H., Samira, Z., Hoda, M., Masoomeh, S-H., Fatemehsadat, J., & Mehdi, R-A. (2018) Recent Advances in Fungal Infections of the Central Nervous System: From Etiology to Diagnosis and Management. *The Microbiology of Central Nervous System Infections*. Elsevier Inc. DOI: 10.1016/B978-0-12-813806-9.00012-3

Govic, Y., Baptiste, D., Julien, C., Yong-Sun, B. & Nicolas, P. (2022). Pathogens infect the central nervous system. *PLoS Pathog.* .DOI: 10.1371/journal.ppat.1010234

Gradidge, K., Casteleijn, D., & Franzsen, D. (2013). Using the Occupational Therapy Practice Framework-ll to treat a rare condition - brain abscess and empyema. *South African Journal of Occupational Therapy*, *43*, 2.

Hoyo-Becerra, C., Schlaak, J. F., & Hermann, D. M. (2014). Insights from interferon-α-related depression for the pathogenesis of depression associated with inflammation. *Brain, Behavior, and Immunity*, *42*, 222–231. DOI: 10.1016/j.bbi.2014.06.200 PMID: 25066466

Hryhorczuk, C., Florea, M., Rodaros, D., Poirier, I., Daneault, C., Des Rosiers, C., Arvanitogiannis, A., Alquier, T., & Fulton, S. (2016). Dampened Mesolimbic Dopamine Function and Signaling by Saturated but not Monounsaturated Dietary Lipids. *Neuropsychopharmacology : Official Publication of the American College ofNeuropsychopharmacology*, *41*(3), 811–821. DOI: 10.1038/npp.2015.207 PMID: 26171719

Iovino, L., Tremblay, M., & Civiero, L. (2020). Glutamate-induced excitotoxicity in Parkinson's disease: The role of glial cells. *Journal of Pharmacological Sciences*, *144*(3), 151–164. DOI: 10.1016/j.jphs.2020.07.011 PMID: 32807662

Jenkins, T. A., Nguyen, J. C., Polglaze, K. E., & Bertrand, P. P. (2016). Influence of Tryptophan and Serotonin on Mood and Cognition with a Possible Role of the Gut-Brain Axis. *Nutrients*, *8*(1), 56. DOI: 10.3390/nu8010056 PMID: 26805875

Leon, M., & Dicks, T. (2022). Gut Bacteria and Neurotransmitters. *Microorganisms*, *10*(9), 1838. Advance online publication. DOI: 10.3390/microorganisms10091838 PMID: 36144440

Liu, Y., Tim, Y., John, C., Ying, C., Sophie, D., Yuen-Shan, H., Gordon, W., & Raymond, C. (2019). The beneficial effects of physical exercise in the brain and related pathophysiological mechanisms in neurodegenerative diseases. *Laboratory Investigation, 99*(7), 943–947. DOI: 10.1038/s41374-019-0232-y PMID: 30808929

Longordo, F., Kopp, C., & Luthi, A. (2009). Consequences of sleep deprivation on neurotransmitter receptor expression and function. Journal Compilation. *The European Journal of Neuroscience, 29*(9), 1810–1819. DOI: 10.1111/j.1460-9568.2009.06719.x PMID: 19492440

Martisova, E., Solas, M., Horrillo, I., Ortega, J. E., Meana, J. J., Tordera, R. M., & Ramírez, M. J. (2012). Long-lasting effects of early-life stress on glutamatergic/GABAergic circuitry in the rat hippocampus. *Neuropharmacology, 62*(5-6), 1944–1953. DOI: 10.1016/j.neuropharm.2011.12.019 PMID: 22245561

Nimgampalle, M., Chakravarthy, H., Sharma, S., Shree, S., Bhat, A. R., Pradeepkiran, J. A., & Devanathan, V. (2023). Neurotransmitter systems in the etiology of major neurological disorders: Emerging insights and therapeutic implications. *Ageing Research Reviews, 89*, 101994. DOI: 10.1016/j.arr.2023.101994 PMID: 37385351

Niyonambaza, S., Kumar, P., Xing, P., Mathault, J., De Koninck, P., Boisselier, E., Boukadoum, M., & Miled, A. (2019). A Review of Neurotransmitters Sensing Methods for Neuro-Engineering Research. *Applied Sciences (Basel, Switzerland), 9*(21), 4719. DOI: 10.3390/app9214719

Ou, Y., Buchanan, A., Witt, C., & Hashemi, P. (2019). Frontiers in electrochemical sensors for neurotransmitter detection: Towards measuring neurotransmitters as chemical diagnostics for brain disorders. *Analytical Methods, 11*(21), 2738–2755. DOI: 10.1039/C9AY00055K PMID: 32724337

Pei, X., Wenjuan, Z., & Haiyang, J. (2021). Food-Origin Mycotoxin-Induced Neurotoxicity: Intend to Break the Rules of Neuroglia Cells. *Oxidative Medicine and Cellular Longevity, 2021*(1), 1–14. DOI: 10.1155/2021/9967334 PMID: 34621467

Prajapati, P., Sripada, L., Singh, K., Bhatelia, K., Singh, R., & Singh, R. (2015). TNF-α regulates miRNA targeting mitochondrial complex-I and induces cell death in dopaminergic cells. *Biochimica et Biophysica Acta, 1852*(3), 451–461. DOI: 10.1016/j.bbadis.2014.11.019 PMID: 25481834

Ramakrishna, A., Giridhar, P., & Ravishankar, G. A. (2011). Phytoserotonin: A review. *Plant Signaling & Behavior, 6*(6), 800–809. DOI: 10.4161/psb.6.6.15242 PMID: 21617371

Sarawagi, A., Soni, N. D., & Patel, A. B. (2021). Glutamate and GABA Homeostasis and Neurometabolism in Major Depressive Disorder. *Frontiers in Psychiatry*, *12*, 637863. DOI: 10.3389/fpsyt.2021.637863 PMID: 33986699

Shinjyo, N. & Kita, K. (2021). Infection and Immunometabolism in the Central Nervous System: A Possible Mechanistic Link Between Metabolic Imbalance and Dementia. *Front Cell Neurosci*. .DOI: 10.3389/fncel.2021.765217

Stojakovic, A., Paz-Filho, G., Arcos-Burgos, M., Licinio, J., Wong, M. L., & Mastronardi, C. A. (2017). Role of the IL-1 Pathway in Dopaminergic Neurodegeneration and Decreased Voluntary Movement. *Molecular Neurobiology*, *54*(6), 4486–4495. DOI: 10.1007/s12035-016-9988-x PMID: 27356916

Teleanu, R., Adelina-Gabriela, N., Eugenia, R., Oana, V., Alexandru, M., Daniel, M., & Nina, K. (2022). Academic Editor Neurotransmitters—Key Factors in Neurological and Neurodegenerative Disorders of the Central Nervous System. *International Journal of Molecular Sciences*, *23*(11), 5954. DOI: 10.3390/ijms23115954 PMID: 35682631

Tennant, D.R. (2018). Review of Glutamate Intake from Both Food Additive and Non-Additive Sources in the European Union. *Ann. Nutr. Metab*. .DOI: 10.1159/000494778

Texel, S., Camandola, S., Ladenheim, B., Rothman, S., Mughal, M., Unger, E. L., Cadet, J. L., & Mattson, M. P. (2012). Ceruloplasmin deficiency results in an anxiety phenotype involving deficits in hippocampal iron, serotonin, and BDNF. *Journal of Neurochemistry*, *120*(1), 125–134. DOI: 10.1111/j.1471-4159.2011.07554.x PMID: 22035068

Valluzzi, R. L., Fierro, V., Arasi, S., Mennini, M., Pecora, V., & Fiocchi, A. (2019). Allergy to food additives. *Current Opinion in Allergy and Clinical Immunology*, *19*(3), 256–262. DOI: 10.1097/ACI.0000000000000528 PMID: 30883393

Wongchitrat, P., Chanmee, T., & Govitrapong, P. (2024). Molecular Mechanisms Associated with Neurodegeneration of Neurotropic Viral Infection. *Molecular Neurobiology*, *61*(5), 2881–2903. DOI: 10.1007/s12035-023-03761-6 PMID: 37946006

Wongchitrat, P., Shukla, M., Sharma, R., Govitrapong, P., & Reiter, R.J. (2021). Role of Melatonin on Virus-Induced Neuropathogenesis-A Concomitant Therapeutic Strategy to Understand SARS-CoV-2 Infection. *Antioxidants*. .DOI: 10.3390/antiox10010047

Yi, M., Li, H., Wu, Z., Yan, J., Liu, Q., Ou, C., & Chen, M. (2018). A promising therapeutic target for metabolic diseases: Neuropeptide Y receptors in humans. *Cellular Physiology and Biochemistry*, *45*(1), 88–107. DOI: 10.1159/000486225 PMID: 29310113

Chapter 9
Automated Segmentation of Brain Tumor MRI Images Using Machine Learning

Senthil Kumar A. V.
https://orcid.org/0000-0002-8587-7017
Nehru Institute of Information Technology and Management, India

N. Kartiga
https://orcid.org/0009-0006-6247-1205
Hindusthan College of Arts and Science, India

Suganya R. V.
VISTAS, India

Gaganpreet Kaur
Chitkara University, India

Ismail Bin Musirin
Universiti Teknologi MARA, Malaysia

G. Jagadamba
https://orcid.org/0000-0002-7379-7925
Siddaganga Institute of Technology, India

G. Vanishree
https://orcid.org/0009-0000-1335-2919
ICFAI Business School, India

Raman Kumar
I.K. Gujral Punjab Technical University, India

Ahmad Fuad Hamadah Bader
Jadara Universty, Jordan

Amit Dutta
All India Council for Technical Education, New Delhi, India

Manjunatha Rao
National Assessment and Accreditation Council, Bangalore, India

G. Sangeetha
https://orcid.org/0000-0002-7138-8888
Christ University, India

DOI: 10.4018/979-8-3693-4070-7.ch009

Vaishali Mishra
https://orcid.org/0009-0008-9850-5758
Expedia Group, USA

ABSTRACT

The field of medical imaging has been revolutionized by intelligent systems, especially those powered by machine learning and artificial intelligence (AI). Among various applications, brain tumor detection and classification stand out due to their critical impact on patient health outcomes. Brain tumors—whether benign or malignant—are among the most serious neurological conditions and often require prompt and accurate diagnosis. Traditionally, identifying brain tumors through imaging has been a manual and expertise-driven process, but with the integration of AI, especially deep learning, the accuracy and speed of diagnosis have improved significantly. This overview explores how machine learning contributes to brain tumor analysis, from the collection and pre-processing of MRI data to model training and classification. Key challenges such as data quality, model explainability, and tumor variability are also addressed, alongside modern advancements in deep learning models that continue to evolve in precision and clinical applicability.

1. INTRODUCTION

The field of medical imaging and healthcare has undergone significant transformation with the introduction of intelligent technologies, particularly machine learning and artificial intelligence (AI). One of the most impactful applications of these advancements is in the detection and classification of brain tumors, which are critical for timely and effective patient care. Brain tumors often present life-threatening challenges and require immediate medical intervention. Traditionally, diagnosing these conditions posed considerable difficulties due to the complexity of brain structures. However, the incorporation of intelligent systems into clinical practice has led to greater accuracy and efficiency in diagnosis.

This overview explores the various stages involved in brain tumor detection, from the acquisition of imaging data to the application of advanced deep learning models. It highlights the importance of early diagnosis, effective data preprocessing, and the selection of meaningful features. Cutting-edge machine learning algorithms play a vital role in enhancing diagnostic precision. The discussion also addresses current challenges such as limited data availability and the difficulty in interpreting model outputs. Finally, it emphasizes recent innovations and ongoing research efforts aimed at improving the reliability and accuracy of brain tumor detection and classification.

1.1 Feature Selection

Hidden deep within the intricate structure of the human brain, a serious medical threat can emerge — the brain tumor. Often undetectable through simple observation, these tumors can have devastating impacts on individuals. The brain, a highly sophisticated and sensitive organ, governs our emotions, thoughts, movements, and essential bodily functions. The presence of a tumor in such a critical organ presents a complex medical challenge that requires immediate attention and advanced intervention strategies.

Brain tumors, whether non-cancerous or malignant, involve the abnormal growth of cells that interfere with normal brain function. These tumors can vary significantly in terms of their location, type, and behaviour, making diagnosis and treatment especially difficult. In many cases, symptoms may develop subtly or resemble less severe conditions, which can delay accurate diagnosis and timely treatment.

This discussion aims to explore the many dimensions of brain tumors — including their classification, potential causes, warning signs, and the unique difficulties they present to healthcare providers. We will also examine current diagnostic tools, treatment options, and the growing importance of research and technological innovation in this field. The fight against brain tumors reflects the continuous drive of science and medicine to understand and overcome some of the most challenging health issues through collaboration and technological progress.

Figure 1. Feature Selection

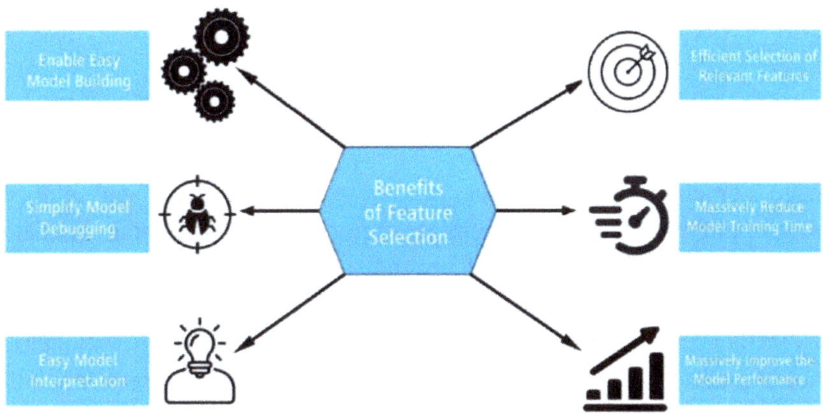

1.2 Image Classification

Image classification is a fundamental technique in the analysis of medical images, especially in detecting abnormalities such as brain tumors. It involves training algorithms to categorize images based on learned features. In the medical domain, this typically means distinguishing between healthy and diseased tissues. Deep learning models, particularly Convolutional Neural Networks (CNNs), are commonly used for this task. CNNs can automatically learn patterns such as shape, intensity, and texture, which are critical for identifying tumors in MRI scans. Their ability to process and classify visual data with high accuracy has made them indispensable in supporting medical diagnoses and improving decision-making in clinical environments.

Figure 2. Image Classification

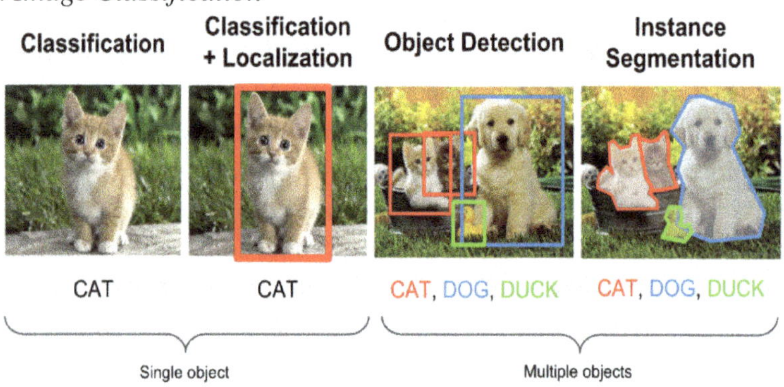

1.3 Image Segmentation

Image segmentation is the process of dividing a digital image into multiple segments to simplify its analysis and highlight regions of interest. In brain MRI analysis, segmentation helps isolate tumors from the surrounding healthy tissue. Accurate segmentation is crucial for determining tumor size, shape, and exact location, which directly influences treatment planning. Traditional segmentation techniques include thresholding and region-based methods, but more advanced approaches like the U-Net deep learning architecture have proven highly effective. U-Net and similar models enable pixel-level classification, allowing for precise delineation of tumor boundaries even in complex or low-contrast images.

1.4 Deep Learning

Deep learning, a subset of machine learning, mimics the human brain through artificial neural networks with many processing layers. These models can automatically learn complex patterns and features from large datasets. In medical imaging, deep learning is transforming how diseases like brain tumors are detected and analyzed. By leveraging architectures such as CNNs and Recurrent Neural Networks (RNNs), these models can process large volumes of MRI data, identify subtle differences between healthy and affected tissue, and reduce the need for manual intervention. Their ability to generalize across datasets makes them powerful tools for enhancing diagnostic accuracy in healthcare.

1.5 Machine Learning

Machine learning involves algorithms that learn from data to make predictions or decisions without being explicitly programmed. In the context of medical diagnostics, machine learning supports the early detection and classification of diseases, including brain tumors. Classical models like decision trees, support vector machines (SVMs), and k-nearest neighbors (KNN) have been used to analyze MRI data. While these models are effective, combining them with deep learning techniques further enhances performance. Machine learning contributes significantly to automating diagnosis, reducing human error, and improving the efficiency of medical image analysis systems.

2. LITERATURE REVIEW

2.1 Brain Tumor Magnetic Resonance Image Classification: A Deep Learning Approach

Lakshmi and Rao (2022) propose that for once a decade, numerous experimenters are concentrated on the brain excrescence discovery medium using glamorous resonance images. The traditional approaches follow the point birth process from nethermost subcaste in the network. This script isn't suitable to the medical images. To address this issue, the proposed model employed Inception- v3 complication neural network model which is a deep literacy medium. This model excerpts themulti-level features and classifies them to find the early discovery of brain excrescence. The proposed model uses the deep literacy approach and hyperactive parameters. The soft maximum classifier is used in the proposed model to classify the images in to multiple classes. It's observed that the delicacy of the commencement- v3 algorithm is recorded as99.34 in training data and 89 delicacies at confirmation data. The developments in the medical field support the medical interpreters to grease the cases effectively. With the application of artificial intelligence (AI) in the health care helps the medical sphere to serve further to the cases. According to the statistics of 2019, utmost of the deaths in the world are happed due to the cardiovascular conditions and in the coming place the cancer conditions are enthralled. Brain excrescence complaint is one of the life threating conditions in the world. glamorous Resonance Imaging (MRI) is one of the safest imaging ways that excerpts the good images and helps in the process of medical opinion. numerous experimenters are concentrated on perfecting the quality of the MR images and also to develop the new styles for quicker and easy medical opinion from the MR images. This study concentrated on the brain excrescence discovery from MR images This paper explained the deep literacy medium for discovery of brain excrescences in MR images. In the proposedpre-trained commencement- V3 deep literacy armature, some of the commencement modules at nethermost layers are removed and concatenated the features from the commencement modules from the top to perform the bracket in the Brain MR Image datasets. The last commencement module in the armature is concatenated with the completely connected layers, global normal pooling and uprooted features of the images from commencement modules. The proposed model excerpts the features from the completely connected subcase and on the uprooted features to the classifier. The soft maximum classifier is used in the proposed model to classify the images in to multiple classes. Tensor inflow and Keros with backend have been used to train the deep literacy model in the proposed armature. The delicacy of the proposed model is recorded as99.34 which is high compared to the VGG- 16 and ResNet50 models. In the future, we're concentrating on the combination of thick Net model and commencement- v3 model to ameliorate the delicacy.

2.2 Brain Tumor Classification Based on Attention Guided Deep Learning Model

In this study, Jun & Liana (2022) highlight that cancer remains the second leading cause of death globally, with brain tumors accounting for a significant proportion—nearly 25%—of all cancer-related fatalities. Ensuring an accurate and prompt diagnosis is essential, as it enables early treatment and can significantly improve outcomes. In recent years, the rapid progress in image classification technologies has greatly supported computer-aided diagnostic systems. Convolutional Neural Networks (CNNs) have become one of the most widely adopted models for image classification tasks. However, a major limitation of traditional CNNs is their inability to precisely locate the lesion's focal point. To overcome this, the authors propose an enhanced brain tumor classification model that incorporates both an attention mechanism and a multipath network architecture. The attention mechanism is designed to prioritize key features from the target region while filtering out irrelevant details. Simultaneously, the multipath network processes data through multiple parallel paths, transforms each path individually, and combines the results. This setup, inspired by grouped convolution techniques, helps to reduce computational complexity while maintaining high performance. The model was evaluated using a dataset comprising 3,064 MRI images and achieved an impressive classification accuracy of 98.61%, outperforming existing models evaluated on the same dataset. According to the World Health Organization, brain cancer continues to claim thousands of lives annually, with over 17,000 deaths reported in the United States in 2019 alone. The five-year survival rates stand at 34% for men and 36% for women post-diagnosis. Early detection and intervention significantly improve recovery chances and life expectancy. Medical imaging, particularly Magnetic Resonance Imaging (MRI), plays a crucial role in diagnosing brain tumours. However, manual analysis of such scans is both time-consuming and highly dependent on expert radiologists, increasing the likelihood of human error. With advancements in artificial intelligence and deep learning, automated diagnostic systems are becoming more prevalent and reliable in the medical field.This paper introduces a novel CNN-based architecture specifically for classifying brain tumors using T1-weighted contrast-enhanced MRI scans. The model focuses on three different types of brain tumors and leverages the power of attention mechanisms and multipath networks to extract rich and relevant features from the images, ultimately enhancing classification performance beyond traditional methods.

2.3 A Deep Learning-Based Framework for Automatic Brain Tumors Classification Using Transfer Learning

In their study, Archie Rehman et al. address the severity of brain tumors, which are among the most aggressive and life-threatening medical conditions, especially in their advanced stages. Misdiagnosis in such cases can lead to inappropriate treatment and significantly reduce patient survival rates. Therefore, achieving accurate diagnosis is crucial for developing effective treatment plans and improving the quality of life for individuals affected by brain tumors. Recent advancements in computer-aided diagnosis systems and convolutional neural networks (CNNs) have shown great promise in enhancing the accuracy and reliability of tumor detection. Deep CNN architectures are particularly effective at automatically extracting strong and relevant features from input images, outperforming traditional neural networks in this domain. In the proposed framework, three separate experimental studies were conducted using well-known CNN architectures: AlexNet, GoogleNet, and VGGNet. These models were employed to classify brain tumors into three categories—meningioma, glioma, and pituitary tumors—using MRI image slices from the Figshare dataset. Transfer learning techniques such as fine-tuning and feature extraction (snap) were applied to improve model efficiency and performance. To enhance generalization and reduce the risk of overfitting, data augmentation techniques were used to expand the dataset and improve the robustness of the models. Among the different approaches tested, the fine-tuned VGG16 model achieved the highest classification accuracy of 98.69% in identifying brain tumor types. Despite tremendous medical advancements over the past few decades, cancer—particularly brain cancer—remains one of the most complex and deadly challenges to humanity. The brain, being the control centre of the human body, governs critical functions such as movement, breathing, and sensory processing. Tumors develop when certain brain cells begin to grow uncontrollably, forming masses of abnormal tissue. Malignant brain tumors are especially dangerous due to their aggressive and uncontrolled growth. In the United States alone, approximately 23,000 new cases of brain tumors are diagnosed each year. According to 2017 cancer statistics, brain tumors remain a major cause of cancer-related illness and death worldwide, affecting both children and adults. In summary, this research presents a pioneering approach in the field of brain tumor classification using deep learning and transfer learning strategies. By leveraging models pre-trained on the ImageNet dataset and applying them to medical imaging data, the study effectively classifies tumor types with high accuracy. The deployment of CNN architectures—Alex Net, Google Net, and VGGNet—on the MRI dataset from Fig share, along with two modes of transfer learning, demonstrates the power of deep neural networks in extracting distinctive features and patterns from medical images. Among all trials, the fine-tuned VGG16 model yielded the best performance with an accuracy of 98.69%.

2.4 Deep Learning for Medical Anomaly Detection - A Survey

Fernando et al. (2022) focus on the critical issue of anomaly detection in medical diagnostics using machine learning techniques. This domain has been extensively researched, with numerous strategies proposed across various areas of medical applications. Although many of these approaches share similar characteristics, there is a noticeable absence of a structured and unified analysis that could help identify their strengths and weaknesses more clearly. The main objective of this review is to offer a comprehensive theoretical examination of prominent deep learning methods used in medical anomaly detection. The authors provide a detailed and systematic comparison of state-of-the-art techniques, focusing on differences in model architectures and training methods. Additionally, the study explores various interpretability methods for deep learning models, which are essential for understanding and trusting the decisions made by these often "black-box" systems in medical contexts. The review also highlights major challenges and limitations in current deep learning approaches to anomaly detection in medicine. It suggests future research directions aimed at improving the detection of data instances that deviate from typical distributions—a core task in anomaly detection. Such anomalies may emerge due to a variety of factors including data noise, shifts in underlying biological processes, or the presence of previously unseen medical conditions.

Anomaly detection plays a vital role in medical signal processing, where identifying unusual patterns or outliers is key to early diagnosis and treatment. The advent of deep learning has significantly advanced the capabilities of machine learning and has been widely adopted in the medical field for this purpose. The resulting surge in research has produced a wide array of deep learning frameworks tailored to anomaly detection in medical datasets. This review paper presents an organized and in-depth summary of existing research, comparing methodologies across different data collection environments and medical applications. It categorizes various deep learning architectures that have been developed in response to specific data characteristics and problem definitions. The authors also discuss multiple training strategies employed in this field and emphasize the importance of model interpretability—essential for validating and explaining diagnostic decisions made by AI systems. In conclusion, this work provides a valuable overview of deep learning-based medical anomaly detection, outlining key methodologies, interpretability techniques, challenges, and future research avenues for improving reliability and performance in real-world medical diagnostics.

2.5 Brain Tumor Segmentation Using Deep Learning on MRI Images

Almetwally M. Mostafa et al. have presented a system addressing the complexities of diagnosing brain tumors (BT), a process that demands significant expertise from radiologists and consumes a considerable amount of time. As patient numbers grow, the volume of medical imaging data increases, making traditional diagnostic methods inefficient and costly. In response, researchers have explored various fast and reliable methods to detect and classify brain tumors effectively. In recent years, deep learning (DL) techniques have emerged as powerful tools for medical diagnostics. These approaches utilize pre-trained convolutional neural networks (CNNs) to identify and classify brain tumors from medical images with high accuracy and speed. In this work, the authors use MRI images from the BT segmentation dataset, which contains 335 annotated scans and serves as a benchmark for developing and evaluating brain tumor detection algorithms. The BraTS dataset—a widely accepted resource for brain tumor segmentation and classification tasks—is used for model training and testing. The authors develop a deep CNN model, employing a categorical cross-entropy loss function and the Adam optimizer to train the network. The model achieves a validation accuracy of 98%, demonstrating its effectiveness in identifying and segmenting tumors. Brain tumors result from the uncontrolled division of abnormal cells, forming a mass that can disrupt normal tissue or organ function. These tumors can be classified based on their origin, structure, and cell type. While primary tumors originate in the brain, secondary tumors spread from other parts of the body. Tumors are further divided into malignant (high-grade) and benign (low-grade). Malignant brain tumors tend to grow rapidly and invade surrounding tissues, severely affecting cognitive abilities and overall quality of life. Even with advanced medical technologies, early diagnosis of certain diseases, including brain tumors, remains a challenge for physicians. Diagnostic imaging methods such as computed tomography (CT) and magnetic resonance imaging (MRI) are commonly used to identify tumors. With a collection of these MRI scans, the researchers trained their model using the U-Net architecture, which is known for its success in image segmentation tasks. The U-Net design integrates convolutional layers, max-pooling, upsampling, and skip connections, allowing it to capture both fine and coarse features from medical images. Through this approach, the proposed deep learning model effectively segments brain tumors and provides a promising tool for enhancing diagnostic accuracy and supporting clinical decision-making.

2.6 Brain Tumor Detection and Classification Using Deep Learning and Sine-Cosine Fitness Grey Wolf Optimization

ZainEldin et al (2022) have developed a system aimed at improving the diagnosis of brain tumors, a task that traditionally relies heavily on radiologist expertise and time. As the number of medical cases and associated imaging data increases, manual diagnosis becomes more time-consuming and costly. To address this, many researchers have turned to advanced algorithms that are faster and more accurate. This study introduces a Brain Tumor Classification Model (BCM-CNN) using deep learning techniques, particularly a Convolutional Neural Network (CNN). The novelty of this work lies in optimizing CNN hyperparameters through an innovative algorithm called Adaptive Dynamic Sine-Cosine Fitness Grey Wolf Optimizer (ADSCFGWO). This algorithm integrates the strengths of sine-cosine and grey wolf optimization techniques to fine-tune the model for better performance. The model uses Inception-ResNetV2, a powerful pre-trained network, and classifies brain tumors with binary output: 0 for normal and 1 for tumor. The method focuses on two sets of hyperparameters—those defining the network architecture and those guiding the training process. Through optimization, the model achieves a remarkable accuracy of 99.98% using the BraTS 2021 Task 1 dataset. The research emphasizes the need for efficient, accurate, and automated diagnostic systems in medical imaging, especially considering that brain tumors rank as the 10th leading cause of death in the U.S. Traditional manual assessments are prone to human error, highlighting the importance of computer-aided diagnostic systems in clinical applications.

2.7 Deep Learning Versus Classical Regression for Brain Tumor Patient Survival Prediction

Suter et al. (2019) explored the use of deep learning (DL) models, specifically 3D Convolutional Neural Networks (3D-CNNs), for predicting survival times in patients with high-grade brain tumors. While DL methods show promise in image-based regression tasks, their success is often limited by the size of the training dataset. This study compares 3D-CNN regression results with classical regression techniques using handcrafted features like intensity, shape, and location. Surprisingly, traditional models—especially Support Vector Classifiers (SVCs)—outperformed the CNNs in survival prediction. The SVC ensemble achieved 72.2% cross-validation accuracy on the BraTS 2018 training set, compared to only 51.5% accuracy for the best CNN approach. The results suggest that CNNs tend to overfit quickly on small datasets and struggle to generalize on unseen data. Additionally, non-imaging clinical data plays a crucial role in enhancing prediction accuracy. The findings align with past studies indicating that simpler regression models often yield better performance on limited datasets due to having fewer learnable parameters. The study underlines the challenges of predicting survival for patients with Grade III or IV gliomas, where the average survival is just 14 months. MRI-based biomarkers could be vital for improving prognosis and treatment planning, but current DL models require more data for reliable results.

2.8 A Low-Resource 3D U-Net Based Deep Learning Model for Medical Image Analysis

Chetty et al. (2022) propose a lightweight deep learning framework for segmenting brain tumors from 3D MRI scans, designed to be effective even in low-resource settings. The motivation stems from the high computational cost and data requirements of existing models, which may not be practical in remote or under-equipped healthcare environments. The method is based on a 3D U-Net architecture—a type of encoder-decoder CNN known for medical image segmentation. The model processes multi-modal, multi-contrast MRI scans without requiring additional data augmentation or high-end hardware. Despite its simplicity, it delivers improved segmentation performance when tested on the BraTS 2018 dataset provided by the MICCAI community. This fully automated system is especially valuable for identifying and analyzing gliomas, which are difficult to detect due to their irregular shape and fuzzy boundaries. Traditional manual segmentation is labor-intensive, subjective, and time-consuming, whereas the proposed system provides a fast and consistent alternative. The integration of lightweight CNNs in this model allows for effective segmentation with minimal resources, making it ideal for use in rural or underdeveloped medical centers. It also opens doors for broader application of AI in global healthcare, especially in diagnostic imaging tasks that require precision and speed.

2.9 A State-of-the-Art Approach for Cloudbased Semantic Segmentation Using Deep Learning and 3D U-Net Architecture

Shaukat et al. (2022) introduced a novel cloud-integrated 3D U-Net model aimed at segmenting glioma, a highly aggressive and life-threatening primary brain tumor with an average survival period of less than 14 months. This study emphasizes the significance of deep learning, particularly 3D U-Net, in conducting semantic segmentation using the BRATS dataset. The model was trained using the Adam optimizer along with varied hyperparameters, achieving a remarkable Dice similarity coefficient of 95%. This score, computed using the Sørensen–Dice metric, represents one of the highest accuracies in a cloud-based framework. An in-depth review of recent literature over the past five years was also conducted to compare various segmentation techniques, confirming that their model surpassed existing architectures in accuracy for glioma segmentation. Gliomas, constituting approximately 16% of central nervous system (CNS) tumors, primarily affect the brain but can also appear in the spinal cord, cerebellum, and brainstem. They occur most frequently in individuals around the age of 64 but can emerge at any age. According to the WHO classification, gliomas are divided into four grades based on malignancy, with Grades III and IV being the most severe. Among all types, glioblastoma is notably the most lethal and fast-spreading, making early detection and accurate diagnosis crucial. The proposed 3D U-Net model is a fully automated, cloud-based solution that allows access across the globe with minimal device requirements—only a stable internet connection and a basic terminal device are needed. The model integrates convolutional layers with max pooling and has proven to be highly effective in semantic segmentation for medical imaging.

2.10 Deep Reinforcement Learning With Automated Label Extraction From Clinical Reports for Accurate Classification of 3D MRI Brain Volumes

Stember & Shalu (2022) explored an efficient method for image classification in radiology, particularly in minimizing the workload of manual dataset labeling. The study introduces a dual-phase framework. In the first phase, sentence-level BERT (SBERT) was fine-tuned on 90 radiology reports to automatically extract labels. These labels were then used to train a reinforcement learning (RL)-based classifier in the second phase. The classifier was trained using 40 images and tested on 24 separate images.To compare, a supervised deep learning (SDL) model was also trained and evaluated on the same dataset using the same labels. While the SDL model quickly overfitted due to the limited training data and performed poorly on the test set with just 50% accuracy, the RL model achieved perfect testing accuracy (100%), with a statistically significant p-value of 4.9×10^{-4}. This study highlights the practicality of automated label extraction and reinforces the value of reinforcement learning in developing data-efficient, generalized classifiers. The process proves beneficial in scenarios where manual annotation is time-consuming and exhaustive.

2.11 Brain Tumor Segmentation and Classification Using 3D U-Net Deep Neural Networks

Agrawal et al. (2022) proposed a deep learning-based framework designed for precise segmentation and classification of brain tumors using 3D MRI scans. Early detection of brain tumors significantly improves the patient's chances of recovery, and MRI is a preferred imaging modality for this purpose. However, manual evaluation of MRI data is often challenging and time-intensive, dependent heavily on a radiologist's expertise.

To address these challenges, the authors employed a 3D U-Net model for volumetric segmentation, followed by classification using Convolutional Neural Networks (CNNs). Performance validation was done using accuracy and loss plots. The framework outperformed existing methods, offering improved efficiency and accuracy. The neural network was trained using an MRI dataset, and segmentation was refined using soft Dice loss functions to correct inaccuracies. The 3D MRI data was subdivided into smaller volumes for processing.

Two distinct datasets were used, collected from different global sources to mitigate dataset bias. The CNN classifier focused on identifying three common tumor types: glioma, meningioma, and pituitary tumors. Unlike other models that rely on region-based pre-processing, this system directly classifies tumors, enhancing efficiency. The results affirm that the proposed model outperforms previous state-of-the-art frameworks in both segmentation and classification tasks.

2.12 Single-Level 3D U-Net With Multipath Residual Attention Block for Brain Tumor Segmentation

Akbar et al. (2022) presented an optimized 3D U-Net-based segmentation model designed to overcome the limitations of manual brain tumor annotation, which is time-consuming, labor-intensive, and prone to human error. Their approach utilizes a single-level down-sampling 3D U-Net architecture integrated with Multipath Residual Attention Blocks (MRAB) to maintain spatial resolution and enhance feature extraction.

Manual segmentation, especially in large MRI datasets, often leads to expert fatigue and inconsistent results. This automated method uses datasets from the Brain Tumor Segmentation (BraTS) competition, which includes 1251 patient scans across four modalities. The segmentation targets are Whole Tumor (WT), Tumor Core (TC), and Enhancing Tumor (ET).

Three key features contribute to the model's superior performance: (1) limiting the network to a single down-sampling level to retain spatial features, (2) employing atrous convolutions within MRABs to capture broader contextual features without increasing computational load, and (3) integrating attention mechanisms in both skip connections and MRABs to enhance focus on relevant features while suppressing noise. The proposed architecture demonstrated competitive results in Dice coefficient and sensitivity, and it holds potential for clinical application due to its robustness and precision.

2.13 Brain Tumor Detection and Classification Using Machine Learning: A Comprehensive Survey

Amin et al. (2022) conducted a detailed survey on brain tumor detection through machine learning techniques, emphasizing MRI (Magnetic Resonance Imaging) as the primary modality. The paper discusses how brain tumors result from uncontrolled cell growth, which, if left untreated at an early stage, can be fatal. Despite significant progress, accurately segmenting and classifying tumors remains challenging due to the diversity in tumor size, shape, and location.

The survey comprehensively covers anatomical information of the brain, public datasets, enhancement techniques, segmentation, feature extraction, classification, and the roles of deep learning, transfer learning, and quantum machine learning in tumor analysis. It also outlines brain anatomy—highlighting key regions such as the cerebrum, cerebellum, and brainstem—and their functions in sensory processing, memory, movement, and coordination. The paper concludes by identifying current limitations in tumor detection models and encourages future researchers to explore improved methods for better segmentation and classification outcomes.

2.14 A Novel Approach for Brain Tumor Classification Using an Ensemble of Deep and Hand-Crafted Features

Kibriya et al. (2023) proposed a hybrid feature-based model for brain tumor detection, combining deep learning and handcrafted feature extraction methods. Given the high fatality rate of brain tumors and the rise in annual cases, rapid and accurate diagnostic systems are critical. The authors introduce an ensemble feature vector (EV) that combines texture-based handcrafted features (using GLCM – Gray Level Co-occurrence Matrix) and deep features extracted from the VGG16 neural network.

This combined feature vector is used in classification models such as Support Vector Machines (SVM) and K-Nearest Neighbors (KNN). The model achieved 99% accuracy on the BT-Large dataset and 96% on the BT-Small dataset. The study emphasizes the reliability of the proposed method and its potential for real-world deployment in clinical MRI-based diagnostics. The authors also suggest expanding the approach to multiple imaging modalities and deeper classification by tumor type in future research.

2.15 A Comprehensive Survey on Brain Tumor Diagnosis Using Deep Learning and Emerging Hybrid Techniques With Multi-Modal MRI

Ali et al. (2022) reviewed recent developments in brain tumor diagnosis using deep learning and hybrid approaches, focusing on MRI-based imaging. The paper highlights the limitations of manual segmentation and the growing need for computer-aided diagnostic systems. The review spans research from 2010 to 2020, noting a paradigm shift from traditional machine learning to deep learning and hybrid models.

The paper categorizes tumor types, such as gliomas, meningiomas, pituitary adenomas, and nerve sheath tumors, and discusses their grades according to the WHO classification. It emphasizes that accurate diagnosis is hindered by low contrast, tumor location variability, and overlapping intensity values. The review identifies trends in classifier usage and imaging modalities, recommending future research in deep, ensemble, and hybrid learning to design more robust and clinically viable computer-aided diagnostic (CAD) systems.

2.16 Deep Learning Based Brain Tumor Segmentation: A Survey

Liu et al. (2023) presented an in-depth study on brain tumor segmentation using deep learning techniques, one of the most complex tasks in medical image analysis. With over 100 referenced papers, the survey explores key areas including network architecture design, handling data imbalance, and processing multi-modal data inputs.The study highlights the effectiveness of deep learning in capturing high-level features for precise segmentation and evaluates various architectures and techniques. Despite advancements, challenges such as tumor location variability, low contrast imaging, and limited data remain significant barriers. The paper concludes by proposing future directions such as improved model robustness and expanded multi-modality training for enhanced performance in real-world scenarios.

2.17 D Deep Learning Based Brain Tumor Segmentation: A Survey of State of the Art

Magadza & Viriri (2021) focused on quantitative brain tumor analysis using advanced segmentation techniques. The authors argue that while manual segmentation is highly accurate, it is impractical for large-scale studies due to time and labor constraints. Therefore, deep learning has emerged as a promising alternative due to its ability to automate and enhance accuracy in segmentation.

The paper reviews several state-of-the-art deep learning architectures applied to medical imaging and discusses their performance in dealing with challenges such as varying image contrast across modalities, lesion heterogeneity, and data imbalance. It emphasizes the critical role of accurate segmentation in clinical treatment planning and prognosis, suggesting that deep learning, although promising, still requires refinement for widespread clinical adoption.

2.18 MRI-Based Brain Tumor Detection Using CNN-Based Deep Learning Approach

In this study, Chattopadhyay & Maître (2022) explore the role of medical imaging—a non-invasive method of examining internal body structures—in improving diagnosis and treatment. Among these, MRI plays a pivotal role in detecting brain tumors. The segmentation of tumors from MRI scans is crucial for accurate image analysis and diagnosis. The researchers focus on segmenting brain tumors using deep learning, aiming to assist medical professionals in locating tumors efficiently. Traditional manual segmentation, involving the examination of multiple MRI slices, is time-consuming and prone to human error. Hence, the study highlights the effectiveness of Convolutional Neural Networks (CNNs) in learning features directly from multi-modal MRI scans to distinguish between healthy tissue and tumor regions.

Initially, the authors used SVM integrated with CNN, but the accuracy achieved was low (20.83%). By modifying the network—changing the final layer to a softmax function and the optimizer to AdaMax—accuracy improved to 98.10%. Further enhancement using the RMSprop optimizer led to a final accuracy of 99.74%. The model used 2,473 training images and 273 testing images, with a 91:9 ratio over 11 training epochs. The CNN architecture includes 9 layers and 14 processing stages, achieving high precision in tumor detection.

2.19 Brain Tumor Segmentation With Deep Learning and Attention Mechanism Using MRI Multimodal Images

Ranjbarzadeh et al. (2021) propose a novel technique for segmenting brain tumors from MRI scans using deep learning with attention mechanisms. Brain tumor analysis using imaging modalities like T1, T1c, T2, and FLAIR provides essential insights, but many existing models are computationally heavy and time-intensive. To overcome this, the study introduces a preprocessing strategy that focuses on analyzing only a smaller region of the MRI slices, which significantly reduces computational load and addresses overfitting in cascade deep learning architectures. A Cascade Convolutional Neural Network (C-CNN) is then developed to extract both local and global features through separate processing paths. To further improve segmentation accuracy, the authors implement a Distance-Wise Attention (DWA) mechanism, which enhances the model's focus on the tumor's central location within the brain. The proposed model is tested on the BRATS 2018 dataset, achieving high average scores for whole tumor (0.9203), enhancing tumor (0.9113), and tumor core (0.8726) segmentations.

This research emphasizes the clinical importance of automated tumor segmentation, which can support radiologists by providing detailed information about tumor volume, shape, and location. Such automation not only aids in treatment planning but may also facilitate earlier diagnosis of related neurological disorders like Alzheimer's disease, schizophrenia, and dementia.

3. EXISTING SYSTEM

Brain is the controlling focal point of our body. With the appearance of time, more current and fresher cerebrum illnesses are being found. Subsequently, on account of the changeability of mind illnesses, existing conclusion or location frameworks are becoming testing and are as yet an open issue for research. Recognition of mind illnesses at a beginning phase can have a colossal effect in endeavoring to fix them. Lately, the utilization of computerized reasoning (man-made intelligence) is flooding through all circles of science, and presumably, it is changing the area of nervous system science. Use of simulated intelligence in clinical science has made cerebrum sickness forecast and discovery more exact and exact. In this review, we present a survey on late AI and profound learning approaches in identifying four mind illnesses like Alzheimer's sickness (Promotion), cerebrum growth, epilepsy, and Parkinson's infection. 147 late articles on four mind illnesses

4. PROPOSED SYSTEM

We present a system that uses cutting-edge machine learning approaches to automate the segmentation of MRI images of brain tumors. To detect tumor locations and healthy tissue, the system first pre-processes and segments raw MRI data. The dataset is then divided into subsets for testing and training in order to construct and assess the model. For classification, we use a deep learning architecture, such as a Long Short-Term Memory (LSTM) network, where the model learns to categorize each pixel or voxel into several classes. The model is used to forecast segmentations for fresh MRI images once training is finished. Ultimately, the segmentation findings are refined by post-processing procedures, producing precise tumor region delineations. The suggested technique provides physicians with a reliable and automated way to diagnose and treat patients with brain tumors more quickly and accurately.

4.1 Brain Image

This module pre-processes and segments the brain's raw MRI images to find areas of interest, such the edges of tumors or healthy tissue. To guarantee consistency across scans, pre-processing techniques including noise reduction, intensity normalization, and image registration may be used. After that, segmentation techniques like region growth, thresholding, or sophisticated deep learning algorithms are used to identify certain abnormalities or structures in the brain pictures.

Figure 3. Original MRI

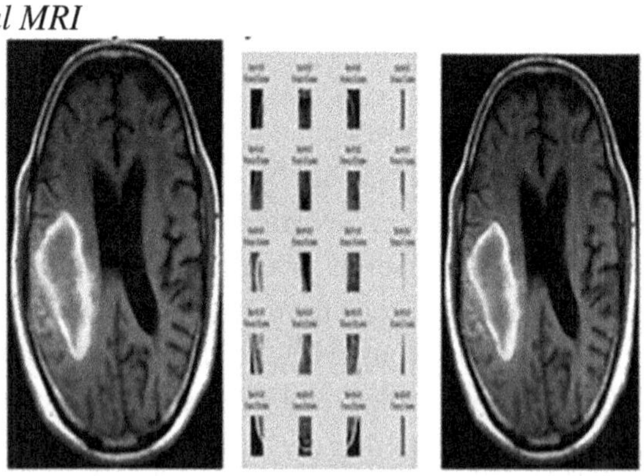

4.2 Segmentation

The technique of dividing a picture into many segments or areas of interest is known as image segmentation. Segmentation, as used in brain tumor analysis, is the process of locating and separating the tumor from the surrounding healthy brain tissue. For this purpose, a variety of segmentation algorithms may be used, including deep learning-based techniques, region-growing, and thresholding.

4.3 Splitting Dataset Into Train and Test Data

The provided dataset is divided into several subsets for the purpose of training and evaluating the machine learning model in this session. Training and testing sets are created by randomly dividing the dataset, which contains brain MRI pictures and the accompanying ground truth annotations, or by using certain techniques (such stratified sampling). In order to enable the model to learn patterns efficiently, most of the data is usually set aside for training, with a smaller amount set aside for assessing the model's performance on unobserved data.

4.4 Classification

This module involves the training of a machine learning algorithm, such as an LSTM network, to categorize individual pixels or voxels in the brain pictures into distinct groups (e.g., tumor, background, healthy tissue). The classification model is trained using the training data, which consists of input MRI pictures and matching ground truth segmentations. Gradient descent and backpropagation are two methods used in iterative parameter optimization that help the model learn to translate input data to the appropriate class labels.

4.5 Prediction

After training, the classification model is used to fresh, unobserved brain MRI data in order to forecast the segmentation masks, or the boundaries between various areas within the pictures. When the raw MRI images are input into the trained model, it produces predictions for every pixel or voxel that show the likelihood or class label connected to the existence of a tumor or other structures. Large amounts of imaging data are often handled effectively by this prediction method with the use of parallel processing techniques.

4.6 Result Generation

In order to produce final outputs and assess the segmentation algorithm's effectiveness, this module post-processes the anticipated segmentation masks. The segmentation results may be improved, artifacts can be eliminated, and the final output mask accuracy can be increased by using post-processing methods as morphological operations, linked component analysis, or probabilistic graphical models. Performance metrics are computed to evaluate the segmentation quality statistically and compare it with ground truth annotations. These metrics include the Hausdorff distance, sensitivity, specificity, and Dice similarity coefficient.

5. RESULT ANALYSIS

The accuracy of two well-known deep learning architectures, Long Short-Term Memory (LSTM) and Convolutional Neural Network (CNN), was assessed in this comparison study of brain tumor picture segmentation techniques. With an accuracy of 90%, the LSTM model outperformed the CNN model, which had an accuracy of 85%. Tumor segmentation became more accurate as a result of the LSTM architecture's greater performance in collecting the complex characteristics and spatial interactions seen in brain MRI images. This architecture is well-known for its capacity to capture temporal dependencies and contextual information. On the other hand, while CNNs are good at identifying hierarchical characteristics in pictures, they may not be as good at capturing temporal dynamics, which might have affected the quality of the segmentation. These results highlight the usefulness of LSTM-based methods for challenges involving the segmentation of images of brain tumors.

Table 1. Comparison graph

Methods	accuracy
LSTM	90
CNN	85

Figure 4. Comparison graph

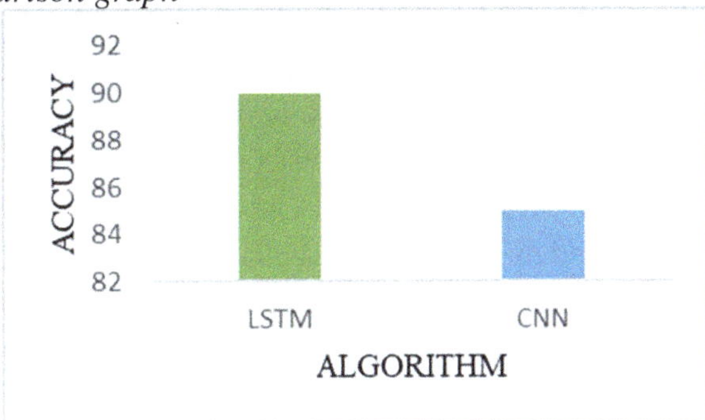

6. ALGORITHM DETAILS

The vanishing gradient issue is notably addressed by the Long Short-Term Memory (LSTM) method, a form of recurrent neural networks (RNNs), which makes it possible for it to capture long-range relationships in sequential data. LSTM units control information flow by combining memory cells with input, forget, and output gates. This allows pertinent information to be retained across longer sequences while unnecessary details are filtered away. Backpropagation across time optimizes the model's capacity to learn and represent intricate temporal patterns by updating its parameters throughout training. LSTM networks are particularly good at capturing temporal and spatial relationships between image slices in the setting of brain tumor MRI image segmentation. This allows for accurate segmentation by using temporal dynamics and contextual information seen in multi-sequence MRI data.

```
Initialize weights and biases for LSTM cells
Initialize hidden state h_t and cell state c_t to zeros
For each time step t:
Concatenate input data x_t with previous hidden state h_{t-1}
Calculate input gate i_t = sigmoid(W_i * [x_t, h_{t-1}] + b_i)
Calculate forget gate f_t = sigmoid(W_f * [x_t, h_{t-1}] + b_f)
Calculate output gate o_t = sigmoid(W_o * [x_t, h_{t-1}] + b_o)
Calculate candidate cell state values ~c_t = tanh(W_c * [x_t, h_{t-1}] + b_c)
Update cell state c_t:
c_t = f_t * c_{t-1} + i_t * ~c_t
Calculate hidden state h_t:
h_t = o_t * tanh(c_t)
End loop
```

7. CONCLUSION

Finally, the LSTM method demonstrates its effectiveness in capturing temporal dynamics and long-range relationships, making it a formidable tool for sequential data processing. LSTM networks are very effective in a number of tasks, such as language modelling, time series prediction, and picture sequence analysis, thanks to its gated mechanism and memory cells. Because LSTM can include both spatial and temporal information, it presents a viable solution for precise and reliable brain tumor MRI picture segmentation. This might pave the way for improved neuro-oncology diagnostics and individualized treatment plans.

8. FUTURE WORK

Subsequent research endeavors in the domain of brain tumor MRI image segmentation may investigate many pathways towards more progress. First off, by offering complementary details regarding tumor properties, the inclusion of multimodal MRI data, such as diffusion-weighted imaging and perfusion-weighted imaging, may improve the segmentation models' resilience and accuracy. Furthermore, investigating the attention processes in LSTM networks may enhance the model's capacity to concentrate on pertinent areas of interest, which may result in a more accurate delineation of tumors. Additionally, the creation of synthetic data or the improvement of segmentation boundaries may be made possible by using generative adversarial networks (GANs) or reinforcement learning approaches. This would increase the dataset and enhance the generalization of the model. Lastly, in order to translate research results into useful clinical practice, it would be crucial to implement and evaluate these sophisticated segmentation algorithms in clinical settings in conjunction with radiologists' knowledge.

REFERENCES

Agrawal, P., Katal, N., & Hooda, N. (2022). 3D U-Net-based segmentation and classification of brain tumors. *International Journal of Cognitive Computing in Engineering, 3*, 199–210. DOI: 10.1016/j.ijcce.2022.11.001

Akbar, A. S., Fatichah, C., & Suciati, N. (2022). UNet3D with residual attention for brain tumor segmentation. *Journal of King Saud University. Computer and Information Sciences, 34*(6), 3247–3258. DOI: 10.1016/j.jksuci.2022.03.022

Ali, S., Li, J., Pei, Y., Khurram, R., & Mahmood, T. (2022). A comprehensive survey on brain tumor diagnosis using deep learning and emerging hybrid techniques with multi-modal MR image. *Archives of Computational Methods in Engineering, 29*(7), 4871–4896. DOI: 10.1007/s11831-022-09758-z

Amin, J., Sharif, M., Haldorai, A., Yasmin, M., & Nayak, R. S. (2022). Brain tumor detection and classification using machine learning: A comprehensive survey. *Complex & Intelligent Systems, 8*(4), 3161–3183. DOI: 10.1007/s40747-021-00563-y

Chattopadhyay, A., & Maître, M. (2022). CNN-based MRI brain tumor image detection technique. *Neuroscience Informatics*, 2.

Chetty, G., Yamin, M., & White, M. (2022). Resource-efficient 3D U-Net model for medical image analysis. *International Journal of Information Technology : an Official Journal of Bharati Vidyapeeth's Institute of Computer Applications and Management, 14*(1), 95–103. DOI: 10.1007/s41870-021-00850-4 PMID: 35005425

Fernando, H., Gamboled, S., Denman, S., Sridharan, S., & Folks, C. (2022). Survey on deep learning for detecting anomalies in medical images. *ACM Computing Surveys, 54*(7), 1–37. DOI: 10.1145/3464423

Jun, W., & Liana, Z. (2022). A deep learning model with attention for classifying brain tumors. *International Journal of Computational Intelligence Systems, 15*(1), 35. DOI: 10.1007/s44196-022-00090-9

Kibriya, H., Amin, R., Kim, J., Nawaz, M., & Gantassi, R. (2023). A novel approach for brain tumor classification using an ensemble of deep and hand-crafted features. *Sensors (Basel), 23*(10), 4693. DOI: 10.3390/s23104693 PMID: 37430604

Lakshmi, M. J., & Rao, S. N. (2022). Classification of brain tumor MRI using deep learning techniques. *Soft Computing, 26*(13), 6245–6253. DOI: 10.1007/s00500-022-07163-z

Liu, Z., Tong, L., Chen, L., Jiang, Z., Zhou, F., Zhang, Q., Zhang, X., Jin, Y., & Zhou, H. (2023). Deep learning based brain tumor segmentation: A survey. *Complex & Intelligent Systems*, *9*(1), 1001–1026. DOI: 10.1007/s40747-022-00815-5

Magadza, T., & Viriri, S. (2021). Deep learning for brain tumor segmentation: A survey of state-of-the-art. *Journal of Imaging*, *7*(2), 19. DOI: 10.3390/jimaging7020019 PMID: 34460618

Ranjbarzadeh, R., Bagherian Kasgari, A., Jafarzadeh Ghoushchi, S., Anari, S., Naseri, M., & Bendechache, M. (2021). Brain tumor segmentation based on deep learning and an attention mechanism using MRI multi-modalities brain images. *Scientific Reports*, *11*(1), 10930. DOI: 10.1038/s41598-021-90428-8 PMID: 34035406

Shaukat, Z., Farooq, Q. U. A., Tu, S., Xiao, C., & Ali, S. (2022). A state-of-the-art technique to perform cloud-based semantic segmentation using deep learning 3D U-Net architecture. *BMC Bioinformatics*, *23*(1), 251. DOI: 10.1186/s12859-022-04794-9 PMID: 35751030

Stember, J. N., & Shalu, H. (2022). Classification of 3D MRI brain volumes using reinforcement learning and clinical reports. *Journal of Digital Imaging*, *35*(5), 1143–1152. DOI: 10.1007/s10278-022-00644-5 PMID: 35562633

Suter, Y., Jungo, A., Rebsamen, M., Knecht, U., Herrmann, E., Wiest, R., & Reyes, M. (2019). Deep learning versus classical regression for brain tumor patient survival prediction. In A. Crimi, S. Bakas, H. Kuijf, F. Keyvan, M. Reyes, & T. van Walsum (Eds.), *Brainlesion: Glioma, multiple sclerosis, stroke and traumatic brain injuries* (pp. 429–440). Springer. DOI: 10.1007/978-3-030-11726-9_38

ZainEldin, H., Gamel, S. A., El-Kenawy, E.-S. M., Alharbi, A. H., Khafaga, D. S., Ibrahim, A., & Talaat, F. M.ZainEldin. (2022). Brain tumor detection and classification using deep learning and sine-cosine fitness grey wolf optimization. *Bioengineering (Basel, Switzerland)*, *10*(1), 18. DOI: 10.3390/bioengineering10010018 PMID: 36671591

Chapter 10
Future Prospective in Therapeutics Approaches in Prevalent Infectious Diseases of CNS

Anmol Kumr
School of Pharmaceutical Science, University Institute of Pharmacy. Chhatrapati Shahu Ji Maharaj University, India

K. Amrutha
CSIR-Central Drug Research Institute, Lucknow, India

Kumar Maurya ARUK
CSIR-Central Drug Research Institute, Lucknow, India

Poonam Verma
CSIR-Central Drug Research Institute, Lucknow, India

Neelam Yadav
https://orcid.org/0000-0002-2245-7824
Dr. Rammanohar Lohia Avadh University, Ayodhya, India

Sarika Singh
CSIR-Central Drug Research Institute, Lucknow, India

ABSTRACT

Central nervous system infections pose a major challenge to modern medicine due to the protective nature of the blood-brain barrier (BBB) towards meningitis, encephalitis, and abscesses treatments. Antimicrobial agents could penetrate the BBB; however, they pose limited effects due to being multi-drug-resistant. Advancements in nanotechnology and targeted drug delivery systems offer promising approaches to overcome including nanoparticle-mediated drug delivery. Additionally, the new antiviral agents targeting specific stages of viral replication cycles, as well as therapies based on host antiviral immune responses may be useful. These include toll-like receptor agonists, interferon preparations, and passive transfer of virus-

DOI: 10.4018/979-8-3693-4070-7.ch010

specific cytotoxic T lymphocytes. Treatment with nanoparticles, exosomes, focused ultrasound, intracerebroventricular delivery, gene therapy, and specific degradomers can contribute to successful treatment though it needs the researcher's attention.

1. INTRODUCTION

The central nervous system (CNS) is a complex structure that consists of the brain, spinal cord, its covering known as meninges and an extensive network of neurons. The CNS pose a highly protected and strong defence mechanism with tight endothelial cell junction against invaders such as pathogens and infection-causing microorganisms through the Blood Brain Barrier (BBB). However, sometimes this protection is breached, leading to CNS infections such as meningitis, encephalitis, and brain abscesses. A wide variety of pathogens, including bacteria, viruses, fungi, and parasites cause these(Faizi & Hassan, 2023; Nath & Tyler, 2013). Prompt recognition and treatment of Central Nervous System (CNS) infections are crucial to overcoming this medical emergency. Globally, the prevalence rate of CNS infection is high and these infections have a high morbidity and mortality rate. This makes them potentially life-threatening and makes them emergency conditions. Recent studies have highlighted the urgent need for effective therapeutics to tackle CNS infections. However, this poses significant challenges due to various factors such as poor BBB penetration, multidrug resistance, lack of awareness, complex pharmacokinetics, and the emergence of new pathogens that can cause a global burden. Therefore, it is imperative to develop and advance therapeutics for CNS infections to address these challenges. In this chapter, will delve into the details of the future prospects of therapeutic approaches for CNS infections (Ang et al., 2023; Le Govic et al., 2022). The future approaches of treating central nervous system (CNS) infections are on the brink of significant transformation, driven by a blend of innovative approaches that are reshaping treatment paradigms. The protective blood-brain barrier (BBB) has historically impeded effective pharmacological interventions, but recent biotechnological advancements and a deeper understanding of CNS infection mechanisms are changing that. Nanotechnology, particularly nanoparticles, is emerging as a promising method for enhancing drug delivery across the BBB, boosting treatment efficacy for various pathogens. Gene therapy is also making strides. Additionally, understanding neuro-immune interactions has unveiled new pharmacological targets, such as the complement system's role in neurodegeneration, suggesting potential for anti-complement drugs. RNA interference (RNAi) technology is being explored to silence disease-causing genes, offering a precise approach to treating CNS infections and neurodegenerative conditions (Aboabdo & Mishkin, 2024; Schwartz et al., 2018; Sigfrid et al., 2019). Despite these advances, challenges remain due to the CNS's complexity, infection intricacies, and the need for precise targeting. The diversity of CNS pathogens and emerging drug-resistant strains also demand ongoing innovation. Nonetheless, the future of CNS infection treatment is promising, with interdisciplinary collaborations and research investments essential to bringing these therapies from the lab to clinical use. Other innovative treatments in targeted drug delivery, immunotherapies, gene therapies, and both invasive and non-invasive techniques. Targeted drug delivery systems, including nanoparticles, liposomes, and polymeric microspheres, aim to transport therapeutic agents directly to infection sites, enhancing efficacy and reducing systemic side effects. Methods such as convection-enhanced delivery and intracerebroventricular delivery are also being explored for direct drug infusion into the CNS (Ciummo et al., 2021; Ng & Solomon, 2015). Immunotherapies, using monoclonal antibodies, checkpoint inhibitors, and therapeutic vaccines, are being developed to boost the immune system's response to CNS pathogens, focusing on neuro-immune interactions and neuroinflammation. Gene therapies, facilitated by advances in viral vector technology like adeno-associated viruses (AAVs), offer potential cures by correcting genetic mutations or altering gene expression to treat CNS disorders at the molecular level. Treatment strategies also include invasive methods, such as surgical implantation of drug-eluting devices, and non-invasive approaches like trans nasal delivery and focused ultrasound, which utilize natural body pathways to deliver therapeutics with reduced surgical risks (Kapoor & Tan, 2020; Ledri et al., 2021).

2. EPIDEMIOLOGICAL SURVEY AND EVIDENCES OF GLOBAL BURDEN

CNS infections are a major public health issue worldwide and affect millions of individuals each year. The epidemiology of CNS infections differs across various regions and populations and is influenced by factors such as access to healthcare, socioeconomic status, and environmental conditions. A recently in 2023 published meta-analysis in the journal Future Medicine has estimated that the occurrence of CNS infections in low- and middle-income countries is approximately 726 and 299 cases per 100,000 populations, respectively. On the other hand, the incidence rate for high-income countries is just 11 cases per 100,000 populations (Faizi & Hassan, 2023).

According to the World Health Organization (WHO) regions, the intracranial abscess had the highest pooled incidence in Southeast Asia (49/100,000 cases), nontuberculous vertebral spondylodiscitis (5/100,000 instances), and bacterial meningitis (65 cases/100,000 people) and *neurocysticercosis* (650/100,000 cases) in Africa (55/100,000 cases (*Meningitis*, n.d.; Sheybani et al., 2023).

A report of CNS infection that the research discovered the root cause of illness in 365 patients, which is 91.0% of the total. CNS tuberculosis was found to be the most frequent cause of the disease, accounting for 51.5%, followed by viral *meningoencephalitis* (13.9%), community-acquired bacterial meningitis (9.7%), *cryptococcal meningitis* (6.2%), *scrub typhus meningoencephalitis* (1.7%), *neurocysticercosis* (1.7%), and fungal brain abscess (1.7%). The study also revealed a mortality rate of 27.9% in patients, with the highest rate being in cases where the root cause of illness could not be identified (64.5%) (Wunrow et al., 2023).

Majorly the occurrence and incidence of CNS infection globally affects millions of people but in the Lancet report of 2019 there were estimated 236000 deaths in 2.51 million cases globally and the incidents of meningitis increased from 2.50 to 2.82 million (Wunrow et al., 2023).

3. CURRENT THERAPEUTICS AND THEIR LIMITATION

3.1 Treatment of Bacterial Meningitis

Bacterial meningitis is an infection with subsequent inflammation of the meninges and the meninges are three layered membranes surrounding the brain and spinal cord. Meningitis is primarily caused by bacteria, fungi, viruses, and parasites; other causes include head trauma, CSF leakage during neurosurgery, sinusitis, and otitis media. Bacterial meningitis is primarily attributed to four types of bacteria namely *Neisseria meningitis (meningococcal), Streptococcus pneumonia, Hemophilic influenza and Streptococcus agalactia* and these bacterial strains are responsible for more than half of deaths due to meningitis. The global annual prevalence of bacterial meningitis is 1.2 million cases, resulting in 100,000 deaths (Gundamraj & Hasbun, 2023; *Meningitis*, n.d.). This highlights the significant threat of this disease, with a high mortality rate affecting individuals of all age groups. The current prompt diagnostic and therapeutic management of bacterial meningitis forces significant limitations, primarily due to the reliance on antimicrobial drugs, these drugs are hindered by poor penetration, resulting from the intricate nature of the blood-brain barrier, which selectively regulates molecular entry so, the choice antibiotics therapies based on different pharmacokinetics and pharmacodynamics factors of the drug such as lipid solubility, molecular structure, molecular size, metabolism and therapeutic concentration that decide the crossing of drug through BBB. Ensuring the adequate concentration of the therapeutic drug at the infection site is essential for effectively treating the infection. However, the blood-brain barrier (BBB) and the blood-cerebrospinal fluid barrier (BCSFB) may pose limitations in achieving the necessary drug levels at the targeted site (Kadry et al., 2020). Meningitis can present with a wide range of clinical signs, depending on the patient's age and immune system condition. Symptoms that are frequently noted include fever, stiffness or soreness in the neck, and light sensitivity. A variety of less focused symptoms, including headaches, *vertigo, delirium, mental disorientation, irritability, and gastrointestinal disturbances* including nausea or vomiting, may also be experienced by patients. A worse prognosis is frequently linked to clinical indicators of increased intracranial pressure, such as altered mental status, neurological deficits, and convulsive events. It is critical to identify these symptoms as soon as possible because they can help in the diagnosis of meningitis patients more quickly and start treating them appropriately, both of which improve patient outcomes. According to recent research, meningeal irritation symptoms like Brudzinski's and Kernig's signs are frequently seen in meningococcal meningitis cases (Palmer et al., 2022). These symptoms are frequently accompanied by unique skin manifestations including purpura and petechia. Furthermore, 10% to 20% of patients have anomalies in their cranial nerves; diseases such as cranial nerve palsy typically appears following bacterial meningitis. The accurate diagnosis of meningitis is crucial for effective treatment and the gold standard technique of diagnosis is lumber puncture (spinal tap) which allows for analysis of the cerebrospinal fluid (CSF) to identify the specific organism. Imaging methods such as CT and MRI are supportive in that they assist rule out other illnesses and screen for consequences like hydrocephalus. Modern developments have further highlighted the importance of neuroimaging in the diagnosis of meningitis, with MRI being especially helpful for its in-depth meninges visualization (Ramachandran & Wilson, 2021; Wunrow et al., 2023). The treatment protocol for bacterial meningitis is highly dependent on accurate and timely diagnosis. Once *bacterial meningitis* is suspected, then empiric antibiotic therapies are initiated. Which is the broad and narrow spectrum treatment aimed at the most likely pathogen based on the patient's age medical history and risk factors. For instance, newborns and young infants may receive a combination of ampicillin and Cefotaxime with different time intervals of administration or *Gentamicin* to cover common pathogens like group *B streptococcus and E. coli*. Older children and adults might be treated with *Ceftriaxone and Cefotaxime plus Vancomycin to cover listeria meningitis and streptococcus pneumonia*. The dose regimen, limitations and adverse effects are described in *table 2.1*.

For the other infections due to skull fractures, penetrating injuries, infections related to shunts, or post-neurosurgical, the pathogens involved are mostly bacteria like *Streptococcus pneumoniae, Hemophilus influenzae, Group B Streptococcus, Staphylococcus aureus, coagulase-negative staphylococci, Enterobacteriaceae, and Pseudomonas spp.* Treatment involves the administration of Vancomycin at 15 mg/kg intravenously every 8 to 12 hours and Ceftriaxone 2 g intravenously every 12 hours for skull fractures, or Cefepime 2 g intravenously every 8 hours for other situations (Chaudhuri et al., 2011; Phar & Bereda G, 2022; Young & Thomas, 2018).

One important tool in the fight against meningitis is vaccination. Novel vaccinations are revolutionary. It is advised that the meningitis belt be mass vaccinated against the five dominant serogroups covered by the WHO-prequalified *Men5CV vaccine*. For those who are 10 years of age or older, the ACIP in the US advises using Pfizer's Pentavalent Meningococcal Vaccine. Due to the vaccines' ability to prevent fatalities and impairments, the disease's economic and societal cost will be reduced, revolutionizing meningitis prevention and care, especially in high-burden areas. A comprehensive global reduction in the incidence of meningitis will require more study in vaccine science and technology. Increasing vaccination coverage and implementing better immunization schedules in healthcare systems are useful strategies (Le et al., 2023; Qu et al., 2023).

Table 1. Empiric antibiotics therapeutics based on Age groups

Age Type	Empiric Treatment with the dose regimen	Antimicrobial Spectrum	Limitation/Adverse effects	References
Neonates (0-28 days)	Ampicillin (50mg/kg IV each after 6hr) + Gentamicin (2.5mg/kg IV each after 8hr) OR Ampicillin (100mg/kg IV every 6hr) + Cefotaxime (50mg/kg every 6hr)	*Listeria monoctogene, E coli, Group B Streptococcus, Streptococcus agalactia*	Antimicrobial resistance and narrow spectrum with ampicillin. Risk of mortality in neonates by third-generation cephalosporin combination. Gentamicin has certain side effects nephrotoxicity and ototoxicity	(Alamarat & Hasbun, 2020; Edwards & Baker, 2013; Li et al., 2017; Ueda et al., 2018)
Infants and Children (1 month-18yrs.)	Ceftriaxone (50mg/kg each after 12hr) + Vancomycin (10mg/kg each after 6hr)	*Neisseria meningitis(meningococcus), Streptococcus pneumoniae, Hemophilus influenzae*	Ceftriaxone is associated with allergic reactions, biliary sludging and resistance. Vancomycin associated with infusion reaction, required therapeutic drug monitoring and nephrotoxicity.	(Holdaway et al., 2018; K. S. Kim, 2010; Shukla et al., 2017)
Adult (18-50 yrs. old)	Dexamethasone (10mg/kg IV/ 6hr) + Cefotaxime (2g IV/12hr) OR Ampicillin (1-2g IV, IM once in day) + Ceftriaxone (2g IV /12hrs)	*Streptococcus pneumoniae, Neisseria meningitis, Hemophilus influenzae*	Ceftriaxone is associated with Pseudomembranous colitis, inflammation in the colon, and Allergic reaction. Dexamethasone having GIT disturbance Cefotaxime is associated with allergic reactions with resistance	(Brouwer & van de Beek, 2023; Garlicki et al., 2023; Nhantumbo et al., 2022)
More than 50yrs.	Ampicillin (2g IV/ 4hr) + Cefotaxime (2g IV/ 12hr) OR Cefotaxime (2g IV/ 6hr) + Vancomycin (15mg/kg IV/12hrs)	*Listeria monoctogene, Aerobic gram-negative bacilli, Hemophilus influenzae, Streptococcus pneumoniae*	Ampicillin has hypersensitivity reactions and resistance. Cefotaxime has hemolytic anaemia. Vancomycin has red men syndrome.	(Domingo et al., 2013; Niemelä et al., 2023; Wunrow et al., 2023)

3.2 Treatment of Viral Meningitis and Encephalitis

Viral Meningitis and encephalitis are a medical emergency condition which has a significantly higher morbidity and mortality rate globally. The occurrence of this infection varies with a different geographical location and seasons. Viral meningitis is characterized by the inflammation of the meninges due to the invasion of viruses in the brain and body various types of viruses are responsible such as Enterovirus, Herpes virus, Rabies, Arbovirus, Mumps, measles and Cryptococcal virus. Viral meningitis can be acute, subacute and chronic with symptoms (Gundamraj & Hasbun, 2023).

Viral encephalitis is a severe inflammatory condition affecting the brain and parenchyma caused the certain viruses. Viral meningitis having a complex medical challenge due to the varied etiology, clinical presentation and having an acute on set of neurological symptoms. Viral meningitis and encephalitis present with a range of neurological and systemic symptoms. Common signs include fever, headache, sensitivity to light, and neck stiffness, indicating meningeal irritation. Neurological issues such as altered mental state, seizures, and localized neurological deficits like hemiparesis or cranial nerve impairment may also occur. Encephalitis can lead to delirium, extreme lethargy, and, in severe instances, coma. Other symptoms may include nausea, vomiting, and signs of increased intracranial pressure. Prompt recognition of these symptoms by healthcare professionals is essential for timely and effective management to prevent complications. Diagnosing viral meningitis and encephalitis involves both clinical evaluation and diagnostic tests (Melhuish & McGill, 2021; Songtao et al., 2023). Viral meningitis is identified through neurological exams and *cerebrospinal fluid (CSF)* analysis obtained via lumbar puncture, with polymerase chain reaction (PCR) testing used to detect viral pathogens in the CSF. For encephalitis, brain imaging techniques like MRI or CT scans help identify swelling or abnormalities, and an electroencephalogram (EEG) can detect brain activity patterns indicative of encephalitis. Additional tests on blood, urine, or throat samples may be performed to pinpoint the specific virus responsible. The current treatment and the management of viral meningitis and encephalitis remains focused on accurate diagnosis, prompt treatment, and thorough supportive care. The treatment strategy is multifaceted, encompassing the use of antiviral medications, additional therapeutic measures, and preventive approaches. Antiviral therapy, particularly with acyclovir, is fundamental in treating herpes simplex virus (HSV) encephalitis ("Encephalitis: Diagnosis, Management and Recent Advances in the Field of Encephalitides.," 2023). Early administration of these medications is vital for improving patient outcomes and lowering mortality rates. When specific viral causes are identified, other targeted antivirals like ganciclovir for cytomegalovirus (CMV) or oseltamivir for the influenza virus may also be used. Another important treatment Supportive Care therapy to managing viral meningitis and encephalitis relies heavily on supportive care, which involves balancing fluids and electrolytes, controlling fever and pain, and preventing secondary infections. In severe instances, patients might need mechanical ventilation and intensive care support. Adjunctive Therapies additional treatments, like corticosteroids, can help reduce brain *swelling and inflammation*. However, their use is debated and usually reserved for specific situations where the potential benefits are greater than the risks. And the prevention is crucial in managing viral CNS infections. Vaccinations for common pathogens such as measles, mumps, rubella, and varicella greatly lower the risk of viral meningitis and encephalitis. Additionally, controlling mosquito populations and using personal protective measures are essential in regions where arboviruses are prevalent. Despite significant advancements in neurology and infectious diseases, treating viral meningitis and encephalitis remains challenging due to diagnostic difficulties, viral diversity, limited antiviral options, individual immune responses, and emerging pathogens. Precisely diagnosing these infections can be tough, often delaying targeted therapy (Hinduja et al., 2019; Shahjin et al., 2019). The wide variety of viruses and their capacity to mutate complicates diagnosis and treatment, with some viruses developing resistance to existing antivirals. Many viral agents lack specific antiviral drugs, leaving supportive care as the primary option, which may not prevent long-term neurological damage. Additionally, individual immune response variability affects treatment effectiveness, particularly in immunocompromised patients. Emerging and re-emerging viral pathogens further complicate treatment efforts, as existing therapies may be ineffective. Preventive measures, including vaccinations and vector control, are not comprehensive for all pathogens, highlighting the need for continued research and improved therapeutic strategies (Nowak et al., 2023; "Virus Prevention, Diagnosis, and Treatment," 2023).

Table 2. The current therapeutic approaches to Viral CNS infection are based on the type of Viruses

Type of Virus	Mode of Pathogenesis/ Transmission	Treatments	Limitation	References
Herpes Simplex Virus	Direct contact with genitals organs, body fluids and contact with sores.	No cure for HSV but supportive care by Antiviral drugs (Acyclovir, Valacyclovir and Famciclovir) and administration of Corticosteroids	No specific cure, Challenge in diagnosis, Persistence in virus, Antiviral resistance and Neurological sequelae	(Aldeen et al., 2014; Burrel et al., 2020; Piperi et al., 2024)
Cytomegalovirus	Direct contact with blood, tears, saliva, semen, urine and breast milk.	Antiviral medication (Ganciclovir) Some analgesic drugs	No specific antiviral medication, Kidney dysfunction, Immunodeficiency and neurological dysfunction.	(Folke et al., 2022; Manan & Manan, 2021)
Measles virus	Transmit through the respiratory tract by airborne droplets	Supportive care and Corticosteroid drugs, Measles-Mumps-Rubella vaccine	Lack of specific therapies, Difficulty in diagnosis, long-term sequelae.	(Drossinos et al., 2021; Haddad et al., 2022)
Respiratory Virus	Transmission through the respiratory tract.	Supportive care (Plenty of fluid and hospitalization), Antiviral medication (Ganciclovir, Foscarnet) and Immunotherapies	Delayed diagnosis, Less specificity with infection and Limited antiviral drugs.	(Aldeen et al., 2014; Simões et al., 2018)
Nipah Virus	Transmit through fruit bats and contact with pigs or infected animals	Supportive care and Antiviral medication (Ribavirin)	Lack of specific antiviral drugs, Challenges in diagnosis	(Ang et al., 2018; Bruno et al., 2023)
Arbovirus (Zika, Japanese encephalitis, tick-borne and Chikungunya virus)	Transmit through the biting of Tick, through the mosquito bite and sand fly	Supportive care (Hospitalization care) Vaccination therapy	Lack of specific antiviral drugs, and having the neurocognitive deficits	(Raksakoon & Potiwat, 2021)
Rabies	Contacted with saliva of infected dog and other infected animal	Antirabies vaccine and Supportive care	No specific medication, Immune system disturbance, or Challenges in diagnosis.	(Jackson et al., 2003; Nath & Tyler, 2013)
Mumps	Spread through the respiratory tract by airborne droplets	No medication cure, Supportive care for management	No target medication, Seizures and cognitive impairment	(Gailson et al., 2021)

3.3 Treatment of Fungal CNS Infection

Fungal infections of the central nervous system (CNS) pose a serious health risk, especially for immunocompromised individuals. These infections can present in several forms, such as *meningitis, encephalitis, meningoencephalitis, ventriculitis, hydrocephalus, cerebral abscesses, orbit-rhino-cerebral syndrome, and spinal infections,* leading to significant morbidity and mortality. Fungal CNS infections, though relatively rare, are becoming more commonly recognized due to the rising number of immunocompromised patients, such as those with HIV/AIDS, transplant recipients, and individuals on immunosuppressive therapies. The primary fungal pathogens affecting the CNS include *Cryptococcus, Candida, Aspergillus, and Coccidioides*. Fungal CNS infections typically begin with the fungus spreading from a primary site, like the lungs, to the brain and spinal cord via the bloodstream, or through direct inoculation during neurosurgical procedures or from contaminated medical devices. These infections are challenging to treat due to difficulties in delivering antifungal agents across the blood-brain barrier and the fungi's ability to form biofilms and evade the immune system. Symptoms can range from mild mental status changes to severe neurological deficits, with common signs including headache, fever, neck stiffness, and localized neurological symptoms. Diagnosing these infections requires a high index of suspicion, especially in at-risk populations, and involves clinical assessments, imaging studies, and laboratory tests like cerebrospinal fluid (CSF) analysis and culture, serological tests, and molecular diagnostics (Brumble et al., 2017; Challa, 2020; Gavito-Higuera et al., 2016; Khaba et al., 2022). Managing fungal infections in the central nervous system (CNS) is a complex task for healthcare professionals. These infections require a thorough approach, often involving long-term antifungal treatment to eliminate the pathogen. Choosing the right antifungal medication is crucial and depends on accurately identifying the fungus. The intensity and duration of treatment are adjusted based on the severity of the infection, considering factors like the pathogen's virulence and its spread within the CNS. Patient immunological health is also a key factor. Immunocompromised patients, such as those with HIV/AIDS or on immunosuppressive therapy, may need more aggressive and prolonged treatment. Conversely, patients with strong immune responses might require a shorter treatment duration. The objective is to balance effectively treating the infection with minimizing side effects, ensuring the best possible outcome. This requires not only the expertise of infectious disease specialists but also a collaborative effort among multidisciplinary teams to continually monitor and adjust the treatment plan as the patient's condition changes. Treating fungal infections in the central nervous system (CNS) is highly challenging, as highlighted in recent research. One major issue is the complex pharmacokinetics of antifungal agents, particularly their ability to penetrate the CNS, which is not well understood. This uncertainty is worsened by the lack of data for many antifungal drugs, making it difficult to predict treatment outcomes (Bloch & Bailin, 2019; Sahu & Katwala, 2022). Clinical responses often do not match drug concentrations in the cerebrospinal fluid or brain tissue, indicating a gap between expected and actual drug efficacy. Additionally, resistance to antifungal treatments further complicates the situation. Despite advancements in diagnostics and new antifungal medications, CNS infections remain highly lethal due to diagnostic delays, poor drug penetration, and difficulties in restoring immune function. The limited number of effective antifungals for CNS infections and variability in drug concentrations across different CNS regions add to the complexity. Thus, while progress has been made in developing new treatments and diagnostic methods, overcoming pharmacokinetic challenges, drug resistance, and achieving timely and accurate diagnoses remain critical for effective treatment (Ashley et al., 2006; Barriere, 1990).

Table 3. The current therapeutics approaches to fungal CNS infection on the basis type of infection

Types of Infection	Dose regimen and Duration of Treatment	Limitation/ Adverse effects	References
Cryptococcal meningoencephalitis	Initial treatment with -Amphotericin B (mg/kg/day) + Flucytosine (100mg/kg/day) For 2 weeks followed by Fluconazole (400-800mg/kg) For 8 weeks	Amphotericin B associated with kidney damage and infusion reaction Flucytosine causes bone marrow suppression	(Wirantara et al., 2023)
Candida Meningitis	Treatment with Fluconazole (6-12mg/kg/day) for about 3 weeks – 3 months as per the immune system condition	Fluconazole is associated with liver toxicity and skin rashes	(Bette et al., 2018; Kelly et al., 2023; Sridharan et al., 2024)
Aspergillosis	Treatment by Voriconazole (6-12mg/kg every 12hrs-24hrs) for 6-12 weeks	Voriconazole is associated with visual disturbance and liver toxicity (enzyme abnormalities)	(Sigera & Denning, 2023; Tang & Li, 2017)
Non-Aspergillus molds	Liposomal Amphotericin B (5 mg/kg/day) or Treatment by Triazole with patient's clinical outcomes	Liposomal Amphotericin B have Kidney dysfunction and infusion reaction	(Nematollahi & Shoham, 2019; Phoompoung & Luong, 2019)

continued on following page

Table 3. Continued

Types of Infection	Dose regimen and Duration of Treatment	Limitation/ Adverse effects	References
Histoplasmosis	Amphotericin B (3-5 mg/kg/ day) for 3-4 Months	Patient compliance due to lengthy treatment, Difficult with immunocompromised patient	(Hage et al., 2010)
Blastomycosis	Amphotericin B (3-5 mg/ kg /day for 1-2 weeks) + Itraconazole (200mg/kg per once or twice daily for 6-12 months)	Itraconazole associated with Nausea, vomiting, Dizziness, stomach pain	(Scolarici et al., 2022)

3.4 Treatment of Parasitic CNS infection

Parasitic infections of the central nervous system (CNS) are complex and often overlooked, posing significant public health challenges, especially for immunocompromised individuals. These infections are caused by various *protozoan and helminthic organisms*, each with unique life cycles, transmission methods, and clinical effects. Protozoan infections such as toxoplasmosis, Chagas disease, and malaria can lead to severe neurological issues. For example, *Toxoplasma gondii,* the parasite responsible for *toxoplasmosis,* can cause encephalitis in individuals with weakened immune systems. Similarly, *Trypanosoma cruzi,* the parasite behind Chagas disease, can result in chronic *meningoencephalitis. Helminthic infections like neurocysticercosis, schistosomiasis, and echinococcosis* also significantly impact CNS health. Neurocysticercosis, caused by the larval stage of the pork tapeworm Taenia solium, is the most common parasitic CNS infection worldwide and a leading cause of acquired epilepsy in endemic regions. Fungal infections of the central nervous system (CNS) are relatively rare but can be life-threatening, especially in immunocompromised individuals. The symptoms vary depending on the specific fungus, the host's immune status, and the infection site within the CNS. Patients with fungal CNS infections might exhibit meningitis symptoms, including headache, fever, neck stiffness, and sensitivity to light. In more severe cases, meningoencephalitis can develop, leading to altered mental status, seizures, and localized neurological deficits (Schlüter & Barragan, 2019; Walker et al., 2006). Brain abscesses and other space-occupying lesions are also common, presenting with symptoms of increased intracranial pressure such as headache, vomiting, and changes in consciousness. Diagnosing parasitic CNS infections requires a high level of clinical suspicion, particularly in patients with neurological symptoms and a history of travel to endemic areas or immunocompromised status. The diagnostic process integrates clinical assessment with laboratory and imaging techniques to identify the causative organism and evaluate the infection's extent. The first step is a thorough clinical evaluation, considering symptoms like headaches, seizures, altered mental status, and focal neurological deficits, along with the patient's travel history, exposure risks, and immune status. Laboratory tests are crucial, with blood tests potentially showing eosinophilia and serological tests detecting specific parasite antibodies. A definitive diagnosis often involves examining cerebrospinal fluid (CSF) obtained via lumbar puncture. Imaging studies, such as CT and MRI, are essential for visualizing the CNS effects of parasitic infections, and detecting lesions, cysts, or structural changes. For instance, neurocysticercosis often presents with cysts visible on CT or MRI scans. Advanced diagnostics may be needed in some cases, including PCR to detect parasitic DNA in CSF or tissue biopsies. Combining imaging with serological tests can provide a conclusive diagnosis for infections like echinococcosis or courses, which produce large cysts in the brain (Chakraborty et al., 2023; Le Govic et al., 2022).

Table 4. The current treatment of parasitic CNS infection

Parasite and Disease	**Mode Transmission of infection**	**Treatment Dose Regimen**	**Limitation / Adverse effects**	**References**
Neurocysticercosis (Taenia Solium)	Transmission via Fecal, oral and Consumption of contaminated eggs	Treatment with Albendazole (15mg/kg/day) for 8-30 days and Praziquantel (50mg/kg/day) for 15 days	Medication associated with potential hepatotoxicity and leukopenia. It requires concurrent administration of corticosteroids to manage inflammation.	(Matthaiou et al., n.d.; Stelzle et al., 2023)
Toxoplasmosis (Toxoplasma gondii)	Ingestion of undercooked contaminated meat and contact with Cat feces	Treatment by Pyrimethamine and Sulfadiazine with folinic acid supplementation. Dose region based on patient weight and severity	Medication associated with risk of bone marrow suppression; regular blood monitoring is required.	(Bollani et al., 2022; Dunay et al., 2018)
Plasmodium falciparum (Cerebral malaria)	Transmit by a mosquito bite.	Treatment through Artemisinin-based combination therapies like Quinine and Artesunate Dose depends on the patient's severity	The limitation delayed in treatment can lead to coma and death.	(Ngasala et al., 2024)
Human African Trypanosomiasis (Trypanosoma brucei).	Transmitted through the biting of a fly.	Pentamidine for early-stage Eflornithine or Melarsoprol for late-stage treatment Dose as per patient severity	It's less toxic but requires a complex administration schedule. Melarsoprol is highly toxic and causes risk of encephalopathy	(Lutumba et al., 2024)

The treatment of parasitic infections, while often effective, faces several significant challenges that can impede patient recovery. One major issue is the development of antimicrobial resistance (AMR), which complicates treatment due to an incomplete understanding of AMR mechanisms in parasitic diseases. Additionally, the complex life cycles of many parasites, involving both human and vector hosts, make controlling and preventing AMR difficult. Antiparasitic medications can also cause a range of side effects, from mild to severe, including fever, fatigue, gastrointestinal issues, and neurological symptoms. For example, treatments for human African trypanosomiasis with drugs like Melarsoprol can risk causing reactive encephalopathy, a potentially fatal condition. Diagnosing parasitic infections is another challenge, often requiring specialized tests and expertise not always available in all healthcare settings. This can delay treatment, leading to severe consequences, such as irreversible neurological damage or death in cases like cerebral malaria. Moreover, the accessibility and availability of treatments are limited, especially in resource-poor areas where parasitic infections are most common(Sheikh et al., 2022; Shields, 2024; Thomas, 2020). The high cost of medication and the need for long-term treatment can make it difficult for patients to complete their treatment courses, increasing the risk of resistance.

3.5 Treatment of Brain Abscesses

A brain abscess is a serious, localized infection within the brain, usually encapsulated, caused by various bacteria, fungi, or parasites. Though uncommon, it can be life-threatening and requires immediate medical intervention. Brain abscesses can develop through direct spread from nearby infections like ear infections, dental issues, or sinusitis, through the bloodstream from distant infections, or following head injuries or brain surgeries. Symptoms vary but often include headache, fever, localized neurological issues, and changes in mental state, depending on the affected brain area and infection severity. Diagnosing a brain abscess involves clinical assessment and advanced imaging techniques. Initially, a neurological exam checks for signs of increased intracranial pressure or localized neurological issues that might indicate an abscess. Symptoms like headache, fever, mental status changes, and focal neurological signs often lead to further investigation (Brouwer & Van De Beek, 2017; Perillo et al., 2024).

Imaging is crucial, with CT and MRI being the main tools used. CT scans, usually performed first, show the abscess as a hypodense area with a ring-enhancing lesion after contrast. MRI offers more detailed views of the abscess capsule and surrounding edema. Blood tests are conducted to detect infection and inflammation, but blood cultures are often negative due to the abscess being encapsulated. Lumbar puncture is generally avoided due to the risk of herniation, but if identifying the causative organism is necessary, stereotactic aspiration of the abscess is performed under CT or MRI guidance for diagnostic and therapeutic purposes (Huang et al., 2021).

Treating brain abscesses usually involves a mix of medical and surgical methods. First, stereotactic-guided needle aspiration is done to drain out the pus and take samples for analysis. If the antimicrobial treatment isn't working or if there are resistant organisms, then an open craniotomy might be needed. Sometimes, just using antimicrobials might be enough, especially if there are only a few small abscesses and the patient's neurological function isn't affected too much. The choice of antimicrobials depends on what bacteria or fungi are causing the abscess and how well those drugs can pass through the blood-brain barrier. For abscesses linked to sinus infections, the treatment usually involves high-dose penicillin and metronidazole. If a dental origin is suspected, then anaerobic cultures are super important. For abscesses caused by chronic ear infections, the treatment is different and involves antibiotics that target anaerobes, Enterobacteriaceae, and Pseudomonas spp. Examples of these antibiotics are cefotaxime, ceftazidime, or ceftriaxone along with metronidazole. The specific drugs used are based on what the cultures show and can change if needed. A 6- to 8-week course of these antibiotics is needed, along with regular imaging for at least 3 months. The doses of these antibiotics are adjusted based on how well the bacteria respond to them in the lab. For Nocardia spp. infections, higher doses of *trimethoprim/sulfamethoxazole* are used, and treatment can last for a long time, especially if the patient is immunocompromised. Surgery is decided based on the patient's overall health and how the abscess looks on imaging tests. Spinal epidural abscesses, which are pus collections between the dura and the vertebral column, are really serious and need to be treated right away because they can cause spinal cord compression and lead to paralysis, especially in older people, people with HIV or IV drug use, or those who have had spinal surgeries or are immunocompromised (Asquier-Khati et al., 2020; Dhar & Pal, 2021; Northfield, 1942).

4. NOVEL THERAPEUTIC APPROACHES

Treating Central Nervous System (CNS) infections is challenging due to limited treatment options and management difficulties. To address these issues, extensive research is underway to improve treatment strategies and reduce the burden. Recent advancements have introduced promising new therapies. Targeted drug delivery systems now enable precise medication delivery to affected CNS areas, enhancing treatment efficacy and minimizing side effects. Innovations in nanotechnology and nanoparticles are helping to overcome the blood-brain barrier, a major hurdle in CNS therapy. Immunotherapies are being developed to modulate the immune response against CNS pathogens, potentially reducing inflammation and preventing neuronal damage. Gene therapies are also being explored to correct genetic mutations that increase susceptibility to severe infections. Additionally, both invasive and non-invasive treatments, such as surgical interventions and transcranial magnetic stimulation, are being investigated to offer a range of individualized treatment options for the complex nature of CNS infections (J. Kim et al., 2022; Leclair & Hersh, 2023).

4.1 Targeted Drug Delivery

One of the biggest challenges in developing treatments for brain diseases is getting drugs to actually reach the brain. Like, 98% of small-molecule drugs can't get there. And it's even harder for larger molecules like antibodies or nucleic acids, with only 0.01% to 0.1% of a dose actually making it in, which isn't enough to be effective. And nucleic acids, like oligonucleotides, can't get in there without some kind of carrier system. The *blood-brain barrier (BBB)* is the main issue. It's like a shield that keeps out most stuff. And it blocks big therapeutic molecules from getting in, so they can't really help. To get around the BBB, scientists have come up with different ways to deliver drugs to the brain, both invasive and non-invasive. One of the significant methods is called receptor-mediated transcytosis (RMT). It's shown promise for getting biotherapeutics, like antibodies and enzyme replacement therapies, into the brain, and it's non-invasive (Meyer et al., 2023).

The innovative approaches in TDDS for CNS infection and the recent studies highlight the development of innovative transdermal drug delivery systems (TDDS) that utilize nanoparticles, nano-formulated drugs, and intranasal administration methods to enhance drug delivery through the blood-brain barrier.

4.2 Nanoparticle-Based Delivery System (NPs)

Nanoparticle-based delivery systems (NPs) are emerging as a promising solution for treating central nervous system (CNS) infections, addressing the challenge of drug delivery across the blood-brain barrier (BBB). NPs can be engineered to cross the BBB through mechanisms like receptor-mediated transcytosis, where NPs target specific receptors on BBB endothelial cells, facilitating their transport into the brain. Another method is adsorptive-mediated transcytosis, which involves the electrostatic interaction between NPs and the BBB. To improve the efficiency of BBB penetration, NPs can be functionalized with ligands, such as antibodies, peptides, or small molecules, that target receptors overexpressed on the BBB during CNS infections. This targeted approach enhances drug delivery to the CNS and reduces systemic side effects. NPs can encapsulate drugs, protecting them from enzymatic degradation in the bloodstream and allowing for controlled release at the infection site. This sustained release maintains therapeutic drug levels in the CNS for extended periods, essential for treating persistent infections. By ensuring that adequate drug concentrations reach the infection site, NPs maximize therapeutic efficacy. They achieve higher local drug concentrations within the CNS compared to traditional systemic administration, improving infection treatment and minimizing systemic exposure. This targeted delivery reduces the risk of adverse effects associated with high-dose systemic therapies, making NPs a highly effective and safer option for CNS infection treatment. Some approved and marketed nanoparticles for disease targeting encompass a variety of types, including nanocrystals, liposomes, lipid nanoparticles, *PEGylated polymeric nanoparticles, protein-based nanoparticles, and metal-based nanoparticles.* These nanoparticles are designed to deliver medication or therapeutic agents directly to the target site, utilizing mechanisms such as enhanced permeability and retention (EPR) or binding to specific target receptors, thereby improving the precision and effectiveness of treatments (Deng et al., 2021; Lashkari & Ranjbar, 2021).

4.3 Extracellular Vesicles as Natural Drug Carrier

Extracellular vesicles (EVs) are emerging as a promising natural drug delivery system for treating central nervous system (CNS) infections. These nano-sized lipid bilayer vesicles, secreted by cells, can carry a variety of biological materials, including nucleic acids, proteins, lipids, and carbohydrates. Their unique ability to cross biological barriers like the blood-brain barrier (BBB) makes them ideal for delivering therapeutic agents directly to the CNS. EVs, derived from various cell types, reflect the physiological and pathological states of their source cells, making them particularly useful for early diagnosis and targeted treatment of CNS infections. Engineered EVs can carry specific therapeutic payloads, such as antimicrobial agents, anti-inflammatory drugs, or nucleic acids that modulate the host's immune response or directly target pathogens. The biocompatibility of EVs significantly reduces the risk of adverse immune reactions often associated with synthetic drug carriers. Additionally, their natural origin helps them evade the immune system, leading to enhanced drug accumulation at infection sites and improved therapeutic outcomes. Recent advancements focus on optimizing EVs for CNS targeting and drug loading through genetic and protein engineering and surface modification. These techniques enhance the specificity and efficiency of EVs as drug carriers, facilitating their binding to specific receptors on the BBB or within the CNS. In vitro and in vivo studies have shown the potential of EVs in treating CNS infections. For instance, EVs loaded with antiviral drugs have been effective in models of viral encephalitis, while those carrying antibiotics have shown promise against bacterial meningitis. The ability of EVs to encapsulate and protect nucleic acids also opens up possibilities for gene therapy approaches to treat CNS infections caused by various pathogens (S. Du et al., 2023; Liang et al., 2023; X. M. Zhang et al., 2024).

4.4 Drug Delivery Through Intranasal and Intrathecal

For treating central nervous system (CNS) infections, intranasal and intrathecal delivery methods offer significant advantages by bypassing the blood-brain barrier (BBB), a major hurdle in effective drug administration.

Intranasal Delivery: This non-invasive technique exploits the close proximity of the nasal passages to the brain. Drugs delivered intranasally can directly reach the CNS via the olfactory and trigeminal nerve pathways, avoiding the BBB. This method is particularly useful for drugs that have poor BBB penetration or are degraded in the gastrointestinal tract. It is also beneficial for rapid drug action, crucial in acute CNS infections (L. Du et al., 2023).

Intrathecal Delivery: This invasive procedure involves administering drugs directly into the cerebrospinal fluid (CSF), completely bypassing the BBB. Intrathecal delivery ensures that therapeutic concentrations of the drug are delivered directly to the CNS, making it highly effective for treating severe infections like bacterial meningitis or fungal encephalitis. This method is often used when other routes are ineffective. Both delivery methods aim to optimize drug availability in the CNS, enhancing local drug concentrations while reducing systemic exposure and minimizing side effects. However, they each present unique challenges. Intranasal delivery may be limited by the small volume that can be administered and mucociliary clearance. In contrast, intrathecal delivery carries risks associated with invasive procedures, such as infection or nerve damage. The intranasal and intrathecal delivery systems are crucial for managing CNS infections, offering the potential for improved therapeutic outcomes. Their use requires careful consideration of the drug's pharmacokinetics and pharmacodynamics, as well as the specific characteristics of the infection being treated (Lv & Liu, 2024).

5. IMMUNOTHERAPIES

Immunotherapies for treating central nervous system (CNS) infections represent a growing field that leverages the body's immune system to combat pathogens in the brain and spinal cord. The CNS environment, along with the protective *blood-brain barrier (BBB)*, presents unique challenges for effective immunotherapy delivery. However, recent advances in immunomodulation show promise in boosting the body's defenses against various CNS infections (von Baumgarten et al., 2023).

Monoclonal Antibodies (mAbs): Monoclonal antibodies are designed to target specific pathogens or infected cells within the CNS. They can recognize and bind to surface antigens on pathogens, facilitating their destruction by immune cells. Additionally, mAbs can target immune checkpoints to enhance T-cell activity against infected cells, thereby boosting the immune response (Mastraccio et al., 2023).

Cytokine Therapy: Cytokines are key mediators of the immune response and can be used to modulate inflammation within the CNS. For example, interferons have antiviral properties and can induce an antiviral state in cells. Administering cytokines like *interleukin-2 (IL-2)* can stimulate the proliferation and activation of *lymphocytes*, aiding in infection clearance (C. Zhang et al., 2024).

Adoptive Cell Transfer: This involves expanding and activating immune cells outside the body before reintroducing them into the patient. This strategy includes transferring T cells that have been primed to recognize CNS pathogens. *Chimeric antigen receptor (CAR) T* cells, which are engineered to target specific antigens, are a promising area of research for treating CNS infections. Immunotherapies are advancing the treatment of CNS infections by enhancing the body's natural defenses, targeting pathogens directly, and modulating the immune environment within the CNS. These innovative approaches are poised to overcome the challenges posed by the BBB and improve therapeutic outcomes for patients with CNS infections (Lambert et al., 2023).

6. GENE THERAPIES

Gene therapy is an innovative treatment approach showing great potential for addressing central nervous system (CNS) infections. It involves introducing, removing, or altering genetic material within a patient's cells to treat or prevent disease. The CNS poses unique challenges for gene therapy due to the blood-brain barrier (BBB), which restricts the entry of many therapeutic agents. However, advancements in gene delivery vectors and techniques have enable the effective targeting of CNS tissues (Perera et al., 2024)

Adeno-Associated Viruses (AAVs) as Delivery Vectors: Adeno-associated viruses (AAVs) are commonly used to deliver gene therapies to the CNS because of their safety, CNS targeting capabilities, and long-lasting effects. AAVs can be engineered to cross the BBB through receptor-mediated transcytosis, allowing them to deliver genetic material directly to affected brain areas. Research has focused on different AAV serotypes, each with unique receptor affinities and transduction efficiencies, to enhance delivery to CNS tissues (Chatterjee et al., 2022).

Genome Editing Technologies: The development of genome editing tools like CRISPR/Cas9 has transformed gene therapy. These technologies enable precise genome modifications, allowing for the correction of mutations that cause CNS infections or the insertion of genes to confer infection resistance. Recent studies have explored CRISPR-based therapies for CNS infections caused by viruses such as HIV and JC virus, which can lead to progressive multifocal leukoencephalopathy (PML). Gene therapy is advancing rapidly, offering new hope for treating CNS infections by overcoming the challenges posed by the BBB and enabling targeted, effective interventions (Stahl et al., 2023).

7. CONCLUSION

The detailed chapter of therapeutic strategies for Central Nervous System (CNS) infections highlights the urgent need for innovative treatments to overcome the significant challenges posed by the blood-brain barrier (BBB), multidrug resistance, and emerging pathogens. Advances in nanotechnology, gene therapy, and immunotherapies offer promising new methods for effective drug delivery and targeted treatment strategies. Epidemiological data show a high global burden of CNS infections, making interdisciplinary research and investment essential to bring these novel therapies from the lab to clinical practice.

Managing CNS infections, including parasitic, bacterial, and fungal infections, is a complex task for healthcare professionals. This complexity necessitates a multifaceted approach that combines laboratory tests, advanced imaging techniques, and a careful mix of medical and surgical interventions to provide optimal patient care. Early and accurate diagnosis, facilitated by a range of laboratory tests such as serological assays and imaging studies like CT and MRI, is crucial in understanding CNS pathology and guiding treatment decisions.

Furthermore, the challenge of delivering therapeutic agents to the CNS due to the BBB underscores the need for innovative strategies to improve drug penetration and effectiveness in this specialized environment. In summary, effective management of CNS infections requires a deep understanding of pathogen characteristics, host immune responses, and the complex dynamics within the CNS. Collaboration among healthcare professionals, researchers, and pharmaceutical companies is vital for advancing diagnostic tools, refining therapeutic methods, and ultimately improving patient outcomes in the treatment of CNS infections.

REFERENCES

Aboabdo, M., & Mishkin, A. (2024). Antifungal therapy for the treatment of CNS infections. In *Current Fungal Infection Reports*. DOI: 10.1007/s12281-024-00492-6

Alamarat, Z., & Hasbun, R. (2020). Management of acute bacterial meningitis in children. In *Infection and Drug Resistance* (Vol. 13). DOI: 10.2147/IDR.S240162

Aldeen, A. Z., Salzman, D. H., Gisondi, M. A., Courtney, D. M., Allard, C. B., Meyer, C. P., Gandaglia, G., Chang, S. L., Chun, F. K. H., Gelpi-Hammerschmidt, F., Hanske, J., Kibel, A. S., Preston, M. A., Trinh, Q.-D., Anderson, C. E., Nicksa, G. A., Stewart, L. L., Anderson, J. B., Beekman, R. H.III, & Brubaker, L. (2014). Influence of Early Surgical Treatment on the Prognosis of Left-Sided Infective Endocarditis: A Multicenter Cohort Study. *Mayo Clinic Proceedings*. Advance online publication. DOI: 10.1016/j.mayocp.2014.12.014 PMID: 25178264

Ang, B. S. P., Lim, T. C. C., & Wang, L. (2018). Nipah virus infection. *Journal of Clinical Microbiology*, *56*(6), e01875-17. Advance online publication. DOI: 10.1128/JCM.01875-17 PMID: 29643201

Ang, B. S. P., Umapathi, T., & Lim, T. (2023). The Changing Epidemiology of Central Nervous System Infection: Can Radiologists Keep Up? In *Neuroimaging Clinics of North America* (Vol. 33, Issue 1). DOI: 10.1016/j.nic.2022.03.002

Ashley, E. S. D., Lewis, R., Lewis, J. S., Martin, C., & Andes, D. (2006). Pharmacology of systemic antifungal agents. In *Clinical Infectious Diseases* (Vol. 43, Suppl. 1). DOI: 10.1086/504492

Asquier-Khati, A., Deschanvres, C., Boutoille, D., Lefebvre, M., Le Turnier, P., Gaborit, B., Lakhal, K., Buffenoir, K., Khatchatourian, L., Asseray, N., Orain, J., Lecomte, R., Brochard, J., Biron, C., Raffi, F., Juvin, M.-E., Roualdes, V., Riem, T., Ngohou, C., & Ngohou, C. (2020). Switch from parenteral to oral antibiotics for brain abscesses: A retrospective cohort study of 109 patients. *The Journal of Antimicrobial Chemotherapy*, *75*(10), 3062–3066. DOI: 10.1093/jac/dkaa285 PMID: 32699907

Barriere, S. L. (1990). Pharmacology and Pharmacokinetics of Traditional Systemic Antifungal Agents. *Pharmacotherapy: The Journal of Human Pharmacology and Drug Therapy, 10*(6P3). DOI: 10.1002/j.1875-9114.1990.tb02598.x

Bette, S., Shpiner, D. S., Singer, C., & Moore, H. (2018). Safinamide in the management of patients with Parkinson's disease not stabilized on levodopa: A review of the current clinical evidence. *Therapeutics and Clinical Risk Management*, *14*, 1737–1745. DOI: 10.2147/TCRM.S139545 PMID: 30271159

Bloch, K. C., & Bailin, S. S. (2019). Update on fungal infections of the central nervous system: Emerging pathogens and emerging diagnostics. *Current Opinion in Infectious Diseases, 32*(3), 277–284. DOI: 10.1097/QCO.0000000000000541 PMID: 30921084

Bollani, L., Auriti, C., Achille, C., Garofoli, F., De Rose, D. U., Meroni, V., Salvatori, G., & Tzialla, C. (2022). Congenital Toxoplasmosis: The State of the Art. *Frontiers in Pediatrics, 10*, 894573. DOI: 10.3389/fped.2022.894573 PMID: 35874584

Brouwer, M. C., & Van De Beek, D. (2017). Epidemiology, diagnosis, and treatment of brain abscesses. *Current Opinion in Infectious Diseases, 30*(1), 129–134. DOI: 10.1097/QCO.0000000000000334 PMID: 27828809

Brouwer, M. C., & van de Beek, D. (2023). Adjunctive dexamethasone treatment in adults with listeria monocytogenes meningitis: A prospective nationwide cohort study. *EClinicalMedicine, 58*, 101922. Advance online publication. DOI: 10.1016/j.eclinm.2023.101922 PMID: 37007737

Brumble, L. M., Reza, M. B., Dhakal, L. P., Cruz, G., Abu Saleh, O. M., Heckman, M. G., Vargas, E. R., Dickson, D. W., Enzler, M. J., Libertin, C. R., & Freeman, W. D. (2017). Fungal Infections of the Central Nervous System: Clinical, Radiographic and Laboratory Manifestations. *Journal of Microbiology & Experimentation, 5*(6). Advance online publication. DOI: 10.15406/jmen.2017.05.00167

Bruno, L., Nappo, M. A., Ferrari, L., Di Lecce, R., Guarnieri, C., Cantoni, A. M., & Corradi, A. (2023). Nipah Virus Disease: Epidemiological, Clinical, Diagnostic and Legislative Aspects of This Unpredictable Emerging Zoonosis. In *Animals* (Vol. 13, Issue 1). DOI: 10.3390/ani13010159

Burrel, S., Topalis, D., & Boutolleau, D. (2020). Herpes simplex virus resistance to antivirals. In *Virologie* (Vol. 24, Issue 5, pp. 325–342). John Libbey. DOI: 10.1684/vir.2020.0864

Chakroborty, N. K., Baksi, S., & Bhattacharya, A. (2023). Cognitive Impairment in Parasitic Protozoan Infection. In *Pathobiology of Parasitic Protozoa*. Dynamics and Dimensions. DOI: 10.1007/978-981-19-8225-5_4

Challa, S. (2020). Invasive Fungal Infections of the Central Nervous System in Immune-Competent Hosts. In *Current Fungal Infection Reports* (Vol. 14, Issue 2). DOI: 10.1007/s12281-020-00384-5

Chatterjee, D., Marmion, D. J., McBride, J. L., Manfredsson, F. P., Butler, D., Messer, A., & Kordower, J. H. (2022). Enhanced CNS transduction from AAV.PHP.eB infusion into the cisterna magna of older adult rats compared to AAV9. *Gene Therapy*, *29*(6), 390–397. DOI: 10.1038/s41434-021-00244-y PMID: 33753910

Chaudhuri, A., Martinez-Martin, P., Kennedy, P. G. E., Seaton, R. A., & Portegie, P. s, Bojar, M., & Steiner, I. (2011). Management of Community-Acquired Bacterial Meningitis. *European Handbook of Neurological Management*, 145–157. DOI: 10.1002/9781444346268.ch11

Ciummo, F., Srinivas, P., & Biedny, J. (2021). Antimicrobial use in central nervous system infections. In *Current Opinion in Infectious Diseases* (Vol. 34, Issue 3). DOI: 10.1097/QCO.0000000000000721

Deng, Y., Huang, R., Huang, S., & Xiong, M. (2021). Nanoparticles Enable Efficient Delivery of Antimicrobial Peptides for the Treatment of Deep Infections. *BIO Integration*, *2*(2), 50. DOI: 10.15212/bioi-2021-0003

Dhar, S., & Pal, B. (2021). *Analysis of 93 Brain Abscess Cases to Review the Effect of Intervention to Determine the Feasibility of the Management Protocol: A Tertiary Care Perspective Original Article.* DOI: 10.4103/ajns.AJNS_467_20

Domingo, P., Pomar, V., de Benito, N., & Coll, P. (2013). The spectrum of acute bacterial meningitis in elderly patients. *BMC Infectious Diseases*, *13*(1), 108. Advance online publication. DOI: 10.1186/1471-2334-13-108 PMID: 23446215

Drossinos, Y., Weber, T. P., & Stilianakis, N. I. (2021). Droplets and aerosols: An artificial dichotomy in respiratory virus transmission. *Health Science Reports*, *4*(2), e275. Advance online publication. DOI: 10.1002/hsr2.275 PMID: 33977157

Du, L., Chen, L., Liu, F., Wang, W., & Huang, H. (2023). Nose-to-brain drug delivery for the treatment of CNS disease: New development and strategies. *International Review of Neurobiology*, *171*, 255–297. DOI: 10.1016/bs.irn.2023.05.014 PMID: 37783558

Du, S., Guan, Y., Xie, A., Yan, Z., Gao, S., Li, W., Rao, L., Chen, X., & Chen, T. (2023). Extracellular vesicles: a rising star for therapeutics and drug delivery. *Journal of Nanobiotechnology*, *21*(1), 1–51. DOI: 10.1186/s12951-023-01973-5

Dunay, I. R., Gajurel, K., Dhakal, R., Liesenfeld, O., & Montoya, J. G. (2018). Treatment of Toxoplasmosis: Historical Perspective, Animal Models, and Current Clinical Practice. *Clinical Microbiology Reviews*, *31*(4), e00057–e17. DOI: 10.1128/CMR.00057-17 PMID: 30209035

Edwards, M. S., & Baker, C. J. (2013). Treatment and outcome of bacterial meningitis in the neonate. *UpToDate*.

Encephalitis: Diagnosis, management and recent advances in the field of encephalitides. (2023). *Postgraduate Medical Journal*. Advance online publication. DOI: 10.1136/POSTMJ/POSTGRADMEDJ-2022-141812

Faizi, N., & Hassan, J. (2023). Etiology and Epidemiology of Central Nervous System Infections. In *Viral and Fungal Infections of the Central Nervous System: A Microbiological Perspective*. DOI: 10.1007/978-981-99-6445-1_1

Folke, J., Ferreira, N., Brudek, T., Borghammer, P., & Van Den Berge, N. (2022). Passive Immunization in Alpha-Synuclein Preclinical Animal Models. *Biomolecules, 12*(2), 168. DOI: 10.3390/biom12020168

Gailson, T., Vohra, V., Saini, A. G., & Bhatia, V. (2021). Mumps infection with meningoencephalitis and cerebellitis. In *BMJ Case Reports* (Vol. 14, Issue 11). DOI: 10.1136/bcr-2021-247306

Garlicki, A., Jawień, M., Pancewicz, S., & Moniuszko-Malinowska, A. (2023). Bacterial meningitis in adults – principles of diagnosis and antibiotic treatment. *Przeglad Epidemiologiczny*, *77*(1), 3–22. Advance online publication. DOI: 10.32394/pe.77.01 PMID: 37283230

Gavito-Higuera, J., Mullins, C., Ramos-Duran, L., Olivas Chacon, C., Hakim, N., & Palacios, E. (2016). Fungal Infections of the Central Nervous System: A Pictorial Review. In *Journal of Clinical Imaging Science* (Vol. 6, Issue 2). DOI: 10.4103/2156-7514.184244

Gundamraj, V., & Hasbun, R. (2023). Viral meningitis and encephalitis: An update. In *Current Opinion in Infectious Diseases* (Vol. 36, Issue 3). DOI: 10.1097/QCO.0000000000000922

Haddad, N., Carr, M., Balian, S., Lannin, J., Kim, Y., Toth, C., & Jarvis, J. (2022). The Blood–Brain Barrier and Pharmacokinetic/Pharmacodynamic Optimization of Antibiotics for the Treatment of Central Nervous System Infections in Adults. In *Antibiotics* (Vol. 11, Issue 12). DOI: 10.3390/antibiotics11121843

Hage, C. A., Bowyer, S., Tarvin, S. E., Helper, D., Kleiman, M. B., & Wheat, L. J. (2010). Recognition, diagnosis, and treatment of histoplasmosis complicating tumor necrosis factor blocker therapy. In *Clinical Infectious Diseases* (Vol. 50, Issue 1). DOI: 10.1086/648724

Hinduja, A., Tariq, A., & Adriance, S. (2019). Intensive Care Management of Meningitis and Encephalitis. *Textbook of Neuroanesthesia and Neurocritical Care*, 131–144. DOI: 10.1007/978-981-13-3390-3_9

Holdaway, I., Reid, I., Young, N., & Thomas, M. (2018). Meningitis in adults: Diagnosis and management. *Internal Medicine Journal*, *48*(11), 1294–1307. DOI: 10.1111/imj.14102 PMID: 30387309

Huang, J., Wu, H., Huang, H., Wu, W., Wu, B., & Wang, L. (2021). Clinical characteristics and outcome of primary brain abscess: A retrospective analysis. *BMC Infectious Diseases*, *21*(1), 1–8. DOI: 10.1186/s12879-021-06947-2 PMID: 34903183

Jackson, A. C., Warrell, M. J., Rupprecht, C. E., Ertl, H. C. J., Dietzschold, B., O'Reilly, M., Leach, R. P., Fu, Z. F., Wunner, W. H., Bleck, T. P., & Wilde, H. (2003). Management of rabies in humans. In *Clinical Infectious Diseases* (Vol. 36, Issue 1). DOI: 10.1086/344905

Kadry, H., Noorani, B., & Cucullo, L. (2020). A blood–brain barrier overview on structure, function, impairment, and biomarkers of integrity. In *Fluids and Barriers of the CNS* (Vol. 17, Issue 1). DOI: 10.1186/s12987-020-00230-3

Kapoor, A., & Tan, C. S. (2020). Immunotherapeutics to Treat HIV in the Central Nervous System. In *Current HIV/AIDS Reports* (Vol. 17, Issue 5). DOI: 10.1007/s11904-020-00519-w

Kelly, L., Walsh, J., Skally, M., Dinesh, B., Burns, K., O'Connell, K., MacNally, S., Humphreys, H., & Fitzpatrick, F. (2023). Candida meningitis/ventriculitis over a decade. Increased morbidity and length of stay a concern. *British Journal of Neurosurgery*, *37*(2), 227–230. Advance online publication. DOI: 10.1080/02688697.2022.2054947 PMID: 35361033

Khaba, M. C., Ngale, T. C., & Makhado, N. A. (2022). Fungal infection of the central nervous system: Autopsy analysis of six cases. *SAGE Open Medical Case Reports*, *10*. Advance online publication. DOI: 10.1177/2050313X221122419 PMID: 36105784

Kim, J., Erice, C., Rohlwink, U. K., & Tucker, E. W. (2022). Infections in the Developing Brain: The Role of the Neuro-Immune Axis. *Frontiers in Neurology*, *13*, 805786. DOI: 10.3389/fneur.2022.805786 PMID: 35250814

Kim, K. S. (2010). Acute bacterial meningitis in infants and children. In *The Lancet Infectious Diseases* (Vol. 10, Issue 1). DOI: 10.1016/S1473-3099(09)70306-8

Lambert, N., El Moussaoui, M., Baron, F., Maquet, P., & Darcis, G. (2023). Virus-Specific T-Cell Therapy for Viral Infections of the Central Nervous System: A Review. *Viruses, 15*(7), 1510. Advance online publication. DOI: 10.3390/v15071510 PMID: 37515196

Lashkari, A., & Ranjbar, R. (2021). Nanoparticles and nanoformulated drugs as promising delivery system in treatment of microbial-induced CNS infection: a systematic review of literature. In *Journal of NeuroVirology* (Vol. 27, Issue 4). DOI: 10.1007/s13365-021-00994-w

Le, N. D., Ricci, S., Grandgirard, D., & Leib, S. L. (2023). Experimental meningitis by Streptococcus pneumoniae and Neisseria meningitidis in rodents. *Handbook of Animal Models in Neurological Disorders*, 329–341. DOI: 10.1016/B978-0-323-89833-1.00050-1

Le Govic, Y., Demey, B., Cassereau, J., Bahn, Y. S., & Papon, N. (2022). Pathogens infecting the central nervous system. *PLoS Pathogens, 18*(2), 1–9. DOI: 10.1371/journal.ppat.1010234 PMID: 35202445

Leclair, N. K., & Hersh, D. S. (2023). Central Nervous System Infections and Their Management. *Pediatric Neurosurgery Board Review: A Comprehensive Guide*, 317–334. DOI: 10.1007/978-3-031-23687-7_19

Ledri, M., Sørensen, A. T., Kokaia, M., Woldbye, D. P. D., & Gøtzsche, C. R. (2021). Editorial: Gene Therapy in the CNS – Progress and Prospects for Novel Therapies. In *Frontiers in Molecular Neuroscience* (Vol. 14). DOI: 10.3389/fnmol.2021.778134

Li, B. D., Bi, Z. Y., Liu, J. F., Si, W. J., Shi, Q. Q., Xue, L. P., & Bai, J. (2017). Adverse effects produced by different drugs used in the treatment of Parkinson's disease: A mixed treatment comparison. *CNS Neuroscience & Therapeutics, 23*(10), 827–842. Advance online publication. DOI: 10.1111/cns.12727 PMID: 28872217

Liang, Y., Iqbal, Z., Lu, J., Wang, J., Zhang, H., Chen, X., Duan, L., & Xia, J. (2023). Cell-derived nanovesicle-mediated drug delivery to the brain: Principles and strategies for vesicle engineering. *Molecular Therapy : the Journal of the American Society of Gene Therapy, 31*(5), 1207–1224. DOI: 10.1016/j.ymthe.2022.10.008 PMID: 36245129

Lutumba, P., Matovu, E., & Boatin, B. A. (2024). *Human African Trypanosomiasis (HAT)*. 73–97. DOI: 10.1007/978-3-031-53901-5_4

Lv, Z., & Liu, Y. (2024). Clinical research progress on intrathecal glucocorticoids in the treatment of infections. *Revista de Medicina (São Paulo), 103*(20), e38123. DOI: 10.1097/MD.0000000000038123 PMID: 38758886

Manan, M. R., & Manan, H. (2021). Congenital Cytomegalovirus Infection: Transmission, Diagnosis and Treatment. *McGill Journal of Medicine : MJM : an International Forum for the Advancement of Medical Sciences by Students*, *20*(1). Advance online publication. DOI: 10.26443/mjm.v20i1.876

Mastraccio, K. E., Huaman, C., Coggins, S. A., Clouse, C., Rader, M., Yan, L., Mandal, P., Hussain, I., Ahmed, A. E., Ho, T., Feasley, A., Vu, B. K., Smith, I. L., Markotter, W., Weir, D. L., Laing, E. D., Broder, C. C., & Schaefer, B. C. (2023). mAb therapy controls CNS-resident lyssavirus infection via a CD4 T cell-dependent mechanism. *EMBO Molecular Medicine*, *15*(10), e16394. Advance online publication. DOI: 10.15252/emmm.202216394 PMID: 37767784

Matthaiou, D. K., Panos, G., Adamidi, E. S., & Falagas, M. E. (n.d.). *Albendazole versus Praziquantel in the Treatment of Neurocysticercosis: A Meta-analysis of Comparative Trials*. DOI: 10.1371/journal.pntd.0000194

Melhuish, A., & McGill, F. (2021). Viral meningitis and encephalitis. *Medicine (Abingdon)*, *49*(11), 675–680. DOI: 10.1016/j.mpmed.2021.08.004

Meningitis. (n.d.). Retrieved June 8, 2024, from https://www.who.int/news-room/fact-sheets/detail/meningitis

Meyer, A. H., Feldsien, T. M., Mezler, M., Untucht, C., Venugopalan, R., & Lefebvre, D. R. (2023). Novel Developments to Enable Treatment of CNS Diseases with Targeted Drug Delivery. *Pharmaceutics, 15*(4), 1100. DOI: 10.3390/pharmaceutics15041100

Nath, A., & Tyler, K. L. (2013). Novel approaches and challenges to treatment of central nervous system viral infections. *Annals of Neurology*, *74*(3), 412–422. DOI: 10.1002/ana.23988 PMID: 23913580

Nematollahi, S., & Shoham, S. (2019). Updates on the Treatment of Non-Aspergillus Hyaline Mold Infections. In *Current Fungal Infection Reports* (Vol. 13, Issue 4). DOI: 10.1007/s12281-019-00364-4

Ng, L. F. P., & Solomon, T. (2015). Decade in review - CNS infections: Major advances against a moving target of CNS infections. In *Nature Reviews Neurology* (Vol. 11, Issue 11). DOI: 10.1038/nrneurol.2015.202

Ngasala, B., Bushukatale, S., Chiduo, M., Makene, T., Mkony, L., Mohamed, A., Molteni, F., Chacky, F., Njau, R. J. A., & Mwaiswelo, R. (2024). Efficacy of artesunate-amodiaquine for treatment of uncomplicated Plasmodium falciparum malaria in mainland Tanzania. *Malaria Journal*, *23*(1), 1–10. DOI: 10.1186/s12936-024-04923-0 PMID: 38553737

Nhantumbo, A. A., Comé, C. E., Maholela, P. I., Munguambe, A. M., da Costa, P., Mott, M., Cunha, G. R., Chambal, L., Dias, C., Cantarelli, V. V., & Gudo, E. S. (2022). Etiology of meningitis among adults in three quaternary hospitals in Mozambique, 2016–2017: The role of HIV. *PLoS ONE, 17*(5 May). DOI: 10.1371/journal.pone.0267949

Niemelä, S., Lempinen, L., Löyttyniemi, E., Oksi, J., & Jero, J. (2023). Bacterial meningitis in adults: A retrospective study among 148 patients in an 8-year period in a university hospital, Finland. *BMC Infectious Diseases*, *23*(1), 45. Advance online publication. DOI: 10.1186/s12879-023-07999-2 PMID: 36690945

Northfield, D. W. C. (1942). The treatment of brain abscess. *Journal of Neurology, Neurosurgery, and Psychiatry*, *5*(1–2), 1–9. DOI: 10.1136/jnnp.5.1-2.1 PMID: 21611397

Nowak, I., Madej, M., Secemska, J., Sarna, R., & Strzalka-Mrozik, B. (2023). Virus-Based Biological Systems as Next-Generation Carriers for the Therapy of Central Nervous System Diseases. *Pharmaceutics*, *15*(7), 1931. Advance online publication. DOI: 10.3390/pharmaceutics15071931 PMID: 37514117

Palmer, M. E., Andrews, L. J., Abbey, T. C., Dahlquist, A. E., & Wenzler, E. (2022). The importance of pharmacokinetics and pharmacodynamics in antimicrobial drug development and their influence on the success of agents developed to combat resistant gram negative pathogens: A review. In *Frontiers in Pharmacology* (Vol. 13). DOI: 10.3389/fphar.2022.888079

Perera, A., Brock, O., Ahmed, A., Shaw, C., & Ashkan, K. (2024). Taking the knife to neurodegeneration: A review of surgical gene therapy delivery to the CNS. *Acta Neurochirurgica*, *166*(1), 136. Advance online publication. DOI: 10.1007/s00701-024-06028-8 PMID: 38483631

Perillo, T., Capasso, R., & Pinto, A. (2024). Neuroimaging of the Most Common Meningitis and Encephalitis of Adults: A Narrative Review. *Diagnostics, 14*(11), 1064. DOI: 10.3390/diagnostics14111064

Phar, & Bereda G. (2022). *Advances in Pharmacology and Clinical Trials Committed to Create Value for Researchers Pathophysiology and Management of Bacterial Meningitis in Pediatrics Adv in Pathophysiology and Management of Bacterial Meningitis in Pediatrics*. DOI: 10.23880/apct-16000198

Phoompoung, P., & Luong, M.-L. (2019). Treatment of Non-Aspergillus Mold Infections: A Focus on Mucormycosis and Fusariosis. *Current Treatment Options in Infectious Diseases*, *11*(4), 401–417. Advance online publication. DOI: 10.1007/s40506-019-00205-5

Piperi, E., Papadopoulou, E., Georgaki, M., Dovrat, S., Bar Illan, M., Nikitakis, N. G., & Yarom, N. (2024). Management of oral herpes simplex virus infections: The problem of resistance. A narrative review. In *Oral Diseases* (Vol. 30, Issue 3, pp. 877–894). John Wiley and Sons Inc. DOI: 10.1111/odi.14635

Qu, C., Wang, Y., Wang, X., He, R., Cao, H., Liu, B., Zhang, H., Zhang, N., Lai, Z., Dai, Z., & Cheng, Q. (2023). Global Burden and Its Association with Socio-economic Development Status of Meningitis Caused by Specific Pathogens over the Past 30 years: A Population-Based Study. *Neuroepidemiology*, *57*(5), 316–335. DOI: 10.1159/000531508 PMID: 37399794

Raksakoon, C., & Potiwat, R. (2021). Current arboviral threats and their potential vectors in Thailand. In *Pathogens* (Vol. 10, Issue 1). DOI: 10.3390/pathogens10010080

Ramachandran, P. S., & Wilson, M. R. (2021). Chronic Meningitis. In *Aminoff's Neurology and General Medicine* (pp. 839–851). Elsevier., DOI: 10.1016/B978-0-12-819306-8.00047-2

Sahu, P. S., & Katwala, J. (2022). Pathogenesis of Fungal Infections in the Central Nervous System: Host and Pathogen Factors in Neurotropism. *Current Fungal Infection Reports*, *16*(4), 221–233. DOI: 10.1007/s12281-022-00444-y

Schlüter, D., & Barragan, A. (2019). Advances and challenges in understanding cerebral toxoplasmosis. In *Frontiers in Immunology* (Vol. 10). Issue FEB. DOI: 10.3389/fimmu.2019.00242

Schwartz, S., Kontoyiannis, D. P., Harrison, T., & Ruhnke, M. (2018). Advances in the diagnosis and treatment of fungal infections of the CNS. In *The Lancet Neurology* (Vol. 17, Issue 4). DOI: 10.1016/S1474-4422(18)30030-9

Scolarici, M. J., King, C., Sterkel, A., Smith, J., Gauthier, G., & Saddler, C. (2022). The Role of Isavuconazonium Sulphate for the Treatment of Blastomycosis: A Case Series and Antifungal Susceptibility. *Open Forum Infectious Diseases*, *9*(7), ofac220. Advance online publication. DOI: 10.1093/ofid/ofac220 PMID: 35821730

Shahjin, F., Chand, S., & Yelamanchili, S. V. (2019). Extracellular Vesicles as Drug Delivery Vehicles to the Central Nervous System. *Journal of Neuroimmune Pharmacology, 15*(3), 443–458. DOI: 10.1007/s11481-019-09875-w

Sheikh, B. A., Bhat, B. A., & Mir, M. A. (2022). Antimicrobial resistance: New insights and therapeutic implications. *Applied Microbiology and Biotechnology*, *106*(19–20), 6427–6440. DOI: 10.1007/s00253-022-12175-8 PMID: 36121484

Sheybani, F., Haddad, M., & Shirazinia, M. (2023). Epidemiology and etiology of community-acquired CNS infections in Iran: a narrative review. In *Future Neurology* (Vol. 18, Issue 4). DOI: 10.2217/fnl-2023-0017

Shields, R. K. (2024). Progress and New Challenges in Combatting the Threat of Antimicrobial Resistance: Perspective From an Infectious Diseases Pharmacist. *The Journal of Infectious Diseases*, *229*(2), 303–306. DOI: 10.1093/infdis/jiad250 PMID: 37487530

Shukla, B., Aguilera, E. A., Salazar, L., Wootton, S. H., Kaewpoowat, Q., & Hasbun, R. (2017). Aseptic meningitis in adults and children: Diagnostic and management challenges. *Journal of Clinical Virology*, *94*, 110–114. Advance online publication. DOI: 10.1016/j.jcv.2017.07.016 PMID: 28806629

Sigera, L. S. M., & Denning, D. W. (2023). Flucytosine and its clinical usage. In *Therapeutic Advances in Infectious Disease* (Vol. 10). DOI: 10.1177/20499361231161387

Sigfrid, L., Perfect, C., Rojek, A., Longuere, K. S., Lipworth, S., Harriss, E., Lee, J., Salam, A., Carson, G., Goossens, H., & Horby, P. (2019). A systematic review of clinical guidelines on the management of acute, community-acquired CNS infections. *BMC Medicine*, *17*(1), 170. Advance online publication. DOI: 10.1186/s12916-019-1387-5 PMID: 31488138

Simões, E. A. F., Bont, L., Manzoni, P., Fauroux, B., Paes, B., Figueras-Aloy, J., Checchia, P. A., & Carbonell-Estrany, X. (2018). Past, Present and Future Approaches to the Prevention and Treatment of Respiratory Syncytial Virus Infection in Children. In *Infectious Diseases and Therapy* (Vol. 7, Issue 1). DOI: 10.1007/s40121-018-0188-z

Songtao, X., Hongzhi, G., & Zhengde, X. (2023). [Expert consensus on the application of pathogenic diagnostic techniques for viral encephalitis and meningitis]. *National Medical Journal of China, 103* 9(9), 648–657. DOI: 10.3760/CMA.J.CN112137-20221014-02154

Sridharan, S., Govindaswamy, A., Rajendran, A., & Roopesh, R. K. (2024). Challenges in management of Candida auris meningitis secondary to infected ventriculoperitoneal shunt – A case report. *Indian Journal of Medical Microbiology*, *48*, 100555. Advance online publication. DOI: 10.1016/j.ijmmb.2024.100555 PMID: 38428528

Stahl, E. C., Sabo, J. K., Kang, M. H., Allen, R., Applegate, E., Kim, S. E., Kwon, Y., Seth, A., Lemus, N., Salinas-Rios, V., Soczek, K. M., Trinidad, M., Vo, L. T., Jeans, C., Wozniak, A., Morris, T., Kimberlin, A., Foti, T., Savage, D. F., & Doudna, J. A. (2023). Genome editing in the mouse brain with minimally immunogenic Cas9 RNPs. *Molecular Therapy : the Journal of the American Society of Gene Therapy, 31*(8), 2422–2438. DOI: 10.1016/j.ymthe.2023.06.019 PMID: 37403358

Stelzle, D., Makasi, C., Schmidt, V., Trevisan, C., Van Damme, I., Ruether, C., Dorny, P., Magnussen, P., Zulu, G., Mwape, K. E., Bottieau, E., Prazeres da Costa, C., Prodjinotho, U. F., Carabin, H., Jackson, E., Fleury, A., Gabriël, S., Ngowi, B. J., & Winkler, A. S. (2023). Efficacy and safety of antiparasitic therapy for neurocysticercosis in rural Tanzania: A prospective cohort study. *Infection, 51*(4), 1127–1139. DOI: 10.1007/s15010-023-02021-y PMID: 36961623

Tang, X., & Li, G. (2017). The interpretation of practice guidelines for the diagnosis and management of aspergillosis: 2016 update by the Infectious Diseases Society of America. In *Chinese Journal of Infection and Chemotherapy* (Vol. 17, Issue 4). DOI: 10.16718/j.1009-7708.2017.04.021

Thomas, S. (2020). Antimicrobial Resistance: Global Challenges and Future Interventions. *Antimicrobial Resistance: Global Challenges and Future Interventions,* 1–230. DOI: 10.1007/978-981-15-3658-8/COVER

Ueda, N. K., Nakamura, K., Go, H., Takehara, H., Kashiwabara, N., Arai, K., Takemura, H., Namai, Y., & Kanemitsu, K. (2018). Neonatal meningitis and recurrent bacteremia with group B Streptococcus transmitted by own mother's milk: A case report and review of previous cases. *International Journal of Infectious Diseases, 74,* 13–15. Advance online publication. DOI: 10.1016/j.ijid.2018.06.016 PMID: 29959094

Virus Prevention, Diagnosis, and Treatment. (2023). *A Guide to Virology for Engineers and Applied Scientists: Epidemiology, Emergency Management, and Optimization,* 57–74. DOI: 10.1002/9781119853169.ch4

von Baumgarten, L., Stauss, H. J., & Lünemann, J. D. (2023). Synthetic Cell-Based Immunotherapies for Neurologic Diseases. *Neurology(R). Neuroimmunology and Neuroinflammation, 10*(5), e200139. Advance online publication. DOI: 10.1212/NXI.0000000000200139 PMID: 37385738

Walker, M., Kublin, J. G., & Zunt, J. B. (2006). Parasitic central nervous system infections in immunocompromised hosts: Malaria, microsporidiosis, leishmaniasis, and African trypanosomiasis. In *Clinical Infectious Diseases* (Vol. 42, Issue 1). DOI: 10.1086/498510

Wirantara, H., Rusli, M., Arfijanto, M. V., & Bramantono, B. (2023). Cryptococcal Meningoencephalitis in HIV/AIDS Patient Coinfected with Tuberculosis. Case Report. *Gaceta Medica de Caracas, 131*(2). Advance online publication. DOI: 10.47307/GMC.2023.131.2.15

Wunrow, H. Y., Bender, R. G., Vongpradith, A., Sirota, S. B., Swetschinski, L. R., Novotney, A., Gray, A. P., Ikuta, K. S., Sharara, F., Wool, E. E., Aali, A., Abd-Elsalam, S., Abdollahi, A., Abdul Aziz, J. M., Abidi, H., Aboagye, R. G., Abolhassani, H., Abu-Gharbieh, E., Adamu, L. H., & Kyu, H. H. (2023). Global, regional, and national burden of meningitis and its aetiologies, 1990–2019: A systematic analysis for the Global Burden of Disease Study 2019. *Lancet Neurology*, *22*(8), 685–711. DOI: 10.1016/S1474-4422(23)00195-3 PMID: 37479374

Young, N., & Thomas, M. (2018). Meningitis in adults: Diagnosis and management. *Internal Medicine Journal*, *48*(11), 1294–1307. Advance online publication. DOI: 10.1111/imj.14102 PMID: 30387309

Zhang, C., Qiu, M., & Fu, H. (2024). Oligodendrocytes in central nervous system diseases: The effect of cytokine regulation. *Neural Regeneration Research*, *19*(10), 2132–2143. DOI: 10.4103/1673-5374.392854 PMID: 38488548

Zhang, X. M., Huang, J., Ni, X. Y., Zhu, H. R., Huang, Z. X., Ding, S., Yang, X. Y., Tan, Y. Di, Chen, J. F., & Cai, J. H. (2024). Current progression in application of extracellular vesicles in central nervous system diseases. *European Journal of Medical Research, 29*(1), 1–14. DOI: 10.1186/s40001-023-01606-5

Compilation of References

Abdullahi, A. M., Sarmast, S. T., & Singh, R. (2020). Molecular biology and epidemiology of neurotropic viruses. *Cureus*, *12*(8), e9674. Advance online publication. DOI: 10.7759/cureus.9674 PMID: 32923269

Aboabdo, M., & Mishkin, A. (2024). Antifungal therapy for the treatment of CNS infections. In *Current Fungal Infection Reports*. DOI: 10.1007/s12281-024-00492-6

Abushaheen, M. A., Fatani, A. J., Alosaimi, M., Mansy, W., George, M., Acharya, S., & Jhugroo, P. (2020). Antimicrobial resistance, mechanisms and its clinical significance. *Disease-a-Month*, *66*(6), 100971. DOI: 10.1016/j.disamonth.2020.100971 PMID: 32201008

Agarwal, D., Gupta, A., & Mehta, V. S. (2005). Role of shunt surgery in pediatric tubercular meningitis with hydrocephalus. *Indian Pediatrics*, *42*(7), 245–249. https://www.indianpediatrics.net/july2005/735.pdf

Agnihotri, S. P. (2019, June). Central nervous system opportunistic infections. *Seminars in Neurology*, *39*(03), 383–390. DOI: 10.1055/s-0039-1687842 PMID: 31378873

Agrawal, P., Katal, N., & Hooda, N. (2022). 3D U-Net-based segmentation and classification of brain tumors. *International Journal of Cognitive Computing in Engineering*, *3*, 199–210. DOI: 10.1016/j.ijcce.2022.11.001

Aguilera, E. R., & Lenz, L. L. (2020). Inflammation as a modulator of host susceptibility to pulmonary influenza, pneumococcal, and co-infections. *Frontiers in Immunology*, *11*, 105. DOI: 10.3389/fimmu.2020.00105 PMID: 32117259

Akbar, A. S., Fatichah, C., & Suciati, N. (2022). UNet3D with residual attention for brain tumor segmentation. *Journal of King Saud University. Computer and Information Sciences*, *34*(6), 3247–3258. DOI: 10.1016/j.jksuci.2022.03.022

Akinyemi, R. O., Ovbiagele, B., Adeniji, O. A., Sarfo, F. S., Abd-Allah, F., Adoukonou, T., Ogah, O. S., Naidoo, P., Damasceno, A., Walker, R. W., Ogunniyi, A., Kalaria, R. N., & Owolabi, M. O. (2021). Stroke in Africa: Profile, progress, prospects and priorities. *Nature Reviews. Neurology*, *17*(10), 634–656. DOI: 10.1038/s41582-021-00542-4 PMID: 34526674

Akter, R., Chowdhury, M. A. R., & Rahman, M. H. (2021). Flavonoids and polyphenolic compounds as potential talented agents for the treatment of Alzheimer's disease and their antioxidant activities. *Current Pharmaceutical Design*, *27*(3), 345–356. DOI: 10.2174/1381612826666200515120047

Akter, R., Rahman, M. H., Behl, T., Chowdhury, M. A. R., Manirujjaman, M., Bulbul, I. J., Elshenaw, S. E., Tit, D. M., & Bungau, S. (2021). Prospective role of polyphenolic compounds in the treatment of neurodegenerative diseases. *CNS & Neurological Disorders - Drug Targets*, *20*(5), 430–450. DOI: 10.2174/18715273 20666210218084449

Alamarat, Z., & Hasbun, R. (2020). Management of acute bacterial meningitis in children. In *Infection and Drug Resistance* (Vol. 13). DOI: 10.2147/IDR.S240162

Alberto, C., Deffert, C., Lambeng, N., Breville, G., Gayet-Ageron, A., Lalive, P., Toutous Trellu, L., & Fontao, L. (2022). Intrathecal synthesis index of specific anti-treponema IgG: A new tool for the diagnosis of neurosyphilis. *Microbiology Spectrum*, *10*(1), e01477–e21. DOI: 10.1128/spectrum.01477-21 PMID: 35138118

Alcántara, R., Fuentes, P., Antiparra, R., Santos, M., Gilman, R. H., & Kirwan, D. E. (2019). MODS-Wayne, a colorimetric adaptation of the microscopic-observation drug susceptibility (MODS) assay for detection of Mycobacterium tuberculosis pyrazinamide resistance from sputum samples. *Journal of Clinical Microbiology*, *57*(2), e01162–e18. https://www.ncbi.nlm.nih.gov/pmc/articles/PMC6355525/

Aldeen, A. Z., Salzman, D. H., Gisondi, M. A., Courtney, D. M., Allard, C. B., Meyer, C. P., Gandaglia, G., Chang, S. L., Chun, F. K. H., Gelpi-Hammerschmidt, F., Hanske, J., Kibel, A. S., Preston, M. A., Trinh, Q.-D., Anderson, C. E., Nicksa, G. A., Stewart, L. L., Anderson, J. B., Beekman, R. H.III, & Brubaker, L. (2014). Influence of Early Surgical Treatment on the Prognosis of Left-Sided Infective Endocarditis: A Multicenter Cohort Study. *Mayo Clinic Proceedings*. Advance online publication. DOI: 10.1016/j.mayocp.2014.12.014 PMID: 25178264

Ali, S., Li, J., Pei, Y., Khurram, R., & Mahmood, T. (2022). A comprehensive survey on brain tumor diagnosis using deep learning and emerging hybrid techniques with multi-modal MR image. *Archives of Computational Methods in Engineering*, *29*(7), 4871–4896. DOI: 10.1007/s11831-022-09758-z

Almubaslat, F., Sanchez-Boluarte, S. S., & Diaz, M. M. (2023). A review of neurological health disparities in Peru. *Frontiers in Public Health*, *11*, 1210238. DOI: 10.3389/fpubh.2023.1210238 PMID: 37744515

Al-Obaidi, M. M. J., & Desa, M. N. M. (2018). Mechanisms of blood brain barrier disruption by different types of bacteria, and bacterial–host interactions facilitate the bacterial pathogen invading the brain. *Cellular and Molecular Neurobiology*, *38*(7), 1349–1368. DOI: 10.1007/s10571-018-0619-z

Amezcua, L., Rivera, V. M., Vazquez, T. C., Baezconde-Garbanati, L., & Langer-Gould, A. (2021). Health disparities, inequities, and social determinants of health in multiple sclerosis and related disorders in the US: A review. *JAMA Neurology*, *78*(12), 1515–1524. DOI: 10.1001/jamaneurol.2021.3416 PMID: 34605866

Amicizia, D., Zangrillo, F., Lai, P. L., Iovine, M., & Panatto, D. (2018). Overview of Japanese encephalitis disease and its prevention. Focus on IC51 vaccine (IXIARO®). *Journal of Preventive Medicine and Hygiene*, *59*(1), E99–E107. DOI: 10.15167/2421-4248/jpmh2018.59.1.962 PMID: 29938245

Amin, J., Sharif, M., Haldorai, A., Yasmin, M., & Nayak, R. S. (2022). Brain tumor detection and classification using machine learning: A comprehensive survey. *Complex & Intelligent Systems*, *8*(4), 3161–3183. DOI: 10.1007/s40747-021-00563-y

Andronikou, S., Wieselthaler, N., Smith, B., Douis, H., Fieggen, A. G., & van Toorn, R. (2005). Value of early follow-up CT in paediatric tuberculous meningitis. *Pediatric Radiology*, *35*(11), 1092–1099. DOI: 10.1007/s00247-005-1549-9

Ang, B. S. P., Umapathi, T., & Lim, T. (2023). The Changing Epidemiology of Central Nervous System Infection: Can Radiologists Keep Up? In *Neuroimaging Clinics of North America* (Vol. 33, Issue 1). DOI: 10.1016/j.nic.2022.03.002

Ang, B. S. P., Lim, T. C. C., & Wang, L. (2018). Nipah virus infection. *Journal of Clinical Microbiology*, *56*(6), e01875-17. Advance online publication. DOI: 10.1128/JCM.01875-17 PMID: 29643201

Archibald, L. K., & Quisling, R. G. (2013). Central Nervous System Infections. *Textbook of Neurointensive Care*, 427–517. DOI: 10.1007/978-1-4471-5226-2_22

Arends, R. M., Nelwan, E. J., Soediro, R., van Crevel, R., Alisjahbana, B., Pohan, H. T., von Borries, A. K. L., Schene, A. H., van der Ven, A. J. A. M., & Schellekens, A. F. A. (2019). Associations between impulsivity, risk behavior and HIV, HBV, HCV and syphilis seroprevalence among female prisoners in Indonesia: A cross-sectional study. *PLoS One*, *14*(2), e0207970. DOI: 10.1371/journal.pone.0207970 PMID: 30768609

Arora, J., Kumar, G., Verma, A. K., Bhalla, M., Sarin, R., & Myneedu, V. P. (2015). Utility of MPT64 antigen detection for rapid confirmation of Mycobacterium tuberculosis complex. *Journal of Global Infectious Diseases*, *7*(2), 66–69. https://www.ncbi.nlm.nih.gov/pmc/articles/PMC4448327/

Arsalane, L., De Microbiologie-virologie, P., Zouhair, S., De Microbiologie-virologie, P., Bourrous, M., Zahlane, K., & De Microbiologie-virologie, P. (2023). *Les méningites de l ' enfant dans la région d ' Agadir.*

Ashley, E. S. D., Lewis, R., Lewis, J. S., Martin, C., & Andes, D. (2006). Pharmacology of systemic antifungal agents. In *Clinical Infectious Diseases* (Vol. 43, Suppl. 1). DOI: 10.1086/504492

Asquier-Khati, A., Deschanvres, C., Boutoille, D., Lefebvre, M., Le Turnier, P., Gaborit, B., Lakhal, K., Buffenoir, K., Khatchatourian, L., Asseray, N., Orain, J., Lecomte, R., Brochard, J., Biron, C., Raffi, F., Juvin, M.-E., Roualdes, V., Riem, T., Ngohou, C., & Ngohou, C. (2020). Switch from parenteral to oral antibiotics for brain abscesses: A retrospective cohort study of 109 patients. *The Journal of Antimicrobial Chemotherapy*, *75*(10), 3062–3066. DOI: 10.1093/jac/dkaa285 PMID: 32699907

Asuku, A. O., Ayinla, M. T., Ajibare, A. J., & Olajide, T. S. (2024b). Mercury chloride causes cognitive impairment, oxidative stress and neuroinflammation in male Wistar rats: The potential protective effect of 6-gingerol-rich fraction of Zingiber officinale via regulation of antioxidant defense system and reversal of pro-inflammatory markers increase. *Brain Research,* 148741: 1826. DOI: 10.1016/j.brainres.2023.148741

Asuku, A. O., Adebayo, P. O., & Ogungbangbe, G. O. (2025). Stress and Gender Differences in Brain Development. In Moradikor, N., & Orish, C. (Eds.), *Stress and the Brain: Evidence from Molecular Mechanisms to Interventions and Therapies.* Elsevier. DOI: 10.1016/bs.pbr.2025.01.013

Asuku, A. O., Ayinla, M. T., & Ajibare, A. J. (2024a). Central Nervous System Regulation of Eating and Brain Functions. In Mohamed, W., & Kobeissy, F. (Eds.), *Nutrition and Psychiatric Disorders. Nutritional Neurosciences.* Springer. DOI: 10.1007/978-981-97-2681-3_4

Autore, G., Bernardi, L., Perrone, S., & Esposito, S. (2021). Update on viral infections involving the central nervous system in pediatric patients. *Children (Basel, Switzerland)*, *8*(9), 782. Advance online publication. DOI: 10.3390/children8090782 PMID: 34572214

Ayinla, M. T., & Asuku, A. O. (2025). The neurotoxic effects of lead acetate and the abrogating actions of 6-gingerol-rich extract of ginger via modulation of antioxidant defence system, pro-inflammatory markers, and apoptotic cascade. *Naunyn-Schmiedeberg's Archives of Pharmacology*, *398*(7), 9341–9356. Advance online publication. DOI: 10.1007/s00210-025-03873-x PMID: 39937255

Ayinla, M. T., Asuku, A. O., Bayo-Olugbami, A., Ayeni, A. O., Abiola, A. A., & Owoyele, B. V. (2020). Melatonin and Vitamin C Modulate Cholinergic Neurotransmission and Oxidative stress in Scopolamine–induced Rat Model of Memory Impairment. *Journal of African Association of Physiological Sciences*, *8*(1), 20.

Azad, A. K., Chakrabarti, S., Xu, Z., Davidge, S. T., & Fu, Y. (2014). Coiled-coil domain containing 3 (CCDC3) represses tumor necrosis factor-α/nuclear factor κB-induced endothelial inflammation. *Cellular Signalling*, *26*(12), 2793–2800. DOI: 10.1016/j.cellsig.2014.08.025 PMID: 25193116

Azak, E., Sertcelik, A., Ersoz, G., Celebi, G., Eser, F., Batirel, A., & Alp, E. (2023). Evaluation of the implementation of WHO infection prevention and control core components in Turkish health care facilities: Results from a WHO infection prevention and control assessment framework (IPCAF)—based survey. *Antimicrobial Resistance and Infection Control*, *12*(1), 11. DOI: 10.1186/s13756-023-01208-0 PMID: 36782267

Azzollini, V., Dalise, S., & Chisari, C. (2021). How does stroke affect skeletal muscle? State of the art and rehabilitation perspective. *Frontiers in Neurology*, *12*, 797559. DOI: 10.3389/fneur.2021.797559 PMID: 35002937

Bagosi, Z., Csabafi, K., Jászberényi, M., & Telegdy, G. (2012). The effects of corticotropin-releasing factor and the urocortin on hypothalamic gamma-aminobutyric acid release – The impacts on the hypothalamic-pituitary-adrenal axis. *Neurochemistry International*, *60*(4), 350–354. DOI: 10.1016/j.neuint.2012.01.007 PMID: 22306347

Bahr, N. C., Marais, S., Caws, M., van Crevel, R., Wilkinson, R. J., & Tyagi, J. S. (2016). GeneXpert MTB/RIF to diagnose tuberculous meningitis: Perhaps the first test but not the last. *Clinical Infectious Diseases*, *62*(9), 1133–1135. https://www.ncbi.nlm.nih.gov/pmc/articles/PMC4826457/

Bahr, N. C., Meintjes, G., & Boulware, D. R. (2019). Inadequate diagnostics: The case to move beyond the bacilli for detection of meningitis due to Mycobacterium tuberculosis. *Journal of Medical Microbiology*, *68*(5), 755–760. https://www.ncbi.nlm.nih.gov/pmc/articles/PMC7176281/

Balaji, S., Chakraborty, R., & Aggarwal, S. (2024). Neurological complications caused by human immunodeficiency virus (HIV) and associated opportunistic co-infections: a review on their diagnosis and therapeutic insights. *CNS & Neurological Disorders-Drug Targets (Formerly Current Drug Targets-CNS & Neurological Disorders), 23*(3), 284-305.

Ball, B., Langille, M., & Geddes-McAlister, J. (2020). Fun(gi)omics: Advanced and Diverse Technologies to Explore Emerging Fungal Pathogens and Define Mechanisms of Antifungal Resistance. *mBio*, *11*(5), e01020-20. Advance online publication. DOI: 10.1128/mBio.01020-20 PMID: 33024032

Barach, P., Fisher, S. D., Adams, M. J., Burstein, G. R., Brophy, P. D., Kuo, D. Z., & Lipshultz, S. E. (2020). Disruption of healthcare: Will the COVID pandemic worsen non-COVID outcomes and disease outbreaks? *Progress in Pediatric Cardiology*, *59*, 101254. DOI: 10.1016/j.ppedcard.2020.101254 PMID: 32837144

Barriere, S. L. (1990). Pharmacology and Pharmacokinetics of Traditional Systemic Antifungal Agents. *Pharmacotherapy: The Journal of Human Pharmacology and Drug Therapy, 10*(6P3). DOI: 10.1002/j.1875-9114.1990.tb02598.x

Baticulon, R. E., & Dewan, M. C. (2021). Endoscopic third ventriculostomy and choroid plexus coagulation in infants: Current concepts and illustrative cases. Neurology India, 69(Suppl. 2). https://journals.lww.com/neur/fulltext/2021/69002/endoscopic_third_ventriculostomy_and_choroid.38.aspx

Bayeh, R., Yampolsky, M. A., & Ryder, A. G. (2021). The social lives of infectious diseases: Why culture matters to COVID-19. *Frontiers in Psychology*, *12*, 648086. DOI: 10.3389/fpsyg.2021.648086 PMID: 34630195

Be, N. A., Bishai, W. R., & Jain, S. K. (2012). Role of Mycobacterium tuberculosis pknD in the pathogenesis of central nervous system tuberculosis. *BMC Microbiology*, *12*, 7. https://www.ncbi.nlm.nih.gov/pmc/articles/PMC3322341/

Berger, R. P. (2006). The use of serum biomarkers to predict outcome after traumatic brain injury in adults and children. *The Journal of Head Trauma Rehabilitation*, *21*(4), 315–333. DOI: 10.1097/00001199-200607000-00010

Berger, R. P., Adelson, P. D., Pierce, M. C., Dulani, T., Cassidy, L. D., & Kochanek, P. M. (2005). Serum neuron-specific enolase, S100B, and myelin basic protein concentrations after inflicted and noninflicted traumatic brain injury in children. *Journal of Neurosurgery. Pediatrics*, *103*(1), 61–68. DOI: 10.3171/ped.2005.103.1.0061

Berger, R. P., Beers, S. R., Richichi, R., Wiesman, D., & Adelson, P. D. (2007). Serum biomarker concentrations and outcome after pediatric traumatic brain injury. *Journal of Neurotrauma*, *24*(12), 1793–1801. DOI: 10.1089/neu.2007.0368

Bernaerts, A., Vanhoenacker, F. M., Parizel, P. M., Van Goethem, J. W. M., van Altena, R., & Laridon, A. (2003). Tuberculosis of the central nervous system: Overview of neuroradiological findings. *European Radiology*, *13*(8), 1876–1890. DOI: 10.1007/s00330-002-1608-7

Bertsch, T., Casarin, W., Kretschmar, M., Zimmer, W., Walter, S., Sommer, C., Muehlhauser, F., Ragoschke, A., Kuehl, S., Schmidt, R., & Pohlmann-Eden, B. (2001). Protein S-100B: A serum marker for ischemic and infectious injury of cerebral tissue. *Clinical Chemistry and Laboratory Medicine*, *39*(4), 319–323. DOI: 10.1515/CCLM.2001.050

Bette, S., Shpiner, D. S., Singer, C., & Moore, H. (2018). Safinamide in the management of patients with Parkinson's disease not stabilized on levodopa: A review of the current clinical evidence. *Therapeutics and Clinical Risk Management*, *14*, 1737–1745. DOI: 10.2147/TCRM.S139545 PMID: 30271159

Bettuzzi, T., Jourdes, A., Robineau, O., Alcaraz, I., Manda, V., Molina, J. M., Mehlen, M., Cazanave, C., Tattevin, P., Mensi, S., Terrier, B., Régent, A., Ghosn, J., Charlier, C., Martin-Blondel, G., & Dupin, N. (2021). Ceftriaxone compared with benzylpenicillin in the treatment of neurosyphilis in France: A retrospective multicentre study. *The Lancet. Infectious Diseases*, *21*(10), 1441–1447. DOI: 10.1016/S1473-3099(20)30857-4 PMID: 34051142

Beviere, M., Reissier, S., Penven, M., Dejoies, L., Guerin, F., & Cattoir, V. (2023). The role of next-generation sequencing (NGS) in the management of tuberculosis: Practical review for implementation in routine. *Pathogens (Basel, Switzerland)*, *12*(8), 978. https://www.ncbi.nlm.nih.gov/pmc/articles/PMC10459500/

Bhattacharya, T., Dey, P. S., Akter, R., Kabir, M. T., Rahman, M. H., & Rauf, A. (2021). Effect of natural leaf extracts as phytomedicine in curing geriatrics. *Experimental Gerontology*, *150*, 111352. Advance online publication. DOI: 10.1016/j.exger.2021.111352

Bidstrup, C., Andersen, P. H., Skinhøj, P., & Andersen, Å. B. (2002). Tuberculous meningitis in a country with a low incidence of tuberculosis: Still a serious disease and a diagnostic challenge. *Scandinavian Journal of Infectious Diseases*, *34*(11), 811–814. DOI: 10.1080/0036554021000026938

Bloch, K. C., & Bailin, S. S. (2019). Update on fungal infections of the central nervous system: Emerging pathogens and emerging diagnostics. *Current Opinion in Infectious Diseases*, *32*(3), 277–284. DOI: 10.1097/QCO.0000000000000541 PMID: 30921084

Bollani, L., Auriti, C., Achille, C., Garofoli, F., De Rose, D. U., Meroni, V., Salvatori, G., & Tzialla, C. (2022). Congenital Toxoplasmosis: The State of the Art. *Frontiers in Pediatrics*, *10*, 894573. DOI: 10.3389/fped.2022.894573 PMID: 35874584

Bonifaz, A., & Tirado-Sánchez, A. (2017). Cutaneous Disseminated and Extracutaneous Sporotrichosis: Current Status of a Complex Disease. *Journal of Fungi (Basel, Switzerland)*, *3*(1), 6. DOI: 10.3390/jof3010006 PMID: 29371525

Bonneh-Barkay, D., & Hayasaka, D. (2011). Biomarkers of encephalitis. In *Pathogenesis of encephalitis*. InTech. DOI: 10.5772/28567

Bonthius, D. J. (2012). Lymphocytic choriomeningitis virus: An underrecognized cause of neurologic disease in the fetus, child, and adult. *Seminars in Pediatric Neurology*, *19*(3), 89–95. DOI: 10.1016/j.spen.2012.02.002 PMID: 22889536

Böttiger, B. W., Möbes, S., Glätzer, R., Bauer, H., Gries, A., Bärtsch, P., Motsch, J., & Martin, E. (2001). Astroglial protein S-100 is an early and sensitive marker of hypoxic brain damage and outcome after cardiac arrest in humans. *Circulation*, *103*(22), 2694–2698. DOI: 10.1161/01.CIR.103.22.2694

Bouvier, D., Castellani, C., Fournier, M., Dauphin, J. B., Ughetto, S., Breton, M., Labbé, A., Weinberg, A. M., & Sapin, V. (2011). Reference ranges for serum S100B protein during the first three years of life. *Clinical Biochemistry*, *44*(10-11), 927–929. DOI: 10.1016/j.clinbiochem.2011.04.012

Brand, H. K., Hermans, P. W. M., & de Groot, R. (2010). Host biomarkers and paediatric infectious diseases: From molecular profiles to clinical application. In *Hot topics in infection and immunity in children VI* (pp. 19–31). Springer.

Brandt, C. T., Lundgren, J. D., Frimodt-Møller, N., Christensen, T., Benfield, T., Espersen, F., Hougaard, D. M., & Østergaard, C. (2005). Blocking of leukocyte accumulation in the cerebrospinal fluid augments bacteremia and increases lethality in experimental pneumococcal meningitis. *Journal of Neuroimmunology*, *166*(1–2), 126–131. DOI: 10.1016/j.jneuroim.2005.05.014 PMID: 15982752

Bransfield, R. C., & Friedman, K. J. (2019, October). Differentiating psychosomatic, somatopsychic, multisystem illnesses and medical uncertainty. *Health Care*, *7*(4), 114. PMID: 31597359

Bremer, M., Kadernani, Y. E., Wasserman, S., Wilkinson, R. J., & Davis, A. G. (2021). Strategies for the diagnosis and management of meningitis in HIV-infected adults in resource limited settings. *Expert Opinion on Pharmacotherapy*, *22*(15), 2053–2070. DOI: 10.1080/14656566.2021.1940954 PMID: 34154509

Brew, B. J., Crowe, S. M., Landay, A., Cysique, L. A., & Guillemin, G. (2009). Neurodegeneration and ageing in the HAART era. *Journal of Neuroimmune Pharmacology*, *4*(2), 163–174. DOI: 10.1007/s11481-008-9143-3

Brinkmann, V. (2018). Neutrophil extracellular traps in the second decade. *Journal of Innate Immunity*, *10*(5–6), 414–421. DOI: 10.1159/000489829 PMID: 29909412

Brooks, J. B., Daneshvar, M. I., Haberberger, R. L., & Mikhail, I. A. (1990). Rapid diagnosis of tuberculous meningitis by frequency-pulsed electron-capture gas-liquid chromatography detection of carboxylic acids in cerebrospinal fluid. *Journal of Clinical Microbiology*, *28*(5), 989–997. https://www.ncbi.nlm.nih.gov/pmc/articles/PMC267852/

Brouwer, M. C., Thwaites, G. E., Tunkel, A. R., & van de Beek, D. (2012). Dilemmas in the diagnosis of acute community-acquired bacterial meningitis. *Lancet*, *380*(9854), 1684–1692. DOI: 10.1016/S0140-6736(12)61185-4 PMID: 23141617

Brouwer, M. C., Tunkel, A. R., & van de Beek, D. (2010). Epidemiology, diagnosis, and antimicrobial treatment of acute bacterial meningitis. *Clinical Microbiology Reviews*, *23*(3), 467–492. DOI: 10.1128/CMR.00070-09 PMID: 20610819

Brouwer, M. C., & Van De Beek, D. (2017). Epidemiology, diagnosis, and treatment of brain abscesses. *Current Opinion in Infectious Diseases*, *30*(1), 129–134. DOI: 10.1097/QCO.0000000000000334 PMID: 27828809

Brouwer, M. C., & van de Beek, D. (2023). Adjunctive dexamethasone treatment in adults with listeria monocytogenes meningitis: A prospective nationwide cohort study. *EClinicalMedicine*, *58*, 101922. Advance online publication. DOI: 10.1016/j.eclinm.2023.101922 PMID: 37007737

Brown, D. L., & Frank, J. E. (2003). Diagnosis and management of syphilis. *American Family Physician*, *68*(2), 283–290. PMID: 12892348

Brumble, L. M., Reza, M. B., Dhakal, L. P., Cruz, G., Abu Saleh, O. M., Heckman, M. G., Vargas, E. R., Dickson, D. W., Enzler, M. J., Libertin, C. R., & Freeman, W. D. (2017). Fungal Infections of the Central Nervous System: Clinical, Radiographic and Laboratory Manifestations. *Journal of Microbiology & Experimentation*, *5*(6). Advance online publication. DOI: 10.15406/jmen.2017.05.00167

Bruno, L., Nappo, M. A., Ferrari, L., Di Lecce, R., Guarnieri, C., Cantoni, A. M., & Corradi, A. (2023). Nipah Virus Disease: Epidemiological, Clinical, Diagnostic and Legislative Aspects of This Unpredictable Emerging Zoonosis. In *Animals* (Vol. 13, Issue 1). DOI: 10.3390/ani13010159

Bryan, J. P., de Silva, H. R., Tavares, A., Rocha, H., & Scheld, W. M. (1990). Etiology and mortality of bacterial meningitis in northeastern Brazil. *Reviews of Infectious Diseases*, *12*(1), 128–135. DOI: 10.1093/clinids/12.1.128 PMID: 2300734

Budreviciute, A., Damiati, S., Sabir, D. K., & Kodzius, R. (2020). Management and prevention strategies for non-communicable diseases (NCDs) and their risk factors. *Frontiers in Public Health*, *8*, 574111. DOI: 10.3389/fpubh.2020.574111 PMID: 33324597

Buitrago-Garcia, D., Martí-Carvajal, A. J., Jimenez, A., Conterno, L. O., & Pardo, R. (2019). Antibiotic therapy for adults with neurosyphilis. *Cochrane Database of Systematic Reviews*, 5. PMID: 31132142

Burrel, S., Topalis, D., & Boutolleau, D. (2020). Herpes simplex virus resistance to antivirals. In *Virologie* (Vol. 24, Issue 5, pp. 325–342). John Libbey. DOI: 10.1684/vir.2020.0864

Buscaglia, C., & Di Noia, J. M. (2003). Trypanosoma cruzi clonal diversity and the epidemiology of Chagas' disease. *Microbes and Infection*, *5*(5), 419–427. DOI: 10.1016/S1286-4579(03)00050-9 PMID: 12737998

Butler, T. (2017). The Jarisch–Herxheimer reaction after antibiotic treatment of spirochetal infections: A review of recent cases and our understanding of pathogenesis. *The American Journal of Tropical Medicine and Hygiene*, *96*(1), 46–52. DOI: 10.4269/ajtmh.16-0434 PMID: 28077740

Butterfield, L. H., Potter, D. M., & Kirkwood, J. M. (2011). Multiplex serum biomarker assessments: Technical and biostatistical issues. *Journal of Translational Medicine*, *9*, 173. Advance online publication. DOI: 10.1186/1479-5876-9-173

Calnan, M., Gadsby, E. W., Kondé, M. K., Diallo, A., & Rossman, J. S. (2018). The response to and impact of the Ebola epidemic: Towards an agenda for interdisciplinary research. *International Journal of Health Policy and Management*, *7*(5), 402–411. DOI: 10.15171/ijhpm.2017.104 PMID: 29764104

Cao, D., Wang, T., Wang, Y., & Han, J. (2022). Analysis of cases with cerebrospinal fluid characteristics similar to tuberculous meningitis. *BioMed Research International*, *2022*, 9692804. https://www.ncbi.nlm.nih.gov/pmc/articles/PMC9825210/

Carlson, J. A., Dabiri, G., Cribier, B., & Sell, S. (2011). The immunopathobiology of syphilis: The manifestations and course of syphilis are determined by the level of delayed-type hypersensitivity. *The American Journal of Dermatopathology*, *33*(5), 433–460. DOI: 10.1097/DAD.0b013e3181e8b587 PMID: 21694502

Carpio, A., Romo, M. L., Parkhouse, R. M. E., Short, B., & Dua, T. (2016). Parasitic diseases of the central nervous system: Lessons for clinicians and policy makers. *Expert Review of Neurotherapeutics*, *16*(4), 401–414. DOI: 10.1586/14737175.2016.1155454 PMID: 26894629

Case, N. T., Berman, J., Blehert, D. S., Cramer, R. A., Cuomo, C., Currie, C. R., Ene, I. V., Fisher, M. C., Fritz-Laylin, L. K., Gerstein, A. C., Glass, N. L., Gow, N. A. R., Gurr, S. J., Hittinger, C. T., Hohl, T. M., Iliev, I. D., James, T. Y., Jin, H., Klein, B. S., & Kronstad, J. W. (2022). The future of fungi: threats and opportunities. *G3 Genes|Genomes|Genetics*, *12*(11). DOI: 10.1093/g3journal/jkac224

Casmiro, M., Maitan, S., De Pasquale, F., Cova, V., Scarpa, E., & Vignatelli, L.NSE Study Group. (2005). Cerebrospinal fluid and serum neuron-specific enolase concentrations in a normal population. *European Journal of Neurology*, *12*(5), 369–374. DOI: 10.1111/j.1468-1331.2004.00985.x

Caviedes, L., Lee, T. S., Gilman, R. H., Sheen, P., Spellman, E., & Lee, E. H. (2000). Rapid, efficient detection and drug susceptibility testing of Mycobacterium tuberculosis in sputum by microscopic observation of broth cultures. *Journal of Clinical Microbiology*, *38*(3), 1203–1208. https://www.ncbi.nlm.nih.gov/pmc/articles/PMC86377/

Centers for Disease Control and Prevention. (2024). Tuberculosis (TB) disease in the United States, 1993–2023 [Slide set]. https://www.cdc.gov/tb-surveillance-report-2023/resources/slide-set.html

Chakravorty, S., Simmons, A. M., Rowneki, M., Parmar, H., Cao, Y., & Ryan, J. (2017). The new Xpert MTB/RIF Ultra: Improving detection of Mycobacterium tuberculosis and resistance to rifampin in an assay suitable for point-of-care testing. *mBio*, *8*(4), e00812–e00817. https://www.ncbi.nlm.nih.gov/pmc/articles/PMC5574709/

Chakroborty, N. K., Baksi, S., & Bhattacharya, A. (2023). Cognitive Impairment in Parasitic Protozoan Infection. In *Pathobiology of Parasitic Protozoa*. Dynamics and Dimensions. DOI: 10.1007/978-981-19-8225-5_4

Challa, S. (2020). Invasive Fungal Infections of the Central Nervous System in Immune-Competent Hosts. In *Current Fungal Infection Reports* (Vol. 14, Issue 2). DOI: 10.1007/s12281-020-00384-5

Chang, J. R., Mukerjee, R., Bagashev, A., Del Valle, L., Chabrashvili, T., Hawkins, B. J., He, J. J., & Sawaya, B. E. (2011). HIV-1 Tat protein promotes neuronal dysfunction through disruption of microRNAs. *The Journal of Biological Chemistry*, *286*(47), 41125–41134. DOI: 10.1074/jbc.M111.268466

Chatterjee, D., Marmion, D. J., McBride, J. L., Manfredsson, F. P., Butler, D., Messer, A., & Kordower, J. H. (2022). Enhanced CNS transduction from AAV.PHP. eB infusion into the cisterna magna of older adult rats compared to AAV9. *Gene Therapy*, *29*(6), 390–397. DOI: 10.1038/s41434-021-00244-y PMID: 33753910

Chattopadhyay, A., & Maître, M. (2022). CNN-based MRI brain tumor image detection technique. *Neuroscience Informatics*, 2.

Chaudhuri, A., Martinez-Martin, P., Kennedy, P. G. E., Seaton, R. A., & Portegie, P. s, Bojar, M., & Steiner, I. (2011). Management of Community-Acquired Bacterial Meningitis. *European Handbook of Neurological Management*, 145–157. DOI: 10.1002/9781444346268.ch11

Chaudhuri, A., & Kennedy, P. G. (2002). Diagnosis and treatment of viral encephalitis. *Postgraduate Medical Journal*, *78*(924), 575–583. DOI: 10.1136/pmj.78.924.575 PMID: 12415078

Chee, S. E. J., & Solito, E. (2021). The impact of ageing on the CNS immune response in Alzheimer's disease. *Frontiers in Immunology*, *12*, 738511. DOI: 10.3389/fimmu.2021.738511 PMID: 34603320

Chen, H., Zhou, Y., Wang, Z.-Y., Yan, B.-X., Zhou, W.-F., Wang, T.-T., Zheng, M., & Man, X.-Y. (2019). Exosomal microRNA profiles from serum and cerebrospinal fluid in neurosyphilis. *Sexually Transmitted Infections*, *95*(4), 246–250. DOI: 10.1136/sextrans-2018-053813 PMID: 30926713

Chen, R., Mukhopadhyay, S., Merits, A., Bolling, B., Nasar, F., Coffey, L. L., Powers, A., & Weaver, S. C.ICTV Report Consortium. (2018). ICTV virus taxonomy profile: Togaviridae. *The Journal of General Virology*, *99*(6), 761–762. DOI: 10.1099/jgv.0.001072 PMID: 29745869

Chen, Y. Z., Sun, L. C., Wen, Y. H., Li, Z. W., Fan, S. J., & Tan, H. K. (2020). Pooled analysis of the Xpert MTB/RIF assay for diagnosing tuberculous meningitis. *Bioscience Reports*, *40*(1), BSR20191312. https://www.ncbi.nlm.nih.gov/pmc/articles/PMC6946622/

Chen, Y., Wang, Y., Liu, X., Li, W., Fu, H., & Liu, X. (2022). Comparative diagnostic utility of metagenomic next-generation sequencing, GeneXpert, modified Ziehl–Neelsen staining, and culture using cerebrospinal fluid for tuberculous meningitis: A multi-center, retrospective study in China. *Journal of Clinical Laboratory Analysis*, *36*(4), e24307. https://www.ncbi.nlm.nih.gov/pmc/articles/PMC8993600/

Cherian, A., & Thomas, S. (2011). Central nervous system tuberculosis. *African Health Sciences*, *11*(1), 116–127. https://www.ncbi.nlm.nih.gov/pmc/articles/PMC3092316/

Chesney, A. M., & Kemp, J. E. (1924). Incidence of Spirochaeta pallida in cerebrospinal fluid during early stage of syphilis. *Journal of the American Medical Association*, *83*(22), 1725–1728. DOI: 10.1001/jama.1924.02660220001001

Chetty, G., Yamin, M., & White, M. (2022). Resource-efficient 3D U-Net model for medical image analysis. *International Journal of Information Technology : an Official Journal of Bharati Vidyapeeth's Institute of Computer Applications and Management*, *14*(1), 95–103. DOI: 10.1007/s41870-021-00850-4 PMID: 35005425

Chitnis, T., & Weiner, H. L. (2017). CNS inflammation and neurodegeneration. *The Journal of Clinical Investigation*, *127*(10), 3577–3587. DOI: 10.1172/JCI90609

Chohan, T., Jain, A., Saeed, M., & Saeed, S. A. (2012). Tuberculous meningitis, an unusual presentation in a young lady. *BMJ Case Reports*, *2012*, bcr1220115370. https://www.ncbi.nlm.nih.gov/pmc/articles/PMC3417028/

Choi, S. H., Kim, Y. S., Bae, I. G., Chung, J. W., Lee, M. S., & Kang, J. M. (2002). The possible role of cerebrospinal fluid adenosine deaminase activity in the diagnosis of tuberculous meningitis in adults. *Clinical Neurology and Neurosurgery*, *104*(1), 10–15. https://www.sciencedirect.com/science/article/pii/S0303846701001597

Choudhri, Y., Miller, J., Sandhu, J., Leon, A., & Aho, J. (2018). Sexually transmitted infections: Infectious and congenital syphilis in Canada, 2010–2015. *Canada Communicable Disease Report = Relevé des Maladies Transmissibles au Canada*, *44*(2), 43. PMID: 29770098

Ciummo, F., Srinivas, P., & Biedny, J. (2021). Antimicrobial use in central nervous system infections. In *Current Opinion in Infectious Diseases* (Vol. 34, Issue 3). DOI: 10.1097/QCO.0000000000000721

Clement, M. E., Okeke, N. L., & Hicks, C. B. (2014). Treatment of syphilis: A systematic review. *Journal of the American Medical Association*, *312*(18), 1905–1917. DOI: 10.1001/jama.2014.13259 PMID: 25387188

Coen, M., O'Sullivan, M., Bubb, W. A., Kuchel, P. W., & Sorrell, T. (2005). Proton nuclear magnetic resonance—Based metabonomics for rapid diagnosis of meningitis and ventriculitis. *Clinical Infectious Diseases, 41*(11), 1582–1590. DOI: 10.1086/497832

Coordination, G., Alastruey-Izquierdo, A., World Health Organization, & World Health Organization. (2022). *WHO fungal priority pathogens list to guide research, development and public health action.* Organización Mundial de la Salud (OMS).

Coovadia, Y. M., Dawood, A., Ellis, M. E., Coovadia, H. M., & Daniel, T. M. (1986). Evaluation of adenosine deaminase activity and antibody to Mycobacterium tuberculosis antigen 5 in cerebrospinal fluid and the radioactive bromide partition test for the early diagnosis of tuberculosis meningitis. *Archives of Disease in Childhood, 61*(5), 428–435. https://www.ncbi.nlm.nih.gov/pmc/articles/PMC1777799/

Cornick, J. E., Everett, D. B., Broughton, C., Denis, B. B., Banda, D. L., Carrol, E. D., & Parry, C. M. (2011). Invasive Streptococcus pneumoniae in children, Malawi, 2004–2006. *Emerging Infectious Diseases, 17*(6), 1107–1109. DOI: 10.3201/eid1706.101404 PMID: 21749782

Corral, I., Quereda, C., Navas, E., Martín-Dávila, P., Pérez-Elías, M. J., & Casado, J. L. (2004). Adenosine deaminase activity in cerebrospinal fluid of HIV-infected patients: Limited value for diagnosis of tuberculous meningitis. *European Journal of Clinical Microbiology & Infectious Diseases, 23*(6), 471–476. DOI: 10.1007/s10096-004-1110-z

Costerus, J. M., Brouwer, M. C., Bijlsma, M. W., Tanck, M. W., van der Ende, A., & van de Beek, D. (2016). Impact of an evidence-based guideline on the management of community-acquired bacterial meningitis: A prospective cohort study. *Clinical Microbiology and Infection, 22*(11), 928–933. DOI: 10.1016/j.cmi.2016.07.026 PMID: 27484018

Costerus, J. M., Brouwer, M. C., Sprengers, M. E. S., Roosendaal, S. D., van der Ende, A., & van de Beek, D. (2018). Cranial computed tomography, lumbar puncture, and clinical deterioration in bacterial meningitis: A nationwide cohort study. *Clinical Infectious Diseases, 67*(6), 920–926. DOI: 10.1093/cid/ciy200 PMID: 29522090

Cottagnoud, P., Pfister, M., Acosta, F., Cottagnoud, M., Flatz, L., Kühn, F., Müller, H.-P., & Stucki, A. (2004). Daptomycin is highly efficacious against penicillin-resistant and penicillin-and quinolone-resistant pneumococci in experimental meningitis. *Antimicrobial Agents and Chemotherapy, 48*(10), 3928–3933. DOI: 10.1128/AAC.48.10.3928-3933.2004 PMID: 15388454

Coyle, C. M. (2021). The returned traveler with neurologic manifestations: Could my patient have a parasite? *Current Opinion in Infectious Diseases, 34*(3), 245–254. DOI: 10.1097/QCO.0000000000000732 PMID: 33769967

Cresswell, F. V., Bangdiwala, A. S., Bahr, N. C., Trautner, E., Nuwagira, E., & Ellis, J. (2018). Tuberculous meningitis diagnosis and outcomes during the Xpert MTB/RIF era: A 6.5-year cohort study in Uganda. *Wellcome Open Research, 3*, 64. https://www.ncbi.nlm.nih.gov/pmc/articles/PMC6039934/

Cristina, M. L., Spagnolo, A. M., Giribone, L., Demartini, A., & Sartini, M. (2021). Epidemiology and prevention of healthcare-associated infections in geriatric patients: A narrative review. *International Journal of Environmental Research and Public Health, 18*(10), 5333. DOI: 10.3390/ijerph18105333 PMID: 34067797

Cui, L., Xu, Z., & Hou, H. (2020). Diagnosis and treatment of spinal syphilitic gumma: A case report. *Frontiers in Neurology, 10*, 490958. DOI: 10.3389/fneur.2019.01352 PMID: 32010040

Curren, E. J., Lindsey, N. P., Fischer, M., & Hills, S. L. (2018). St. Louis encephalitis virus disease in the United States, 2003–2017. *The American Journal of Tropical Medicine and Hygiene, 99*(4), 1074–1079. DOI: 10.4269/ajtmh.18-0420 PMID: 30182919

Curto, M., Reali, C., Palmieri, G., Scintu, F., Schivo, M. L., & Sogos, V. (2004). Inhibition of cytokines expression in human microglia infected by virulent and non-virulent mycobacteria. *Neurochemistry International, 44*(6), 381–392. https://www.sciencedirect.com/science/article/pii/S0197018603002031

Czarniak, N., Kamińska, J., Matowicka-Karna, J., & Koper-Lenkiewicz, O. M. (2023). Cerebrospinal fluid–basic concepts review. *Biomedicines, 11*(5), 1461. DOI: 10.3390/biomedicines11051461 PMID: 37239132

Dai, T., Li, K., Lu, H., Gu, X., Wang, Q., & Zhou, P. (2012). Molecular typing of Treponema pallidum: A 5-year surveillance in Shanghai, China. *Journal of Clinical Microbiology, 50*(11), 3674–3677. DOI: 10.1128/JCM.01195-12 PMID: 22972832

Dando, S. J., Mackay-Sim, A., Norton, R., Currie, B. J., St John, J. A., Ekberg, J. A. K., Batzloff, M., Ulett, G. C., & Beacham, I. R. (2014). Pathogens penetrating the central nervous system: Infection pathways and the cellular and molecular mechanisms of invasion. *Clinical Microbiology Reviews, 27*(4), 691–726. DOI: 10.1128/CMR.00118-13 PMID: 25278572

Daniel, B. D., Grace, G. A., & Natrajan, M. (2019). Tuberculous meningitis in children: Clinical management & outcome. *The Indian Journal of Medical Research, 150*(2), 117–130. https://www.ncbi.nlm.nih.gov/pmc/articles/PMC6829784/

Dash, S., Shakyawar, S. K., Sharma, M., & Kaushik, S. (2019). Big data in healthcare: Management, analysis and future prospects. *Journal of Big Data, 6*(1), 1–25. DOI: 10.1186/s40537-019-0217-0

Dastur, D. K., Manghani, D. K., & Udani, P. M. (1995). Pathology and pathogenetic mechanisms in neurotuberculosis. *Radiologic Clinics of North America, 33*(4), 733–752.

David, S., & Abraham, A. (2016). Epidemiological and clinical aspects on West Nile virus, a globally emerging pathogen. *Infectious Diseases, 48*(8), 571–586. DOI: 10.3109/23744235.2016.1164890 PMID: 27207312

Davis, A. G., Rohlwink, U. K., Proust, A., Figaji, A. A., & Wilkinson, R. J. (2019). The pathogenesis of tuberculous meningitis. *Journal of Leukocyte Biology, 105*(2), 267–280. https://www.ncbi.nlm.nih.gov/pmc/articles/PMC6355360/

Davis, A., Meintjes, G., & Wilkinson, R. J. (2018). Treatment of tuberculous meningitis and its complications in adults. *Current Treatment Options in Neurology, 20*(3), 5. Advance online publication. DOI: 10.1007/s11940-018-0490-9

Dawi, J., Mohan, A. S., Misakyan, Y., Affa, S., Gonzalez, E., & Hajjar, K. (2024). The role of oxidative stress in TB meningitis and therapeutic options. *Diseases (Basel, Switzerland), 12*(3), 50. https://www.mdpi.com/2079-9721/12/3/50

de Buhr, N., Reuner, F., Neumann, A., Stump-Guthier, C., Tenenbaum, T., Schroten, H., Ishikawa, H., Müller, K., Beineke, A., Hennig-Pauka, I., Gutsmann, T., Valentin-Weigand, P., Baums, C. G., & von Köckritz-Blickwede, M. (2017). Neutrophil extracellular trap formation in the Streptococcus suis-infected cerebrospinal fluid compartment. *Cellular Microbiology, 19*(2), e12649. DOI: 10.1111/cmi.12649 PMID: 27450700

DeCrom, S. C., Rossen, J. W. A., van Furth, A. M., & Obihara, C. C. (2016). Enterovirus and parechovirus infection in children: A brief overview. *European Journal of Pediatrics, 175*(8), 1023–1029. DOI: 10.1007/s00431-016-2725-7 PMID: 27156106

Deghmane, A. E., & Taha, M. K. (2021). Invasive bacterial infections in subjects with genetic and acquired susceptibility and impacts on recommendations for vaccination: A narrative review. *Microorganisms, 9*(3), 467. DOI: 10.3390/microorganisms9030467 PMID: 33668334

Deigendesch, N., Costa Nunez, J., & Stenzel, W. (2017). Parasitic and fungal infections. *Handbook of Clinical Neurology*, *145*, 245–262. DOI: 10.1016/B978-0-12-802395-2.00018-3 PMID: 28987173

Deng, Y., Huang, R., Huang, S., & Xiong, M. (2021). Nanoparticles Enable Efficient Delivery of Antimicrobial Peptides for the Treatment of Deep Infections. *BIO Integration*, *2*(2), 50. DOI: 10.15212/bioi-2021-0003

Deutschman, C. S., & Tracey, K. J. (2014). Sepsis: Current dogma and new perspectives. *Immunity*, *40*(4), 463–475. DOI: 10.1016/j.immuni.2014.04.001

DeVincenzo, J. P., Berning, S. E., Peloquin, C. A., & Husson, R. N. (1999). Multidrug-resistant tuberculous meningitis: Clinical problems and concentrations of second-line antituberculous medications. *The Annals of Pharmacotherapy*, *33*(11), 1184–1188. DOI: 10.1345/aph.19008

Dhar, S., & Pal, B. (2021). *Analysis of 93 Brain Abscess Cases to Review the Effect of Intervention to Determine the Feasibility of the Management Protocol: A Tertiary Care Perspective Original Article.* DOI: 10.4103/ajns.AJNS_467_20

Ding, C., Wu, Y., Chen, X., Chen, Y., Wu, Z., Lin, Z., Kang, D., Fang, W., & Chen, F. (2022). Global, regional, and national burden and attributable risk factors of neurological disorders: The Global Burden of Disease study 1990–2019. *Frontiers in Public Health*, *10*, 952161. DOI: 10.3389/fpubh.2022.952161 PMID: 36523572

Dodd, P. J., Osman, M., Cresswell, F. V., Stadelman, A. M., Lan, N. H., & Thuong, N. T. T. (2021). The global burden of tuberculous meningitis in adults: A modelling study. *PLOS Global Public Health*, *1*(12), e0000069. https://www.ncbi.nlm.nih.gov/pmc/articles/PMC10021871/

Domingo, P., Pomar, V., de Benito, N., & Coll, P. (2013). The spectrum of acute bacterial meningitis in elderly patients. *BMC Infectious Diseases*, *13*(1), 108. Advance online publication. DOI: 10.1186/1471-2334-13-108 PMID: 23446215

Donald, P. R., Schaaf, H. S., & Schoeman, J. F. (2005). Tuberculous meningitis and miliary tuberculosis: The Rich focus revisited. *The Journal of Infection*, *50*(3), 193–195. DOI: 10.1016/j.jinf.2004.02.010

Donovan, J., Phu, N. H., Mai, N. T. H., Dung, L. T., Imran, D., & Burhan, E. (2018). Adjunctive dexamethasone for the treatment of HIV-infected adults with tuberculous meningitis (ACT HIV): Study protocol for a randomised controlled trial. *Wellcome Open Research*, *3*, 31. https://www.ncbi.nlm.nih.gov/pmc/articles/PMC6143919/

Donovan, J., & Thwaites, G. E. (2020). Tuberculous meningitis: Where to from here? *Current Opinion in Infectious Diseases, 33*(3), 259–266. https://www.ncbi.nlm.nih.gov/pmc/articles/PMC7259381/

Dorovini-Zis, K., Schmidt, K., Huynh, H., Fu, W., Whitten, R. O., Milner, D., Kamiza, S., Molyneux, M., & Taylor, T. E. (2011). The Neuropathology of Fatal Cerebral Malaria in Malawian Children. *American Journal of Pathology, 178*(5), 2146–2158. DOI: 10.1016/j.ajpath.2011.01.016 PMID: 21514429

Drago, F., Javor, S., & Parodi, A. (2016). Neurosyphilis: From infection to autoinflammation? []. SAGE Publications Sage UK: London, England.]. *International Journal of STD & AIDS, 27*(4), 327–328. DOI: 10.1177/0956462415590710 PMID: 26873161

Drossinos, Y., Weber, T. P., & Stilianakis, N. I. (2021). Droplets and aerosols: An artificial dichotomy in respiratory virus transmission. *Health Science Reports, 4*(2), e275. Advance online publication. DOI: 10.1002/hsr2.275 PMID: 33977157

du Preez, K., Jenkins, H. E., Donald, P. R., Solomons, R. S., Graham, S. M., Schaaf, H. S., Starke, J. R., Hesseling, A. C., & Seddon, J. A. (2022). Tuberculous meningitis in children: A forgotten public health emergency. *Frontiers in Neurology, 13*, 751133. DOI: 10.3389/fneur.2022.751133 PMID: 35370901

Du, S., Guan, Y., Xie, A., Yan, Z., Gao, S., Li, W., Rao, L., Chen, X., & Chen, T. (2023). Extracellular vesicles: a rising star for therapeutics and drug delivery. *Journal of Nanobiotechnology, 21*(1), 1–51. DOI: 10.1186/s12951-023-01973-5

Dudley, M. Z., Salmon, D. A., Halsey, N. A., Orenstein, W. A., Limaye, R. J., O'Leary, S. T., ... & Omer, S. B. (2018). Do Vaccines Cause Meningitis or Encephalitis/Encephalopathy?. *The Clinician's Vaccine Safety Resource Guide: Optimizing Prevention of Vaccine-Preventable Diseases Across the Lifespan*, 281-289.

Du, F. Z., Zhang, X., Zhang, R. L., & Wang, Q. Q. (2023). CARE-NS, a research strategy for neurosyphilis. *Frontiers in Medicine, 9*(January), 1–7. DOI: 10.3389/fmed.2022.1040133 PMID: 36687428

Dugger, B. N., & Dickson, D. W. (2017). Pathology of neurodegenerative diseases. *Cold Spring Harbor Perspectives in Biology, 9*(7), a028035. Advance online publication. DOI: 10.1101/cshperspect.a028035

Du, L., Chen, L., Liu, F., Wang, W., & Huang, H. (2023). Nose-to-brain drug delivery for the treatment of CNS disease: New development and strategies. *International Review of Neurobiology, 171*, 255–297. DOI: 10.1016/bs.irn.2023.05.014 PMID: 37783558

Dunay, I. R., Gajurel, K., Dhakal, R., Liesenfeld, O., & Montoya, J. G. (2018). Treatment of Toxoplasmosis: Historical Perspective, Animal Models, and Current Clinical Practice. *Clinical Microbiology Reviews*, *31*(4), e00057–e17. DOI: 10.1128/CMR.00057-17 PMID: 30209035

Edelmann, M. J., & Maegawa, G. H. (2020). CNS-targeting therapies for lysosomal storage diseases: Current advances and challenges. *Frontiers in Molecular Biosciences*, *7*, 559804. DOI: 10.3389/fmolb.2020.559804 PMID: 33304924

Edwards, M. S., & Baker, C. J. (2013). Treatment and outcome of bacterial meningitis in the neonate. *UpToDate*.

Ehsanifar, M., Reihane, R., Akram, G., & Joseph, P. (2023). Mold and Mycotoxin Exposure and Brain Disorders. *Journal of Integrative Neuroscience*, *22*(6), 137. DOI: 10.31083/j.jin2206137 PMID: 38176924

Ekloh, W., Asafu-Adjaye, A., & Nii, C. (2024). A comprehensive exploration of schistosomiasis: Global impact, molecular characterization, drug discovery, artificial intelligence and future prospects. *Heliyon*, *10*(12), e33070–e33070. DOI: 10.1016/j.heliyon.2024.e33070 PMID: 38988508

El Aidy, S., Dinan, T. G., & Cryan, J. F. (2014). Immune modulation of the brain-gut-microbe axis. *Frontiers in Microbiology*, *5*, 146. Advance online publication. DOI: 10.3389/fmicb.2014.00146

Elmakrini, N. (2014). *Méningites Infectieuses Communautaires: Profil Microbiologique et Épidémiologique à l'Hôpital Militaire Moulay Ismaïl de Meknès (De 2011 à 2013).*

El-Mansoury, B., Smimih, K., Hamdan, Y. A., El Khiat, A., Elouali, S., El Fatimi, H., Draoui, A., El Hiba, O., & Jayakumar, A. R. (2023). The Interplay Between Environmental Pollutants, Gut Microbiota, and Infections: Current Concepts and Therapies. *Ecological and Evolutionary Perspectives on Infections and Morbidity*, 173–207.

Encephalitis: Diagnosis, management and recent advances in the field of encephalitides. (2023). *Postgraduate Medical Journal*. Advance online publication. DOI: 10.1136/POSTMJ/POSTGRADMEDJ-2022-141812

Erdem, H., Inan, A., Guven, E., Hargreaves, S., Larsen, L., Shehata, G., Pernicova, E., Khan, E., Bastakova, L., Namani, S., Harxhi, A., Roganovic, T., Lakatos, B., Uysal, S., Sipahi, O. R., Crisan, A., Miftode, E., Stebel, R., Jegorovic, B., & Nassar, M. (2017). The burden and epidemiology of community-acquired central nervous system infections: A multinational study. *European Journal of Clinical Microbiology & Infectious Diseases*, *36*(9), 1595–1611. DOI: 10.1007/s10096-017-2973-0 PMID: 28397100

Erni, S. T., Fernandes, G., Buri, M., Perny, M., Rutten, R. J., Van Noort, J. M., Senn, P., Grandgirard, D., Roccio, M., & Leib, S. L. (2019). Anti-inflammatory and oto-protective effect of the small heat shock protein alpha B-crystallin (HspB5) in experimental pneumococcal meningitis. *Frontiers in Neurology*, *10*, 570. DOI: 10.3389/fneur.2019.00570 PMID: 31244750

Fahn, S. (2018). The 200-year journey of Parkinson disease: Reflecting on the past and looking towards the future. *Parkinsonism & Related Disorders*, *46*(Suppl. 1), S1–S5. DOI: 10.1016/j.parkreldis.2017.07.020

Faizi, N., & Hassan, J. (2023). Etiology and Epidemiology of Central Nervous System Infections. In *Viral and Fungal Infections of the Central Nervous System: A Microbiological Perspective*. DOI: 10.1007/978-981-99-6445-1_1

Fancourt, D., & Finn, S. (2019). *What is the evidence on the role of the arts in improving health and well-being? A scoping review*. World Health Organization. Regional Office for Europe.

Fathilah, J., & Choo, M. M. (2003). The Jarisch-Herxheimer reaction in ocular syphilis. *The Medical Journal of Malaysia*, *58*(3), 437–439. PMID: 14750386

Feigin, V. L., Vos, T., Nichols, E., Owolabi, M. O., Carroll, W. M., Dichgans, M., Deuschl, G., Parmar, P., Brainin, M., & Murray, C. (2020). The global burden of neurological disorders: Translating evidence into policy. *Lancet Neurology*, *19*(3), 255–265. DOI: 10.1016/S1474-4422(19)30411-9 PMID: 31813850

Fernando, H., Gamboled, S., Denman, S., Sridharan, S., & Folks, C. (2022). Survey on deep learning for detecting anomalies in medical images. *ACM Computing Surveys*, *54*(7), 1–37. DOI: 10.1145/3464423

Filho, V. W., de Castilho, E. A., Rodrigues, L. C., & Huttly, S. R. A. (n.d.). *Effectiveness of BCG vaccination against tuberculous meningitis: A case-control study in São Paulo*.

Fisher, M. C., Alastruey-Izquierdo, A., Berman, J., Bicanic, T., Bignell, E. M., Bowyer, P., Bromley, M., Brüggemann, R., Garber, G., Cornely, O. A., Gurr, S. J., Harrison, T. S., Kuijper, E., Rhodes, J., Sheppard, D. C., Warris, A., White, P. L., Xu, J., Zwaan, B., & Verweij, P. E. (2022). Tackling the emerging threat of antifungal resistance to human health. *Nature Reviews. Microbiology*, *20*(9), 557–571. DOI: 10.1038/s41579-022-00720-1 PMID: 35352028

Flores-Maldonado, O., González, G. M., Enríquez-Bañuelos, J. F., Andrade, Á., Treviño-Rangel, R., & Becerril-García, M. A. (2023). Candida albicans causes brain regional invasion and necrosis, and activation of microglia during lethal neonatal neurocandidiasis. *Microbes and Infection*, *25*(6), 105119. DOI: 10.1016/j.micinf.2023.105119 PMID: 36758890

Folke, J., Ferreira, N., Brudek, T., Borghammer, P., & Van Den Berge, N. (2022). Passive Immunization in Alpha-Synuclein Preclinical Animal Models. *Biomolecules, 12*(2), 168. DOI: 10.3390/biom12020168

Fong, T. H., Shi, W., Ruan, G., Li, S., Liu, G., & Yang, L. (2023). Tuberculostearic acid incorporated predictive model contributes to the clinical diagnosis of tuberculous meningitis. *iScience*, *26*(10), 107858. https://www.ncbi.nlm.nih.gov/pmc/articles/PMC10520543/

Forrestel, A. K., Kovarik, C. L., & Katz, K. A. (2020). Sexually acquired syphilis: Historical aspects, microbiology, epidemiology, and clinical manifestations. *Journal of the American Academy of Dermatology*, *82*(1), 1–14. DOI: 10.1016/j.jaad.2019.02.073 PMID: 30986477

Franceschi, C., Garagnani, P., Parini, P., Giuliani, C., & Santoro, A. (2018). Inflammaging: A new immune–metabolic viewpoint for age-related diseases. *Nature Reviews. Endocrinology*, *14*(10), 576–590. DOI: 10.1038/s41574-018-0059-4

Fu, R., Wang, C., Shi, C., Lu, M., Fang, Z., & Lu, J. (2009). An improved whole-blood gamma interferon assay based on the CFP21-MPT64 fusion protein. *Clinical and Vaccine Immunology; CVI*, *16*(5), 686–691. https://www.ncbi.nlm.nih.gov/pmc/articles/PMC2681596/

Fu, Y., Phan, Q. T., Luo, G., Solis, N. V., Liu, Y., Cormack, B. P., Edwards, J. E.Jr, Ibrahim, A. S., & Filler, S. G. (2013). Investigation of the Function of Candida albicans Als3 by Heterologous Expression in Candida glabrata. *Infection and Immunity*, *81*(7), 2528–2535. DOI: 10.1128/IAI.00013-13 PMID: 23630968

Gailson, T., Vohra, V., Saini, A. G., & Bhatia, V. (2021). Mumps infection with meningoencephalitis and cerebellitis. In *BMJ Case Reports* (Vol. 14, Issue 11). DOI: 10.1136/bcr-2021-247306

Gambhir, I. S., Mehta, M., Singh, D. S., & Khanna, H. D. (1999). Evaluation of CSF-adenosine deaminase activity in tubercular meningitis. *The Journal of the Association of Physicians of India*, *47*(2), 192–194.

Garcia, H. H. (2021). Parasitic Infections of the Nervous System. *Continuum (Minneapolis, Minn.)*, *27*(4), 943–962. DOI: 10.1212/CON.0000000000000986 PMID: 34623099

Garcia, H. H., Nash, T. E., & Del Brutto, O. H. (2014). Clinical symptoms, diagnosis, and treatment of neurocysticercosis. *Lancet Neurology*, *13*(12), 1202–1215. DOI: 10.1016/S1474-4422(14)70094-8 PMID: 25453460

Garg, D., Radhakrishnan, D. M., Agrawal, U., Vanjare, H. A., Gandham, E. J., & Manesh, A. (2023). Tuberculosis of the spinal cord. *Annals of Indian Academy of Neurology*, *26*(2). https://journals.lww.com/annalsofian/fulltext/2023/26020/tuberculosis_of_the_spinal_cord.5.aspx

Garlicki, A., Jawień, M., Pancewicz, S., & Moniuszko-Malinowska, A. (2023). Bacterial meningitis in adults – principles of diagnosis and antibiotic treatment. *Przeglad Epidemiologiczny*, *77*(1), 3–22. Advance online publication. DOI: 10.32394/pe.77.01 PMID: 37283230

Garnier, Y., Frigiola, A., Li Volti, G., Florio, P., Frulio, R., Berger, R., Alm, S., Von Duering, M. U., Coumans, A. B., Reis, F. M., Petraglia, F., & Huppertz, B. (2009). Increased maternal/fetal blood S100B levels following systemic endotoxin administration and periventricular white matter injury in preterm fetal sheep. *Reproductive Sciences (Thousand Oaks, Calif.)*, *16*(8), 758–766. DOI: 10.1177/1933719109335801

Gasmi, A., Aniqa, N., Alain, M., & Asma, G. (2022, December 26). Benahmed, Lyudmila, P., Sàdaf, N., Massimilian, P., Salvatore, C., & Geir, B. (2023). Neurotransmitters Regulation and Food Intake: The Role of Dietary Sources in Neurotransmission. *Molecules (Basel, Switzerland)*, *28*(1), 210. Advance online publication. DOI: 10.3390/molecules28010210 PMID: 36615404

Gaur, P., Kachramanoglou, C., Lyall, H., & Jan, W. (2020). Is it not time for international guidelines to combat congenital cytomegalovirus infection? A review of central nervous system manifestations. *Clinical Radiology*, *75*(8), 644–e7. DOI: 10.1016/j.crad.2020.02.009 PMID: 32216960

Gavito-Higuera, J., Mullins, C., Ramos-Duran, L., Olivas Chacon, C., Hakim, N., & Palacios, E. (2016). Fungal Infections of the Central Nervous System: A Pictorial Review. In *Journal of Clinical Imaging Science* (Vol. 6, Issue 2). DOI: 10.4103/2156-7514.184244

Gazzolo, D., Bruschettini, M., Corvino, V., Oliva, R., Sarli, R., Lituania, M., Bruschettini, P., & Michetti, F. (2001). S100B protein concentrations in amniotic fluid correlate with gestational age and with cerebral ultrasound scanning results in healthy fetuses. *Clinical Chemistry*, *47*(5), 954–956. DOI: 10.1093/clinchem/47.5.954

Gazzolo, D., Frulio, R., Bruschettini, P., Lituania, M., & Michetti, F. (2004). Effects of temperature on pre-analytical stability of S100B protein concentrations in urine of healthy full-term infants. *Clinica Chimica Acta*, *350*(1-2), 231–232. DOI: 10.1016/j.cccn.2004.08.001

Gazzolo, D., Michetti, F., Bruschettini, M., Marchese, N., Lituania, M., Mangraviti, S., Pedrazzi, E., & Bruschettini, P. (2003). Pediatric concentrations of S100B protein in blood: Age- and sex-related changes. *Clinical Chemistry*, *49*(6), 967–970. DOI: 10.1373/49.6.967

Gerber, P., Stucki, A., Acosta, F., Cottagnoud, M., & Cottagnoud, P. (2006). Daptomycin is more efficacious than vancomycin against a methicillin-susceptible Staphylococcus aureus in experimental meningitis. *The Journal of Antimicrobial Chemotherapy*, *57*(4), 720–723. DOI: 10.1093/jac/dkl007 PMID: 16459345

Ghanem, K. G. (2010). Neurosyphilis: A historical perspective and review. *CNS Neuroscience & Therapeutics*, *16*(5), e157–e168. DOI: 10.1111/j.1755-5949.2010.00183.x PMID: 20626434

Ghanem, K. G., Ram, S., & Rice, P. A. (2020). The modern epidemic of syphilis. *The New England Journal of Medicine*, *382*(9), 845–854. DOI: 10.1056/NEJMra1901593 PMID: 32101666

Ghani, S., Murthy, P., Jain, S., & Sarin, A. (2018). Syphilis and psychiatry at the Mysore Government Mental Hospital (NIMHANS) in the early 20th century. *Indian Journal of Psychiatry*, *60*(6, Suppl 2), S270–S276. DOI: 10.4103/psychiatry.IndianJPsychiatry_449_17 PMID: 29527060

Ghavami, S., Shojaei, S., Yeganeh, B., Ande, S. R., Jangamreddy, J. R., Mehrpour, M., Christoffersson, J., Chaabane, W., Moghadam, A. R., Kashani, H. H., Hashemi, M., Owji, A. A., & Łos, M. J. (2014). Autophagy and apoptosis dysfunction in neurodegenerative disorders. *Progress in Neurobiology*, *112*, 24–49. DOI: 10.1016/j.pneurobio.2013.10.004

Gholami-Shabani, M. H., Samira, Z., Hoda, M., Masoomeh, S-H., Fatemehsadat, J., & Mehdi, R-A. (2018) Recent Advances in Fungal Infections of the Central Nervous System: From Etiology to Diagnosis and Management. *The Microbiology of Central Nervous System Infections*. Elsevier Inc. DOI: 10.1016/B978-0-12-813806-9.00012-3

Girgis, N. I., Sultan, Y., Farid, Z., Mansour, M. M., Erian, M. W., & Hanna, L. S. (1998). Tuberculosis meningitis, Abbassia Fever Hospital-Naval Medical Research Unit No. 3-Cairo, Egypt, from 1976 to 1996. *The American Journal of Tropical Medicine and Hygiene*, *58*(1), 28–34. https://www.ajtmh.org/view/journals/tpmd/58/1/article-p28.xml

Girometti, N., Junejo, M. H., Nugent, D., McOwan, A., Whitlock, G., Gedela, K., Patel, S., Suchak, T., & Tittle, V. (2021). Clinical and serological outcomes in patients treated with oral doxycycline for early neurosyphilis. *The Journal of Antimicrobial Chemotherapy*, *76*(7), 1916–1919. DOI: 10.1093/jac/dkab100 PMID: 33783506

Giussani, D. A., Thakor, A. S., Frulio, R., & Gazzolo, D. (2005). Acute hypoxia increases S100β protein in association with blood flow redistribution away from peripheral circulations in fetal sheep. *Pediatric Research*, *58*(2), 179–184. DOI: 10.1203/01.PDR.0000169993.39867.5B

Glimåker, M., Sjölin, J., Åkesson, S., & Naucler, P. (2018). Lumbar puncture performed promptly or after neuroimaging in acute bacterial meningitis in adults: A prospective national cohort study evaluating different guidelines. *Clinical Infectious Diseases*, *66*(3), 321–328. DOI: 10.1093/cid/cix806 PMID: 29020334

Golde, T. E., & Miller, V. M. (2009). Proteinopathy-induced neuronal senescence: A hypothesis for brain failure in Alzheimer's and other neurodegenerative diseases. *Alzheimer's Research & Therapy*, *1*(1), 5. Advance online publication. DOI: 10.1186/alzrt5

Gold, S. M., Köhler-Forsberg, O., Moss-Morris, R., Mehnert, A., Miranda, J. J., Bullinger, M., Steptoe, A., Whooley, M. A., & Otte, C. (2020). Comorbid depression in medical diseases. *Nature Reviews. Disease Primers*, *6*(1), 69. DOI: 10.1038/s41572-020-0200-2 PMID: 32820163

Goldschneider, B. Y. I., Gotschlich, E. C., & Artenstein, M. S. (1969). Immunity in the Adult : The Carrier State as an Immunizing Process. *Serum, 2191*.

Gomes, T., Reis-Santos, B., Bertolde, A., Johnson, J. L., Riley, L. W., & Maciel, E. L. (2014). Epidemiology of extrapulmonary tuberculosis in Brazil: A hierarchical model. *BMC Infectious Diseases*, *14*, 9. https://www.ncbi.nlm.nih.gov/pmc/articles/PMC3893400/

Gonzalez, H., Koralnik, I. J., & Marra, C. M. (2019). Neurosyphilis. *Seminars in Neurology*, *39*(4), 448–455. DOI: 10.1055/s-0039-1688942 PMID: 31533185

Goonetilleke, U. R., Scarborough, M., Ward, S. A., & Gordon, S. B. (2010). Proteomic analysis of cerebrospinal fluid in pneumococcal meningitis reveals potential biomarkers associated with survival. *The Journal of Infectious Diseases*, *202*(4), 542–550. DOI: 10.1086/654819

Góralska, K., Blaszkowska, J., & Dzikowiec, M. (2018). Neuroinfections caused by fungi. *Infection*, *46*(4), 443–459. DOI: 10.1007/s15010-018-1152-2 PMID: 29785613

Gordon, S. M., Eaton, M. E., George, R., Larsen, S., Lukehart, S. A., Kuypers, J., Marra, C. M., & Thompson, S. (1994). The response of symptomatic neurosyphilis to high-dose intravenous penicillin G in patients with human immunodeficiency virus infection. *The New England Journal of Medicine*, *331*(22), 1469–1473. DOI: 10.1056/NEJM199412013312201 PMID: 7969296

Gotlieb, E. G., Blank, L., Willis, A. W., Agarwal, P., & Jette, N. (2023). Health equity integrated epilepsy care and research: A narrative review. *Epilepsia*, *64*(11), 2878–2890. DOI: 10.1111/epi.17728 PMID: 37725065

Gradidge, K., Casteleijn, D., & Franzsen, D. (2013). Using the Occupational Therapy Practice Framework-ll to treat a rare condition - brain abscess and empyema. *South African Journal of Occupational Therapy*, *43*, 2.

Grahn, A., Hagberg, L., Nilsson, S., Blennow, K., Zetterberg, H., & Studahl, M. (2013). Cerebrospinal fluid biomarkers in patients with varicella-zoster virus CNS infections. *Journal of Neurology*, *260*(7), 1813–1821. DOI: 10.1007/s00415-013-6883-5

Gray, L. D., & Fedorko, D. P. (1992). Laboratory diagnosis of bacterial meningitis. *Clinical Microbiology Reviews*, *5*(2), 130–145. DOI: 10.1128/CMR.5.2.130 PMID: 1576585

Green, J. A., Thi Hong Chau, T., Farrar, J. J., Friedland, J. S., & Thwaites, G. E. (2011). CNS infection, CSF matrix metalloproteinase concentrations, and clinical/laboratory features. *Neurology*, *76*(6), 577–579. DOI: 10.1212/WNL.0b013e31820b7600 PMID: 21300974

Green, J. A., Tran, C. T. H., Farrar, J. J., Nguyen, M. T. H., Nguyen, P. H., Dinh, S. X., Ho, N. D. T., Ly, C. V., Tran, H. T., Friedland, J. S., & Thwaites, G. E. (2009). Dexamethasone, cerebrospinal fluid matrix metalloproteinase concentrations and clinical outcomes in tuberculous meningitis. *PLoS One*, *4*(9), e7277. DOI: 10.1371/journal.pone.0007277 PMID: 19789647

Guadarrama-Ortiz, P., Choreno-Parra, J. A., Sanchez-Martinez, C. M., Pacheco-Sanchez, F. J., Rodriguez-Nava, A. I., & Garcia-Quintero, G. (2020). Neurological aspects of SARS-CoV-2 infection: Mechanisms and manifestations. *Frontiers in Neurology*, *11*, 1039. DOI: 10.3389/fneur.2020.01039 PMID: 33013675

Gubler, D. J., Vasilakis, N., & Musso, D. (2017). History and emergence of Zika virus. *The Journal of Infectious Diseases*, *216*(Suppl. 10), S860–S867. DOI: 10.1093/infdis/jix451 PMID: 29267917

Güémez, A., & García, E. (2021). Primary Amoebic Meningoencephalitis by Naegleria fowleri: Pathogenesis and Treatments. *Biomolecules*, *11*(9), 1320. DOI: 10.3390/biom11091320 PMID: 34572533

Gundamraj, V., & Hasbun, R. (2023). Viral meningitis and encephalitis: An update. In *Current Opinion in Infectious Diseases* (Vol. 36, Issue 3). DOI: 10.1097/QCO.0000000000000922

Gupta, M., Tobin, E. H., & Munakomi, S. (2024). CNS tuberculosis. In *StatPearls*. StatPearls Publishing. https://www.ncbi.nlm.nih.gov/books/NBK585138/

Gupta, R., Thakur, R., Gupta, P., Jalan, N., Kushwaha, S., & Gupta, M. (2015). Evaluation of GenoType MTBDRplus line probe assay for early detection of drug resistance in tuberculous meningitis patients in India. *Journal of Global Infectious Diseases*, *7*(1), 5–10. https://www.ncbi.nlm.nih.gov/pmc/articles/PMC4338458/

Gutiérrez-Bugallo, G., Piedra, L. A., Rodriguez, M., Bisset, J. A., Lourenço-de-Oliveira, R., Weaver, S. C., Vasilakis, N., & Vega-Rúa, A. (2019). Vector-borne transmission and evolution of Zika virus. *Nature Ecology & Evolution*, *3*(4), 561–569. DOI: 10.1038/s41559-019-0836-z PMID: 30886369

Gutierrez, M., & Emmanuel, P. J. (2018). Expanding molecular diagnostics for central nervous system infections. *Advances in Pediatrics*, *65*(1), 209–227. DOI: 10.1016/j.yapd.2018.04.005 PMID: 30053925

Haddad, N., Carr, M., Balian, S., Lannin, J., Kim, Y., Toth, C., & Jarvis, J. (2022). The blood–brain barrier and pharmacokinetic/pharmacodynamic optimization of antibiotics for the treatment of central nervous system infections in adults. *Antibiotics (Basel, Switzerland)*, *11*(12), 1843. DOI: 10.3390/antibiotics11121843 PMID: 36551500

Hage, C. A., Bowyer, S., Tarvin, S. E., Helper, D., Kleiman, M. B., & Wheat, L. J. (2010). Recognition, diagnosis, and treatment of histoplasmosis complicating tumor necrosis factor blocker therapy. In *Clinical Infectious Diseases* (Vol. 50, Issue 1). DOI: 10.1086/648724

Hahn, A., Podbielski, A., Meyer, T., Zautner, A. E., Loderstädt, U., Schwarz, N. G., Krüger, A., Cadar, D., & Frickmann, H. (2020). On detection thresholds–a review on diagnostic approaches in the infectious disease laboratory and the interpretation of their results. *Acta Tropica*, *205*, 105377. DOI: 10.1016/j.actatropica.2020.105377 PMID: 32007448

Hamed, S. A., Hamed, E. A., & Zakary, M. M. (2009). Oxidative stress and S-100B protein in children with bacterial meningitis. *BMC Neurology*, *9*, 51. Advance online publication. DOI: 10.1186/1471-2377-9-51

Hamill, M. M., Ghanem, K. G., & Tuddenham, S. (2024). State-of-the-Art Review: Neurosyphilis. *Clinical Infectious Diseases*, *78*(5), e57–e68. DOI: 10.1093/cid/ciad437 PMID: 37593890

Hampel, H., O'Bryant, S. E., Molinuevo, J. L., Zetterberg, H., Masters, C. L., Lista, S., Kiddle, S. J., Batrla, R., & Blennow, K. (2018). Blood-based biomarkers for Alzheimer disease: Mapping the road to the clinic. *Nature Reviews. Neurology*, *14*(11), 639–652. DOI: 10.1038/s41582-018-0079-7

Hansson, O. (2021). Biomarkers for neurodegenerative diseases. *Nature Medicine*, *27*(6), 954–963. DOI: 10.1038/s41591-021-01382-x

Haran, H., Santos, I. C., Batista, R. L., & Silva-Vergara, M. L. (2024). Congestive heart failure associated with itraconazole in a patient with paracoccidioidomycosis. *The Brazilian Journal of Infectious Diseases : an Official Publication of the Brazilian Society of Infectious Diseases*, *28*(5), 103868–103868. DOI: 10.1016/j.bjid.2024.103868 PMID: 39276794

Harausz, E. P., Garcia-Prats, A. J., Law, S., Schaaf, H. S., Kredo, T., & Seddon, J. A. (2018). Treatment and outcomes in children with multidrug-resistant tuberculosis: A systematic review and individual patient data meta-analysis. *PLoS Medicine*, *15*(7), e1002591. https://www.ncbi.nlm.nih.gov/pmc/articles/PMC6040687/

Hårdemark, H. G., Persson, L., Bolander, H. G., Hillered, L., Olsson, Y., & Påhlman, S. (1988). Neuron-specific enolase is a marker of cerebral ischemia and infarct size in rat cerebrospinal fluid. *Stroke*, *19*(9), 1140–1144. DOI: 10.1161/01.STR.19.9.1140

Ha, S., Ho, S. H., Bae, Y. H., Lee, M., Kim, J. H., Kim, J. H., & Lee, J. (2023). Digital Health Equity and Tailored Health Care Service for People With Disability: User-Centered Design and Usability Study. *Journal of Medical Internet Research*, *25*, e50029. DOI: 10.2196/50029 PMID: 38015589

Hasbun, R., Abrahams, J., Jekel, J., & Quagliarello, V. J. (2001). Computed tomography of the head before lumbar puncture in adults with suspected meningitis. *The New England Journal of Medicine*, *345*(24), 1727–1733. DOI: 10.1056/NEJMoa010399 PMID: 11742046

Ha, T., Tadi, P., Leslie, S., & Dubensky, L. (2024). *Neurosyphilis*. StatPearls.

Hawker, J., Begg, N., Reintjes, R., Ekdahl, K., Edeghere, O., & Van Steenbergen, J. E. (2019). *Communicable disease control and health protection handbook*. John Wiley & Sons. DOI: 10.1002/9781119328070

Heemskerk, D., Day, J., Chau, T. T. H., Dung, N. H., Yen, N. T. B., & Bang, N. D. (2011). Intensified treatment with high dose rifampicin and levofloxacin compared to standard treatment for adult patients with tuberculous meningitis (TBM-IT): Protocol for a randomized controlled trial. *Trials*, *12*, 25. https://www.ncbi.nlm.nih.gov/pmc/articles/PMC3041687/

Heidary, M., Khosravi, A. D., Khoshnood, S., Nasiri, M. J., Soleimani, S., & Goudarzi, M. (2018). Daptomycin. *The Journal of Antimicrobial Chemotherapy*, *73*(1), 1–11. DOI: 10.1093/jac/dkx349 PMID: 29059358

Henao-Martínez, A. F., & Vela-Duarte, D. (2018). Cryptococcal meningitis and other opportunistic fungal infections of the central nervous system: epidemiology, pathogenesis, diagnosis, and treatment. In *The Microbiology of Central Nervous System Infections* (pp. 261–278). Academic Press. DOI: 10.1016/B978-0-12-813806-9.00013-5

He, T., Kaplan, S., Kamboj, M., & Tang, Y.-W. (2016). Laboratory diagnosis of central nervous system infection. *Current Infectious Disease Reports*, *18*(11), 35. Advance online publication. DOI: 10.1007/s11908-016-0545-6 PMID: 27686677

Hinduja, A., Tariq, A., & Adriance, S. (2019). Intensive Care Management of Meningitis and Encephalitis. *Textbook of Neuroanesthesia and Neurocritical Care*, 131–144. DOI: 10.1007/978-981-13-3390-3_9

Holbrook, M. R. (2017). Historical perspectives on flavivirus research. *Viruses*, *9*(5), 97. Advance online publication. DOI: 10.3390/v9050097 PMID: 28468299

Holdaway, I., Reid, I., Young, N., & Thomas, M. (2018). Meningitis in adults: Diagnosis and management. *Internal Medicine Journal*, *48*(11), 1294–1307. DOI: 10.1111/imj.14102 PMID: 30387309

Honoré-Bouakline, S., Vincensini, J. P., Giacuzzo, V., Lagrange, P. H., & Herrmann, J. L. (2003). Rapid diagnosis of extrapulmonary tuberculosis by PCR: Impact of sample preparation and DNA extraction. *Journal of Clinical Microbiology*, *41*(6), 2323–2329. https://www.ncbi.nlm.nih.gov/pmc/articles/PMC156509/

Hooshmand, H., Escobar, M. R., & Kopf, S. W. (1972). Neurosyphilis: A study of 241 patients. *Journal of the American Medical Association*, *219*(6), 726–729. DOI: 10.1001/jama.1972.03190320032011 PMID: 5066697

Hotson, J. R. (1981). Modern neurosyphilis: A partially treated chronic meningitis. *The Western Journal of Medicine*, *135*(3), 191. PMID: 7340118

Hoyo-Becerra, C., Schlaak, J. F., & Hermann, D. M. (2014). Insights from interferon-α-related depression for the pathogenesis of depression associated with inflammation. *Brain, Behavior, and Immunity*, *42*, 222–231. DOI: 10.1016/j.bbi.2014.06.200 PMID: 25066466

Hryhorczuk, C., Florea, M., Rodaros, D., Poirier, I., Daneault, C., Des Rosiers, C., Arvanitogiannis, A., Alquier, T., & Fulton, S. (2016). Dampened Mesolimbic Dopamine Function and Signaling by Saturated but not Monounsaturated Dietary Lipids. *Neuropsychopharmacology : Official Publication of the American College of Neuropsychopharmacology*, *41*(3), 811–821. DOI: 10.1038/npp.2015.207 PMID: 26171719

Huang, J., Wu, H., Huang, H., Wu, W., Wu, B., & Wang, L. (2021). Clinical characteristics and outcome of primary brain abscess: A retrospective analysis. *BMC Infectious Diseases*, *21*(1), 1–8. DOI: 10.1186/s12879-021-06947-2 PMID: 34903183

Hughes, A. J., & Biggs, B. A. (2002). Parasitic worms of the central nervous system: An Australian perspective. *Internal Medicine Journal*, *32*(11), 541–553. DOI: 10.1046/j.1445-5994.2002.00265.x PMID: 12412938

Huppert, J., Closhen, D., Croxford, A., White, R., Kulig, P., Pietrowski, E., Bechmann, I., Becher, B., Luhmann, H. J., Waisman, A., & Kuhlmann, C. R. W. (2010). Cellular mechanisms of IL-17-induced blood-brain barrier disruption. *The FASEB Journal*, *24*(4), 1023–1034. DOI: 10.1096/fj.09-141978 PMID: 19940258

Husain, M., Jha, D. K., Rastogi, M., Husain, N., & Gupta, R. K. (2005). Role of neuroendoscopy in the management of patients with tuberculous meningitis hydrocephalus. *Neurosurgical Review*, *28*(4), 278–283. DOI: 10.1007/s10143-005-0397-2

Hussein, A. S., & Shafran, S. D. (2000). Acute bacterial meningitis in adults: A 12-year review. *Medicine*, *79*(6), 360–368. DOI: 10.1097/00005792-200011000-00002 PMID: 11144034

Imperato, A., Consales, A., Ravegnani, M., Castagnola, E., Bandettini, R., & Rossi, A. (2016). Primary Hydatid Cyst of the Brain in a Child: A Case Report. *Polish Journal of Radiology / Polish Medical Society of Radiology*, *81*, 578–582. DOI: 10.12659/PJR.898619 PMID: 27994696

Infante, J. R., Martínez, A., Ochoa, J., Cañadillas, F., Torres-Avisbal, M., Vallejo, J. A., González, F. M., Pacheco, C., & Latre, J. M. (2003). Cerebrospinal fluid S-100 protein levels in neurological pathologies. *Journal of Physiology and Biochemistry*, *59*(4), 255–261. DOI: 10.1007/BF03179892

Iovino, L., Tremblay, M., & Civiero, L. (2020). Glutamate-induced excitotoxicity in Parkinson's disease: The role of glial cells. *Journal of Pharmacological Sciences*, *144*(3), 151–164. DOI: 10.1016/j.jphs.2020.07.011 PMID: 32807662

Isabel, B. E., & Rogelio, H. P. (2014). Pathogenesis and immune response in tuberculous meningitis. *The Malaysian Journal of Medical Sciences : MJMS*, *21*(1), 4–10. https://www.ncbi.nlm.nih.gov/pmc/articles/PMC3952336/

Ito, Y., Ofengeim, D., Najafov, A., Das, S., Saberi, S., Li, Y., Hitomi, J., Zhu, H., Chen, H., Mayo, L., Geng, J., Elliott, J. L., & Yuan, J. (2016). RIPK1 mediates axonal degeneration by promoting inflammation and necroptosis in ALS. *Science*, *353*(6299), 603–608. DOI: 10.1126/science.aaf6803

Jackson, A. C., Warrell, M. J., Rupprecht, C. E., Ertl, H. C. J., Dietzschold, B., O'Reilly, M., Leach, R. P., Fu, Z. F., Wunner, W. H., Bleck, T. P., & Wilde, H. (2003). Management of rabies in humans. In *Clinical Infectious Diseases* (Vol. 36, Issue 1). DOI: 10.1086/344905

Jacquier, M., & Piroth, L. (2018). Vertebral Hydatidosis. *The New England Journal of Medicine*, *379*(2). Advance online publication. DOI: 10.1056/NEJMicm1714206 PMID: 29996078

Jakka, S., Veena, S., Rao, A. R. M., & Eisenhut, M. (2005). Cerebrospinal fluid adenosine deaminase levels and adverse neurological outcome in pediatric tuberculous meningitis. *Infection*, *33*(4), 264–266. DOI: 10.1007/s15010-005-5005-4

Janier, M., Unemo, M., Dupin, N., Tiplica, G. S., Potočnik, M., & Patel, R. (2021). 2020 European guideline on the management of syphilis. *Journal of the European Academy of Dermatology and Venereology*, *35*(3), 574–588. DOI: 10.1111/jdv.16946 PMID: 33094521

Jellinger, K. A. (2009). Recent advances in our understanding of neurodegeneration. *Journal of Neural Transmission (Vienna, Austria)*, *116*(9), 1111–1162. DOI: 10.1007/s00702-009-0240-y

Jeltsch-David, H., & Muller, S. (2014). Neuropsychiatric systemic lupus erythematosus: Pathogenesis and biomarkers. *Nature Reviews. Neurology*, *10*(10), 579–596. DOI: 10.1038/nrneurol.2014.148

Jenkins, T. A., Nguyen, J. C., Polglaze, K. E., & Bertrand, P. P. (2016). Influence of Tryptophan and Serotonin on Mood and Cognition with a Possible Role of the Gut-Brain Axis. *Nutrients*, *8*(1), 56. DOI: 10.3390/nu8010056 PMID: 26805875

Ji, H., Rabbi, M. F., Labis, B., Pavlov, V. A., Tracey, K. J., & Ghia, J. E. (2014). Central cholinergic activation of a vagus nerve-to-spleen circuit alleviates experimental colitis. *Mucosal Immunology*, *7*(2), 335–347. DOI: 10.1038/mi.2013.52

Jochems, S. P., Marcon, F., Carniel, B. F., Holloway, M., Mitsi, E., Smith, E., Gritzfeld, J. F., Solórzano, C., Reiné, J., Pojar, S., Nikolaou, E., German, E. L., Hyder-Wright, A., Hill, H., Hales, C., de Steenhuijsen Piters, W. A. A., Bogaert, D., Adler, H., Zaidi, S., & Ferreira, D. M. (2018). Inflammation induced by influenza virus impairs human innate immune control of pneumococcus. *Nature Immunology*, *19*(12), 1299–1308. DOI: 10.1038/s41590-018-0231-y PMID: 30374129

Johnson, R. T. (1996). Acute encephalitis. *Clinical Infectious Diseases*, *23*(2), 219–226. DOI: 10.1093/clinids/23.2.219 PMID: 8842253

Johnston, J. C., Chiang, L., & Elwood, K. (2017). Mycobacterium kansasii. *Microbiology Spectrum*, *5*(1). Advance online publication. DOI: 10.1128/microbiolspec.TNMI7-0011-2016

Jung, Y. J., Tweedie, D., Scerba, M. T., & Greig, N. H. (2019). Neuroinflammation as a factor of neurodegenerative disease: Thalidomide analogs as treatments. *Frontiers in Cell and Developmental Biology*, *7*, 313. Advance online publication. DOI: 10.3389/fcell.2019.00313

Jun, W., & Liana, Z. (2022). A deep learning model with attention for classifying brain tumors. *International Journal of Computational Intelligence Systems*, *15*(1), 35. DOI: 10.1007/s44196-022-00090-9

Kadambari, S., Braccio, S., Ribeiro, S., Allen, D. J., Pebody, R., Brown, D., Cunney, R., Sharland, M., & Ladhani, S. (2019). Enterovirus and parechovirus meningitis in infants younger than 90 days old in the UK and Republic of Ireland: A British Paediatric Surveillance Unit study. *Archives of Disease in Childhood*, *104*(6), 552–557. DOI: 10.1136/archdischild-2018-315643 PMID: 30530486

Kadry, H., Noorani, B., & Cucullo, L. (2020). A blood–brain barrier overview on structure, function, impairment, and biomarkers of integrity. In *Fluids and Barriers of the CNS* (Vol. 17, Issue 1). DOI: 10.1186/s12987-020-00230-3

Kakooza-Mwesige, A., Tshala-Katumbay, D., & Juliano, S. L. (2019). Viral infections of the central nervous system in Africa. *Brain Research Bulletin, 145*, 2–17. DOI: 10.1016/j.brainresbull.2018.12.019 PMID: 30658129

Kanakaraj, L., Mamtani, H., Dahale, A. B., Netravathi, M., Nagarathna, S., Sinha, S., & Thippeswamy, H. (2024). Psychiatric manifestations of neurosyphilis over past two decades: Findings from a tertiary care neuropsychiatric hospital in south India. *Asian Journal of Psychiatry*, *94*, 103952. DOI: 10.1016/j.ajp.2024.103952 PMID: 38364749

Kanungo, R., & Anupurba, S. (2023). Association of Viral and Fungal Infections of the CNS During Immunosuppression. In *Viral and Fungal Infections of the Central Nervous System: A Microbiological Perspective* (pp. 465–482). Springer Nature Singapore. DOI: 10.1007/978-981-99-6445-1_20

Kapila, R., & Schwartz, R. A. (2021). Neurosyphilis and the Jarisch-Herxheimer reaction: A therapy concern with HIV disease. *Dermatologic Therapy*, *34*(2), e14839. DOI: 10.1111/dth.14839 PMID: 33527658

Kapoor, A., & Tan, C. S. (2020). Immunotherapeutics to Treat HIV in the Central Nervous System. In *Current HIV/AIDS Reports* (Vol. 17, Issue 5). DOI: 10.1007/s11904-020-00519-w

Karthika, C., Hari, B., Rahman, M. H., Akter, R., Najda, A., Albadrani, G. M., Sayed, A. A., Akhtar, M. F., & Abdel-Daim, M. M. (2021). Multiple strategies with the synergistic approach for addressing colorectal cancer. *Biomedicine and Pharmacotherapy*, *140*, 111704. Advance online publication. DOI: 10.1016/j.biopha.2021.111704

Karvouniaris, M., Brotis, A., Tsiakos, K., Palli, E., & Koulenti, D. (2022). Current perspectives on the diagnosis and management of healthcare-associated ventriculitis and meningitis. *Infection and Drug Resistance*, *15*, 697–721. DOI: 10.2147/IDR.S326456 PMID: 35250284

Kaslow, R. A., & Bell, D. M. (2022). Epidemiology and Control: From Principles to Pandemics. In *Viral Infections of Humans: Epidemiology and Control* (pp. 1–80). Springer US. DOI: 10.1007/978-1-4939-9544-8_1-1

Kataria, J., Rukmangadachar, L. A., Hariprasad, G., Jithesh, O., Tripathi, M., & Srinivasan, A. (2011). Two dimensional difference gel electrophoresis analysis of cerebrospinal fluid in tuberculous meningitis patients. *Journal of Proteomics*, *74*(10), 2194–2203. DOI: 10.1016/j.jprot.2011.06.020

Katti, M. K. (2004). Pathogenesis, diagnosis, treatment, and outcome aspects of cerebral tuberculosis. *Medical Science Monitor*, *10*(9), RA215–RA229. www.medscimonit.com/abstract/index/idArt/11749

Kayal, A. K., Goswami, M., Das, M., & Paul, B. (2011). Clinical spectrum of neurosyphilis in North East India. *Neurology India*, *59*(3), 344–350. DOI: 10.4103/0028-3886.82719 PMID: 21743160

Keidel, A. (1921). Studies in asymptomatic neurosyphilis: I. A tentative classification of early asymptomatic neurosyphilis. *Archives of Neurology and Psychiatry*, *6*(3), 286–291. DOI: 10.1001/archneurpsyc.1921.02190030033004

Kelly, L., Walsh, J., Skally, M., Dinesh, B., Burns, K., O'Connell, K., MacNally, S., Humphreys, H., & Fitzpatrick, F. (2023). Candida meningitis/ventriculitis over a decade. Increased morbidity and length of stay a concern. *British Journal of Neurosurgery*, *37*(2), 227–230. Advance online publication. DOI: 10.1080/02688697.2022.2054947 PMID: 35361033

Kennedy, P. G. (2021). An overview of viral infections of the nervous system in the immunosuppressed. *Journal of Neurology*, *268*(8), 3026–3030. DOI: 10.1007/s00415-020-10265-z PMID: 33048220

Kesidou, E., Theotokis, P., Damianidou, O., Boziki, M., Konstantinidou, N., Taloumtzis, C., Sintila, S.-A., Grigoriadis, P., Evangelopoulos, M. E., Bakirtzis, C., & Simeonidou, C. (2023). CNS Ageing in health and neurodegenerative disorders. *Journal of Clinical Medicine*, *12*(6), 2255. DOI: 10.3390/jcm12062255 PMID: 36983254

Khaba, M. C., Ngale, T. C., & Makhado, N. A. (2022). Fungal infection of the central nervous system: Autopsy analysis of six cases. *SAGE Open Medical Case Reports*, *10*. Advance online publication. DOI: 10.1177/2050313X221122419 PMID: 36105784

Khalaf, S. A., Patel, P., Caruso, C. R., Parrett, T., & Bran, A. (2022). CNS Histoplasmosis as a Gliosarcoma mimicker: The diagnostic dilemma of solitary brain lesions. *IDCases*, *27*, e01364. DOI: 10.1016/j.idcr.2021.e01364 PMID: 35024338

Khan, F., & Amatya, B. (2020). Medical rehabilitation in pandemics: Towards a new perspective. *Journal of Rehabilitation Medicine*, *52*(4), 1–4. DOI: 10.2340/16501977-2676 PMID: 32271393

Kibriya, H., Amin, R., Kim, J., Nawaz, M., & Gantassi, R. (2023). A novel approach for brain tumor classification using an ensemble of deep and hand-crafted features. *Sensors (Basel)*, *23*(10), 4693. DOI: 10.3390/s23104693 PMID: 37430604

Kim, K. S. (2010). Acute bacterial meningitis in infants and children. In *The Lancet Infectious Diseases* (Vol. 10, Issue 1). DOI: 10.1016/S1473-3099(09)70306-8

Kim, J., Erice, C., Rohlwink, U. K., & Tucker, E. W. (2022). Infections in the Developing Brain: The Role of the Neuro-Immune Axis. *Frontiers in Neurology*, *13*, 805786. DOI: 10.3389/fneur.2022.805786 PMID: 35250814

Kim, K. S. (2003). Pathogenesis of bacterial meningitis: From bacteraemia to neuronal injury. *Nature Reviews. Neuroscience*, *4*(5), 376–385. DOI: 10.1038/nrn1103 PMID: 12728265

Kimuda, S., Kasozi, D., Namombwe, S., Gakuru, J., Mugabi, T., & Kagimu, E. (2023). Advancing diagnosis and treatment in people living with HIV and tuberculosis meningitis. *Current HIV/AIDS Reports*, *20*(6), 379–393. https://www.ncbi.nlm.nih.gov/pmc/articles/PMC10719136/

King, J., McManus, H., Gray, R., & McGregor, S. (2022). *HIV, viral hepatitis and sexually transmissible infections in Australia Annual surveillance report 2021.*

Kissani, N., Nafia, S., Zahlane, S., & Louhab, N. (2021). Neurosyphilis: A series of 178 cases at the 3rd-level hospital of Marrakesh (Morocco). *European Journal of Clinical Microbiology & Infectious Diseases*, *40*(10), 2129–2135. DOI: 10.1007/s10096-021-04253-y PMID: 33942164

Knoester, M., Helfferich, J., Poelman, R., Van Leer-Buter, C., Brouwer, O. F., & Niesters, H. G. M. (2016). EV-D68 AFM Working Group. (2019). Twenty-nine cases of enterovirus-D68-associated acute flaccid myelitis in Europe 2016: A case series and epidemiologic overview. *The Pediatric Infectious Disease Journal*, *38*(1), 16–21. DOI: 10.1097/INF.0000000000002188 PMID: 30234793

Knopman, D. S., Amieva, H., Petersen, R. C., Chételat, G., Holtzman, D. M., Hyman, B. T., Nixon, R. A., & Jones, D. T. (2021). Alzheimer disease. *Nature Reviews. Disease Primers*, *7*, 33. Advance online publication. DOI: 10.1038/s41572-021-00269-y

Kobeissi, Z. A., & Zanotti-Cavazzoni, S. L. (2010). Biomarkers of sepsis. *The Year Book of Critical Care Medicine*, *227–228*. Advance online publication. DOI: 10.1016/S0733-8627(10)28015-5

Koedel, U., Scheld, W. M., & Pfister, H.-W. (2002). Pathogenesis and pathophysiology of pneumococcal meningitis. *The Lancet. Infectious Diseases*, *2*(12), 721–736. DOI: 10.1016/S1473-3099(02)00450-4 PMID: 12467688

Kovacs, G. G., Robinson, J. L., Xie, S. X., Lee, E. B., Grossman, M., Wolk, D. A., Irwin, D. J., Weintraub, D., Kim, C. F., Schuck, T., Yousef, A., Wagner, J. A., Trojanowski, J. Q., & Lee, V. M.-Y. (2017). Evaluating the patterns of aging-related tau astrogliopathy unravels novel insights into brain aging and neurodegenerative diseases. *Journal of Neuropathology and Experimental Neurology*, *76*(4), 270–288. DOI: 10.1093/jnen/nlx007

Kozyolkin, O. A., Vizir, I. V., & Sikorskay, M. V. (2023). Infectious and parasitic disease of the nervous system: Textbook for students-foreign citizen IV course of medical faculties of the speciality. *Medicine*.

Kuhle, J., & Petzold, A. (2011). What makes a prognostic biomarker in CNS diseases: Strategies for targeted biomarker discovery? Part 1: Acute and monophasic diseases. *Expert Opinion on Medical Diagnostics*, *5*(4), 333–346. DOI: 10.1517/17530059.2011.586072

Kumar, A., Mudassir, S., Ranjan, A., Wankhade, B., Rai, A. K., & Kumar, S. (2023). Clinical profile and mortality predictors in hospitalised patients of tuberculous meningitis. *Neurology Asia*, *28*(1), 149–157. http://www.neurology-asia.org/articles/neuroasia-2023-28(1)-149.pdf

Kumar, P., Benny, P., Jain, M., & Singh, S. (2014). Comparison of an in-house multiplex PCR with two commercial immuno-chromatographic tests for rapid identification and differentiation of MTB from NTM isolates. *International Journal of Mycobacteriology*, *3*(1), 50–56. https://www.sciencedirect.com/science/article/pii/S2212553114000028

Kumar, R., Pandey, C., Bose, N., & Sahay, S. (2002). Tuberculous brain abscess: Clinical presentation, pathophysiology and treatment (in children). *Child's Nervous System*, *18*(3), 118–123. DOI: 10.1007/s00381-002-0575-2

Kurien, R., & Sudarsanam, T. D. S., & Thomas, K. (2013). Tuberculous meningitis: A comparison of scoring systems for diagnosis. Oman Medical Journal, 28(3), 163–166. http://www.omjournal.org/fultext_PDF.aspx?DetailsID=372&type=fultext

Lakshmi, M. J., & Rao, S. N. (2022). Classification of brain tumor MRI using deep learning techniques. *Soft Computing*, *26*(13), 6245–6253. DOI: 10.1007/s00500-022-07163-z

Lambert, N., El Moussaoui, M., Baron, F., Maquet, P., & Darcis, G. (2023). Virus-Specific T-Cell Therapy for Viral Infections of the Central Nervous System: A Review. *Viruses*, *15*(7), 1510. Advance online publication. DOI: 10.3390/v15071510 PMID: 37515196

Lamers, K. J. B., van Engelen, B. G. M., Gabreels, F. J. M., Hommes, O. R., Borm, G. F., & Wevers, R. A. (1995). Cerebrospinal neuron-specific enolase, S-100 and myelin basic protein in neurological disorders. *Acta Neurologica Scandinavica, 92*(3), 247–251. DOI: 10.1111/j.1600-0404.1995.tb01694.x

Lamers, K. J. B., Vos, P., Verbeek, M. M., Rosmalen, F., van Geel, W. J. A., & van Engelen, B. G. (2003). Protein S-100B, neuron-specific enolase (NSE), myelin basic protein (MBP) and glial fibrillary acidic protein (GFAP) in cerebrospinal fluid (CSF) and blood of neurological patients. *Brain Research Bulletin, 61*(3), 261–264. DOI: 10.1016/S0361-9230(03)00033-X

Lamridi, O. (2017). *Les facteurs pronostiques des méningites bactériennes communautaires de l'adulte.*

Landry, T., Smyczek, P., Cooper, R., Gratrix, J., Bertholet, L., Read, R., Romanowski, B., & Singh, A. E. (2019). Retrospective review of tertiary and neurosyphilis cases in Alberta, 1973–2017. *BMJ Open, 9*(6), e025995. DOI: 10.1136/bmjopen-2018-025995 PMID: 31230001

Lan, Y., Chen, W., Yan, Q., & Liu, W. (2020). Interferon-γ release assays for tuberculous meningitis diagnosis: A meta-analysis. *Archives of Medical Science : AMS, 17*(5), 1241–1250. https://www.ncbi.nlm.nih.gov/pmc/articles/PMC8425237/

Lashkari, A., & Ranjbar, R. (2021). Nanoparticles and nanoformulated drugs as promising delivery system in treatment of microbial-induced CNS infection: a systematic review of literature. In *Journal of NeuroVirology* (Vol. 27, Issue 4). DOI: 10.1007/s13365-021-00994-w

Le Govic, Y., Demey, B., Cassereau, J., Bahn, Y. S., & Papon, N. (2022). Pathogens infecting the central nervous system. *PLoS Pathogens, 18*(2), e1010234. DOI: 10.1371/journal.ppat.1010234 PMID: 35202445

Le, N. D., Ricci, S., Grandgirard, D., & Leib, S. L. (2023). Experimental meningitis by Streptococcus pneumoniae and Neisseria meningitidis in rodents. *Handbook of Animal Models in Neurological Disorders*, 329–341. DOI: 10.1016/B978-0-323-89833-1.00050-1

Leclair, N. K., & Hersh, D. S. (2023). Central Nervous System Infections and Their Management. *Pediatric Neurosurgery Board Review: A Comprehensive Guide*, 317–334. DOI: 10.1007/978-3-031-23687-7_19

Ledri, M., Sørensen, A. T., Kokaia, M., Woldbye, D. P. D., & Gøtzsche, C. R. (2021). Editorial: Gene Therapy in the CNS – Progress and Prospects for Novel Therapies. In *Frontiers in Molecular Neuroscience* (Vol. 14). DOI: 10.3389/fnmol.2021.778134

Leib, S. L., Clements, J. M., Lindberg, R. L. P., Heimgartner, C., Loeffler, J. M., Pfister, L.-A., Täuber, M. G., & Leppert, D. (2001). Inhibition of matrix metalloproteinases and tumour necrosis factor α converting enzyme as adjuvant therapy in pneumococcal meningitis. *Brain, 124*(9), 1734–1742. DOI: 10.1093/brain/124.9.1734 PMID: 11522576

Leib, S. L., Leppert, D., Clements, J., & Täuber, M. G. (2000). Matrix metalloproteinases contribute to brain damage in experimental pneumococcal meningitis. *Infection and Immunity, 68*(2), 615–620. DOI: 10.1128/IAI.68.2.615-620.2000 PMID: 10639424

Leib, S. L., & Tauber, M. G. (1999). Pathogenesis of Bacterial meningitis. *Infectious Disease Clinics of North America, 13*(3), 527–548. DOI: 10.1016/S0891-5520(05)70093-3 PMID: 10470554

Lemkhoudem, M. A. (2022). *évolutif et préventif des méningites à Haemophilus à Marrakech.*

Leonard, J. M. (2017). Central nervous system tuberculosis. *Microbiology Spectrum, 5*(2). Advance online publication. DOI: 10.1128/microbiolspec.TNMI7-0044-2017

Leon, M., & Dicks, T. (2022). Gut Bacteria and Neurotransmitters. *Microorganisms, 10*(9), 1838. Advance online publication. DOI: 10.3390/microorganisms10091838 PMID: 36144440

Leung, A. K., Hon, K. L., Leong, K. F., & Sergi, C. M. (2018). Measles: A disease often forgotten but not gone. *Hong Kong Medical Journal, 24*(5), 512–520. DOI: 10.12809/hkmj187470 PMID: 30245481

Liang, Y., Iqbal, Z., Lu, J., Wang, J., Zhang, H., Chen, X., Duan, L., & Xia, J. (2023). Cell-derived nanovesicle-mediated drug delivery to the brain: Principles and strategies for vesicle engineering. *Molecular Therapy : the Journal of the American Society of Gene Therapy, 31*(5), 1207–1224. DOI: 10.1016/j.ymthe.2022.10.008 PMID: 36245129

Li, B. D., Bi, Z. Y., Liu, J. F., Si, W. J., Shi, Q. Q., Xue, L. P., & Bai, J. (2017). Adverse effects produced by different drugs used in the treatment of Parkinson's disease: A mixed treatment comparison. *CNS Neuroscience & Therapeutics, 23*(10), 827–842. Advance online publication. DOI: 10.1111/cns.12727 PMID: 28872217

Liechti, F. D., Grandgirard, D., Leppert, D., & Leib, S. L. (2014). Matrix metalloproteinase inhibition lowers mortality and brain injury in experimental pneumococcal meningitis. *Infection and Immunity, 82*(4), 1710–1718. DOI: 10.1128/IAI.00073-14 PMID: 24491581

Lima, J. E., Takayanagui, O. M., Garcia, L. V., & Leite, J. P. (2004). Use of neuron-specific enolase for assessing the severity and outcome of neurological disorders in patients. *Brazilian Journal of Medical and Biological Research = Revista Brasileira de Pesquisas Médicas e Biológicas*, *37*(1), 19–26. DOI: 10.1590/S0100-879X2004000100003

Lima, M. A., Freitas, D. F. S., Oliveira, R. V. C., Fichman, V., Varon, A. G., Freitas, A. D., Lamas, C. C., Andrade, H. B., Veloso, V. G., Almeida-Paes, R., Almeida-Silva, F., Zancopé-Oliveira, R. M., de Macedo, P. M., Valle, A. C. F., Silva, M. T. T., Araújo, A. Q. C., & Gutierrez-Galhardo, M. C. (2022). Meningeal Sporotrichosis Due to Sporothrix brasiliensis: A 21-Year Cohort Study from a Brazilian Reference Center. *Journal of Fungi (Basel, Switzerland)*, *9*(1), 17. DOI: 10.3390/jof9010017 PMID: 36675837

Lindsey, N. P., Lehman, J. A., Staples, J. E., & Fischer, M. (2014). West Nile virus and other arboviral diseases—United States, 2013. *MMWR. Morbidity and Mortality Weekly Report*, *63*(24), 521–526. PMID: 24941331

Lin, L.-R., Lin, D.-H., Tong, M.-L., Liu, L.-L., Fan, J.-Y., Zhu, X.-Z., Gao, K., Chen, M.-J., Zheng, W.-H., Zhang, H.-L., Li, S.-L., Lin, H.-L., Lin, Z.-F., Niu, J.-J., & Yang, T.-C. (2016). Macrophage migration inhibitory factor as a novel cerebrospinal fluid marker for neurosyphilis among HIV-negative patients. *Clinica Chimica Acta*, *463*, 103–108. DOI: 10.1016/j.cca.2016.10.018 PMID: 27751728

Lino, R., Guimarães, A. R., Sousa, E., Azevedo, M., & Santos, L. (2024). Emerging Fungal Infections of the Central Nervous System in the Past Decade: A Literature Review. *Infectious Disease Reports*, *16*(5), 952–976. DOI: 10.3390/idr16050076 PMID: 39452161

Lins, H., Wallesch, C. W., & Wunderlich, M. T. (2005). Sequential analyses of neurobiochemical markers of cerebral damage in cerebrospinal fluid and serum in CNS infections. *Acta Neurologica Scandinavica*, *112*(5), 303–308. DOI: 10.1111/j.1600-0404.2005.00491.x

Li, P., Lee, G. H., Kim, S. Y., Kwon, S. Y., Kim, H. R., & Park, S. (2021). From diagnosis to treatment: Recent advances in patient-friendly biosensors and implantable devices. *ACS Nano*, *15*(2), 1960–2004. DOI: 10.1021/acsnano.0c06688 PMID: 33534541

Li, S., Nguyen, I. P., & Urbanczyk, K. (2020). Common infectious diseases of the central nervous system—Clinical features and imaging characteristics. *Quantitative Imaging in Medicine and Surgery*, *10*(12), 2227–2259. DOI: 10.21037/qims-20-886 PMID: 33269224

Littera, R., Campagna, M., Deidda, S., Angioni, G., Cipri, S., Melis, M., Firinu, D., Santus, S., Lai, A., Porcella, R., Lai, S., Rassu, S., Scioscia, R., Meloni, F., Schirru, D., Cordeddu, W., Kowalik, M. A., Serra, M., Ragatzu, P., & Chessa, L. (2020). Human leukocyte antigen complex and other immunogenetic and clinical factors influence susceptibility or protection to SARS-CoV-2 infection and severity of the disease course. The Sardinian experience. *Frontiers in Immunology*, *11*, 605688. DOI: 10.3389/fimmu.2020.605688 PMID: 33343579

Liu, K., Sun, Y.-C., Pan, R.-T., Xu, A.-L., Xue, H., Tian, N., Zheng, J.-X., Shi, F.-Y., Lu, Y., & Li, L.-H. (2024). Infection and biogeographical characteristics of Paragonimus westermani and P. skrjabini in humans and animal hosts in China: A systematic review and meta-analysis. *PLoS Neglected Tropical Diseases*, *18*(8), e0012366–e0012366. DOI: 10.1371/journal.pntd.0012366 PMID: 39102441

Liu, L.-L., Liu, W.-N., Jiang, X.-Y., Chen, M.-H., Liu, Z.-J., Lin, Y., Zhu, S.-G., Lin, L.-R., Zheng, W.-H., & Yan, J.-H. (2019). Changes of T lymphocyte subsets in patients with HIV-negative symptomatic neurosyphilis. *Microbial Pathogenesis*, *130*, 213–218. DOI: 10.1016/j.micpath.2019.03.008 PMID: 30862559

Liu, Q., Wang, Z.-D., Huang, S.-Y., & Zhu, X.-Q. (2015). Diagnosis of toxoplasmosis and typing of Toxoplasma gondii. *Parasites & Vectors*, *8*(1), 292. Advance online publication. DOI: 10.1186/s13071-015-0902-6 PMID: 26017718

Liu, Y., Tim, Y., John, C., Ying, C., Sophie, D., Yuen-Shan, H., Gordon, W., & Raymond, C. (2019). The beneficial effects of physical exercise in the brain and related pathophysiological mechanisms in neurodegenerative diseases. *Laboratory Investigation*, *99*(7), 943–947. DOI: 10.1038/s41374-019-0232-y PMID: 30808929

Liu, Z., Tong, L., Chen, L., Jiang, Z., Zhou, F., Zhang, Q., Zhang, X., Jin, Y., & Zhou, H. (2023). Deep learning based brain tumor segmentation: A survey. *Complex & Intelligent Systems*, *9*(1), 1001–1026. DOI: 10.1007/s40747-022-00815-5

Li, W., Jiang, M., Xu, D., Kou, C., Zhang, L., Gao, J., Qin, K., Wu, W., & Zhang, X. (2019). Clinical and Laboratory Characteristics of Symptomatic and Asymptomatic Neurosyphilis in HIV-Negative Patients: A Retrospective Study of 264 Cases. *BioMed Research International*, *2019*(1), 2426313. DOI: 10.1155/2019/2426313 PMID: 31198783

Loh, E., Kugelberg, E., Tracy, A., Zhang, Q., Gollan, B., Ewles, H., Chalmers, R., Pelicic, V., & Tang, C. M. (2013). Temperature triggers immune evasion by Neisseria meningitidis. *Nature*, *502*(7470), 237–240. DOI: 10.1038/nature12616 PMID: 24067614

Long, J. M., & Holtzman, D. M. (2019). Alzheimer disease: An update on pathobiology and treatment strategies. *Cell, 179*(2), 312–339. DOI: 10.1016/j.cell.2019.09.001

Longordo, F., Kopp, C., & Luthi, A. (2009). Consequences of sleep deprivation on neurotransmitter receptor expression and function. Journal Compilation. *The European Journal of Neuroscience, 29*(9), 1810–1819. DOI: 10.1111/j.1460-9568.2009.06719.x PMID: 19492440

Lucchinetti, C. F., Guo, Y., Popescu, B. F., Fujihara, K., Itoyama, Y., & Misu, T. (2014). The pathology of an autoimmune astrocytopathy: Lessons learned from neuromyelitis optica. *Brain Pathology (Zurich, Switzerland), 24*(1), 83–97. DOI: 10.1111/bpa.12099

Ludden, C., Raven, K. E., Jamrozy, D., Gouliouris, T., Blane, B., Coll, F., de Goffau, M., Naydenova, P., Horner, C., Hernandez-Garcia, J., Wood, P., Hadjirin, N., Radakovic, M., Brown, N. M., Holmes, M., Parkhill, J., & Peacock, S. J. (2019). One health genomic surveillance of Escherichia coli demonstrates distinct lineages and mobile genetic elements in isolates from humans versus livestock. *mBio, 10*(1), 10–1128. DOI: 10.1128/mBio.02693-18 PMID: 30670621

Lukehart, S. A. (2008). Biology of treponemes. *Sexually Transmitted Diseases, 4*, 647–659.

Lukehart, S. A., Hook, E. W.III, Baker-Zander, S. A., Collier, A. C., Critchlow, C. W., & Handsfield, H. H. (1988). Invasion of the central nervous system by Treponema pallidum: Implications for diagnosis and treatment. *Annals of Internal Medicine, 109*(11), 855–862. DOI: 10.7326/0003-4819-109-11-855 PMID: 3056164

Luo, M., Wang, W., Zeng, Q., Luo, Y., Yang, H., & Yang, X. (2018). Tuberculous meningitis diagnosis and treatment in adults: A series of 189 suspected cases. *Experimental and Therapeutic Medicine, 16*(3), 2770–2776. https://www.ncbi.nlm.nih.gov/pmc/articles/PMC6122581/

Lu, S., Wang, J., He, Z., He, S., Zheng, K., Xu, M., Yuan, S., & Wu, Y. (2022). Treponema pallidum Tp0751 alters the expression of tight junction proteins by promoting bEnd3 cell apoptosis and IL-6 secretion. *International Journal of Medical Microbiology, 312*(4), 151553. DOI: 10.1016/j.ijmm.2022.151553 PMID: 35358795

Lutumba, P., Matovu, E., & Boatin, B. A. (2024). *Human African Trypanosomiasis (HAT)*. 73–97. DOI: 10.1007/978-3-031-53901-5_4

Lv, Z., & Liu, Y. (2024). Clinical research progress on intrathecal glucocorticoids in the treatment of infections. *Revista de Medicina (São Paulo), 103*(20), e38123. DOI: 10.1097/MD.0000000000038123 PMID: 38758886

Magadza, T., & Viriri, S. (2021). Deep learning for brain tumor segmentation: A survey of state-of-the-art. *Journal of Imaging*, *7*(2), 19. DOI: 10.3390/jimaging7020019 PMID: 34460618

Mahmoudinezhad Dezfouli, S. M., & Khosravi, S. (2021). Impact of Meningitis on Cognitive Skills and Development in Children. *Indian Journal of Forensic Medicine Toxicology*, *15*(1).

Majeed, S., Radotra, B. D., & Sharma, S. (2016). Adjunctive role of MMP-9 inhibition along with conventional anti-tubercular drugs against experimental tuberculous meningitis. *International Journal of Experimental Pathology*, *97*(3), 230–237. DOI: 10.1111/iep.12191 PMID: 27385155

Mak, A., Cheung, M. W. L., Chiew, H. J., Liu, Y., & Ho, R. C. M. (2012). Global trend of survival and damage of systemic lupus erythematosus: Meta-analysis and meta-regression of observational studies from the 1950s to 2000s. *Seminars in Arthritis and Rheumatism*, *41*(6), 830–839. DOI: 10.1016/j.semarthrit.2011.11.002

Manan, M. R., & Manan, H. (2021). Congenital Cytomegalovirus Infection: Transmission, Diagnosis and Treatment. *McGill Journal of Medicine : MJM : an International Forum for the Advancement of Medical Sciences by Students*, *20*(1). Advance online publication. DOI: 10.26443/mjm.v20i1.876

Mandal, S., Rao, R., & Joshi, R. (2023). Estimating the burden of tuberculosis in India: A modelling study. *Indian Journal of Community Medicine : Official Publication of Indian Association of Preventive & Social Medicine*, *48*(3), 436–442. https://www.ncbi.nlm.nih.gov/pmc/articles/PMC10353668/

Mannebach, K., Dressel, A., & Eason, L. (2022). Pediatric tuberculosis in India: Justice and human rights. *Public Health Nursing (Boston, Mass.)*, *39*(5), 1058–1064. DOI: 10.1111/phn.13061 PMID: 35152480

Manyelo, C. M., Solomons, R. S., Walzl, G., & Chegou, N. N. (2021). Tuberculous meningitis: Pathogenesis, immune responses, diagnostic challenges, and the potential of biomarker-based approaches. *Journal of Clinical Microbiology*, *59*(3), e01771–e20. https://www.ncbi.nlm.nih.gov/pmc/articles/PMC8106718/

Marks, M., Lawrence, D., Kositz, C., & Mabey, D. (2018). Diagnostic performance of PCR assays for the diagnosis of neurosyphilis: A systematic review. *Sexually Transmitted Infections*, *94*(8), 585–588. DOI: 10.1136/sextrans-2018-053666 PMID: 30061192

Marra, C. M. (2015). Neurosyphilis. *Continuum (Minneapolis, Minn.)*, *21*(6), 1714–1728. DOI: 10.1212/CON.0000000000000250 PMID: 26633785

Marra, C. M., Longstreth, W. T.Jr, Maxwell, C. L., & Lukehart, S. A. (1996). Resolution of serum and cerebrospinal fluid abnormalities after treatment of neurosyphilis: Influence of concomitant human immunodeficiency virus infection. *Sexually Transmitted Diseases*, *23*(3), 184–189. DOI: 10.1097/00007435-199605000-00005 PMID: 8724507

Marra, C. M., Maxwell, C. L., Tantalo, L., Eaton, M., Rompalo, A. M., Raines, C., Stoner, B. P., Corbett, J. J., Augenbraun, M., Zajackowski, M., Kee, R., & Lukehart, S. A. (2004). Normalization of cerebrospinal fluid abnormalities after neurosyphilis therapy: Does HIV status matter? *Clinical Infectious Diseases*, *38*(7), 1001–1006. DOI: 10.1086/382532 PMID: 15034833

Marra, C. M., Sahi, S. K., Tantalo, L. C., Ho, E. L., Dunaway, S. B., Jones, T., & Hawn, T. R. (2014). Toll-like receptor polymorphisms are associated with increased neurosyphilis risk. *Sexually Transmitted Diseases*, *41*(7), 440–446. DOI: 10.1097/OLQ.0000000000000149 PMID: 24922103

Marra, C. M., Tantalo, L. C., Sahi, S. K., Maxwell, C. L., & Lukehart, S. A. (2010). CXCL13 as a cerebrospinal fluid marker for neurosyphilis in HIV-infected patients with syphilis. *Sexually Transmitted Diseases*, *37*(5), 283–287. DOI: 10.1097/OLQ.0b013e3181d877a1 PMID: 20393380

Martín-Noguerol, T., Paulano-Godino, F., Riascos, R. F., Calabia-del-Campo, J., Márquez-Rivas, J., & Luna, A. (2019). Hybrid computed tomography and magnetic resonance imaging 3D printed models for neurosurgery planning. *Annals of Translational Medicine*, *7*(22), 684. DOI: 10.21037/atm.2019.10.109 PMID: 31930085

Martisova, E., Solas, M., Horrillo, I., Ortega, J. E., Meana, J. J., Tordera, R. M., & Ramírez, M. J. (2012). Long-lasting effects of early-life stress on glutamatergic/GABAergic circuitry in the rat hippocampus. *Neuropharmacology*, *62*(5-6), 1944–1953. DOI: 10.1016/j.neuropharm.2011.12.019 PMID: 22245561

Marx, G. E., & Chan, E. D. (2011). Tuberculous meningitis: Diagnosis and treatment overview. *Tuberculosis Research and Treatment*, *2011*, 798764. https://www.ncbi.nlm.nih.gov/pmc/articles/PMC3335590/

Mastraccio, K. E., Huaman, C., Coggins, S. A., Clouse, C., Rader, M., Yan, L., Mandal, P., Hussain, I., Ahmed, A. E., Ho, T., Feasley, A., Vu, B. K., Smith, I. L., Markotter, W., Weir, D. L., Laing, E. D., Broder, C. C., & Schaefer, B. C. (2023). mAb therapy controls CNS-resident lyssavirus infection via a CD4 T cell-dependent mechanism. *EMBO Molecular Medicine*, *15*(10), e16394. Advance online publication. DOI: 10.15252/emmm.202216394 PMID: 37767784

Matthaiou, D. K., Panos, G., Adamidi, E. S., & Falagas, M. E. (n.d.). *Albendazole versus Praziquantel in the Treatment of Neurocysticercosis: A Meta-analysis of Comparative Trials*. DOI: 10.1371/journal.pntd.0000194

Mauffrey, P., Tchitchek, N., Barroca, V., Bemelmans, A. P., Firlej, V., Allory, Y., Roméo, P. H., & Magnon, C. (2019). Progenitors from the central nervous system drive neurogenesis in cancer. *Nature*, *569*(7758), 672–678. DOI: 10.1038/s41586-019-1219-y

Mazumder, R., & Lee, J. K. (2022). Epileptogenesis in Common Parasitic Infections. *Current Neurology and Neuroscience Reports*, *22*(4), 285–291. DOI: 10.1007/s11910-022-01187-6 PMID: 35332514

Mazzini, G. S., Souza, D. O., & Portela, L. V. (2009). The ischemic heart as an extracerebral source for S100B. *Resuscitation*, *80*(1), 144. DOI: 10.1016/j.resuscitation.2008.09.015

McGill, F., Griffiths, M. J., Bonnett, L. J., Geretti, A. M., Michael, B. D., Beeching, N. J., McKee, D., Scarlett, P., Hart, I. J., Mutton, K. J., Jung, A., Adan, G., Gummery, A., Sulaiman, W. A. W., Ennis, K., Martin, A. P., Haycox, A., Miller, A., Solomon, T., & Martin, W. (2018). Incidence, aetiology, and sequelae of viral meningitis in UK adults: A multicentre prospective observational cohort study. *The Lancet. Infectious Diseases*, *18*(9), 992–1003. DOI: 10.1016/S1473-3099(18)30245-7 PMID: 30153934

McMaughan, D. J., Oloruntoba, O., & Smith, M. L. (2020). Socioeconomic status and access to healthcare: Interrelated drivers for healthy aging. *Frontiers in Public Health*, *8*, 512143. DOI: 10.3389/fpubh.2020.00231 PMID: 32626678

Medical Research Council. (1948). Streptomycin treatment of tuberculous meningitis. *Lancet*, *251*(6503), 582–596. https://linkinghub.elsevier.com/retrieve/pii/S0140673648920030

Mehrdadi, S. (2019). Acute Bacterial Meningitis: Diagnosis, Treatment and Prevention. *Journal of Archives in Military Medicine*. Advance online publication. DOI: 10.5812/jamm.84749

Melhuish, A., & McGill, F. (2021). Viral meningitis and encephalitis. *Medicine (Abingdon)*, *49*(11), 675–680. DOI: 10.1016/j.mpmed.2021.08.004

Meli, D. N., Loeffler, J. M., Baumann, P., Neumann, U., Buhl, T., Leppert, D., & Leib, S. L. (2004). In pneumococcal meningitis a novel water-soluble inhibitor of matrix metalloproteinases and TNF-α converting enzyme attenuates seizures and injury of the cerebral cortex. *Journal of Neuroimmunology*, *151*(1–2), 6–11. DOI: 10.1016/j.jneuroim.2004.01.026 PMID: 15145598

Mendez, O. A., & Koshy, A. A. (2017). Toxoplasma gondii: Entry, association, and physiological influence on the central nervous system. *PLoS Pathogens, 13*(7), e1006351. DOI: 10.1371/journal.ppat.1006351 PMID: 28727854

Meningitis. (n.d.). Retrieved June 8, 2024, from https://www.who.int/news-room/fact-sheets/detail/meningitis

Menzies, D., Pai, M., & Comstock, G. (2007). Meta-analysis: New tests for the diagnosis of latent tuberculosis infection: Areas of uncertainty and recommendations for research. *Annals of Internal Medicine, 146*(5), 340–354. https://www.acpjournals.org/doi/abs/10.7326/0003-4819-146-5-200703060-00006

Meyer, A. H., Feldsien, T. M., Mezler, M., Untucht, C., Venugopalan, R., & Lefebvre, D. R. (2023). Novel Developments to Enable Treatment of CNS Diseases with Targeted Drug Delivery. *Pharmaceutics, 15*(4), 1100. DOI: 10.3390/pharmaceutics15041100

Miceli, I., de Kantor, I. N., Colaiácovo, D., Peluffo, G., Cutillo, I., & Gorra, R. (1988). Evaluation of the effectiveness of BCG vaccination using the case control method in Buenos Aires, Argentina. *International Journal of Epidemiology, 17*(3), 629–634. DOI: 10.1093/ije/17.3.629

Michael, B., Menezes, B. F., Cunniffe, J., Miller, A., Kneen, R., Francis, G., Beeching, N. J., & Solomon, T. (2010). Effect of delayed lumbar punctures on the diagnosis of acute bacterial meningitis in adults. *Emergency Medicine Journal : EMJ, 27*(6), 433–438. DOI: 10.1136/emj.2009.075598 PMID: 20360497

Milburn, J., Suresh, R., Doyle, R., & Jarvis, J. N. (2024). The diagnosis of central nervous system infections in resource-limited settings and the use of novel and molecular diagnostic platforms to improve diagnosis. *Expert Review of Molecular Diagnostics, 24*(3), 1–12. DOI: 10.1080/14737159.2024.2317414 PMID: 38369939

Mishra, O. (1996). Cerebrospinal fluid adenosine deaminase activity for the diagnosis of tuberculous meningitis in children. *Journal of Tropical Pediatrics, 42*(3), 129–132. https://academic.oup.com/tropej/article-lookup/doi/10.1093/tropej/42.3.129

Mohanty, T., Fisher, J., Bakochi, A., Neumann, A., Cardoso, J. F. P., Karlsson, C. A. Q., Pavan, C., Lundgaard, I., Nilson, B., Reinstrup, P., Bonnevier, J., Cederberg, D., Malmström, J., Bentzer, P., & Linder, A. (2019). Neutrophil extracellular traps in the central nervous system hinder bacterial clearance during pneumococcal meningitis. *Nature Communications, 10*(1), 1667. DOI: 10.1038/s41467-019-09040-0 PMID: 30971685

Mohebalizadeh, M., Babapour, G., Maleki Aghdam, M., Mohammadi, T., Jafari, R., & Shafiei-Irannejad, V. (2023). Role of Maternal Immune Factors in Neuroimmunology of Brain Development. *Molecular Neurobiology*, 1–13. PMID: 38057641

Mohr, J. A., Griffiths, W., Jackson, R., Saadah, H., Bird, P., & Riddle, J. (1976). Neurosyphilis and penicillin levels in cerebrospinal fluid. *Journal of the American Medical Association, 236*(19), 2208–2209. DOI: 10.1001/jama.1976.03270200046031 PMID: 989815

Molloy, S. F., Kanyama, C., Heyderman, R. S., Loyse, A., Kouanfack, C., Chanda, D., Mfinanga, S., Temfack, E., Lakhi, S., Lesikari, S., Chan, A. K., Stone, N., Kalata, N., Karunaharan, N., Gaskell, K., Peirse, M., Ellis, J., Chawinga, C., Lontsi, S., & Harrison, T. S. (2018). Antifungal combinations for treatment of cryptococcal meningitis in Africa. *The New England Journal of Medicine*, *378*(11), 1004–1017. DOI: 10.1056/NEJMoa1710922 PMID: 29539274

Montgomery, J. M., Hossain, M. J., Gurley, E., Carroll, D. S., Croisier, A., Bertherat, E., Asgari, N., Formenty, P., Keeler, N., Comer, J., Bell, M. R., Akram, K., Molla, A. R., Zaman, K., Islam, M. R., Wagoner, K., Mills, J. N., Rollin, P. E., Ksiazek, T. G., & Breiman, R. F. (2008). Risk factors for Nipah virus encephalitis in Bangladesh. *Emerging Infectious Diseases*, *14*(10), 1526–1532. DOI: 10.3201/eid1410.060507 PMID: 18826814

Mook-Kanamori, B. B., Rouse, M. S., Kang, C.-I., van de Beek, D., Steckelberg, J. M., & Patel, R. (2009). Daptomycin in experimental murine pneumococcal meningitis. *BMC Infectious Diseases*, *9*(1), 1–9. DOI: 10.1186/1471-2334-9-50 PMID: 19405978

Moore, J. E. (1945). The chemotherapy of syphilis. *Bulletin of the New York Academy of Medicine*, *21*(1), 3. PMID: 19312421

Moore, J. E.MOORE. (1928). Asymptomatic neurosyphilis: V. A comparison of early and late asymptomatic neurosyphilis. *Archives of Dermatology and Syphilology*, *18*(1), 99–108. DOI: 10.1001/archderm.1928.02380130102009

Moro, P., & Schantz, P. M. (2009). Echinococcosis: A review. *International Journal of Infectious Diseases*, *13*(2), 125–133. DOI: 10.1016/j.ijid.2008.03.037 PMID: 18938096

Moseman, E. A., Blanchard, A. C., Nayak, D., & McGavern, D. B. (2020). T cell engagement of cross-presenting microglia protects the brain from a nasal virus infection. *Science Immunology, 5*(48), Article eabb1817. DOI: 10.1126/sciimmunol.abb1817

Moxon, C. A., Heyderman, R. S., & Wassmer, S. C. (2009). Dysregulation of coagulation in cerebral malaria. *Molecular and Biochemical Parasitology*, *166*(2), 99–108. DOI: 10.1016/j.molbiopara.2009.03.006 PMID: 19450727

Muri, L., Grandgirard, D., Buri, M., Perny, M., & Leib, S. L. (2018). Combined effect of non-bacteriolytic antibiotic and inhibition of matrix metalloproteinases prevents brain injury and preserves learning, memory and hearing function in experimental paediatric pneumococcal meningitis. *Journal of Neuroinflammation*, *15*(1), 1–14. DOI: 10.1186/s12974-018-1272-8 PMID: 30131074

Muri, L., Leppert, D., Grandgirard, D., & Leib, S. L. (2019). MMPs and ADAMs in neurological infectious diseases and multiple sclerosis. *Cellular and Molecular Life Sciences : CMLS*, *76*(16), 3097–3116. DOI: 10.1007/s00018-019-03174-6 PMID: 31172218

Muschol, N., Giugliani, R., Jones, S. A., Muenzer, J., Smith, N. J., Whitley, C. B., Donnell, M., Drake, E., Elvidge, K., Melton, L., & O'Neill, C.MPS III Guideline Development Group. (2022). Sanfilippo syndrome: Consensus guidelines for clinical care. *Orphanet Journal of Rare Diseases*, *17*(1), 391. DOI: 10.1186/s13023-022-02484-6 PMID: 36303195

Nagafuchi, M., Nagafuchi, Y., Sato, R., Imaizumi, T., Ayabe, M., Shoji, H., & Ichiyama, T. (2006). Adult meningism and viral meningitis, 1997-2004: Clinical data and cerebrospinal fluid cytokines. *Internal Medicine (Tokyo, Japan)*, *45*(21), 1209–1212. DOI: 10.2169/internalmedicine.45.1769 PMID: 17139119

Nagai, S., Wiker, H. G., Harboe, M., & Kinomoto, M. (1991). Isolation and partial characterization of major protein antigens in the culture fluid of Mycobacterium tuberculosis. *Infection and Immunity*, *59*(1), 372–382. https://www.ncbi.nlm.nih.gov/pmc/articles/PMC257751/

Nahid, P., Dorman, S. E., Alipanah, N., Barry, P. M., Brozek, J. L., & Cattamanchi, A. (2016). Official American Thoracic Society/Centers for Disease Control and Prevention/Infectious Diseases Society of America clinical practice guidelines: Treatment of drug-susceptible tuberculosis. *Clinical Infectious Diseases*, *63*(7), e147–e195. https://academic.oup.com/cid/article/63/7/e147/2196792

Nanda, E. (2024). The brain pathobiome in Alzheimer's disease. *Neurotherapeutics; the Journal of the American Society for Experimental NeuroTherapeutics*, *21*(6), e00475–e00475. DOI: 10.1016/j.neurot.2024.e00475 PMID: 39510900

Nath, A., & Tyler, K. L. (2013). Novel approaches and challenges to treatment of central nervous system viral infections. *Annals of Neurology*, *74*(3), 412–422. DOI: 10.1002/ana.23988 PMID: 23913580

Nathan, C. L., Emmert, B. E., Nelson, E., & Berger, J. R. (2021). CNS fungal infections: A review. *Journal of the Neurological Sciences*, *422*, 117325. DOI: 10.1016/j.jns.2021.117325 PMID: 33516057

National Center for Sexually Transmitted Disease Control, C. C. for D. C. and P., Committee of Sexually Transmitted Disease Chinese Medical Association, B. of D., & Committee of Sexually Transmitted Disease Chinese Medical Doctor Association, B. of D. (2020). (2019). Chinese expert consensus statement on diagnosis and treatment of syphilis. *Chinese Medical Journal*, *133*(19), 2335–2337. PMID: 32852386

Nauseef, W. M., & Borregaard, N. (2014). Neutrophils at work. *Nature Immunology*, *15*(7), 602–611. DOI: 10.1038/ni.2921 PMID: 24940954

Nematollahi, S., & Shoham, S. (2019). Updates on the Treatment of Non-Aspergillus Hyaline Mold Infections. In *Current Fungal Infection Reports* (Vol. 13, Issue 4). DOI: 10.1007/s12281-019-00364-4

Ng, L. F. P., & Solomon, T. (2015). Decade in review - CNS infections: Major advances against a moving target of CNS infections. In *Nature Reviews Neurology* (Vol. 11, Issue 11). DOI: 10.1038/nrneurol.2015.202

Ngarka, L., Siewe Fodjo, J. N., Aly, E., Masocha, W., & Njamnshi, A. K. (2022). The interplay between neuroinfections, the immune system and neurological disorders: A focus on Africa. *Frontiers in Immunology*, *12*, 803475. DOI: 10.3389/fimmu.2021.803475 PMID: 35095888

Ngasala, B., Bushukatale, S., Chiduo, M., Makene, T., Mkony, L., Mohamed, A., Molteni, F., Chacky, F., Njau, R. J. A., & Mwaiswelo, R. (2024). Efficacy of artesunate-amodiaquine for treatment of uncomplicated Plasmodium falciparum malaria in mainland Tanzania. *Malaria Journal*, *23*(1), 1–10. DOI: 10.1186/s12936-024-04923-0 PMID: 38553737

Nguyen, D. T., Agarwal, S., & Graviss, E. A. (2019). Trends of tuberculosis meningitis and associated mortality in Texas, 2010-2017, a large population-based analysis. *PLoS One*, *14*(2), e0212729. https://www.ncbi.nlm.nih.gov/pmc/articles/PMC6395025/

Nhantumbo, A. A., Comé, C. E., Maholela, P. I., Munguambe, A. M., da Costa, P., Mott, M., Cunha, G. R., Chambal, L., Dias, C., Cantarelli, V. V., & Gudo, E. S. (2022). Etiology of meningitis among adults in three quaternary hospitals in Mozambique, 2016–2017: The role of HIV. *PLoS ONE, 17*(5 May). DOI: 10.1371/journal.pone.0267949

Nhantumbo, A. A., Gudo, E. S., Caierão, J., Munguambe, A. M., Comé, C. E., Zimba, T. F., Moraes, M. O., Dias, C., & Cantarelli, V. V. (2016). Serotype distribution and antimicrobial resistance of Streptococcus pneumoniae in children with acute bacterial meningitis in Mozambique: Implications for a national immunization strategy. *BMC Microbiology, 16*(1), 1–9. DOI: 10.1186/s12866-016-0747-y PMID: 27357587

Niemelä, S., Lempinen, L., Löyttyniemi, E., Oksi, J., & Jero, J. (2023). Bacterial meningitis in adults: A retrospective study among 148 patients in an 8-year period in a university hospital, Finland. *BMC Infectious Diseases, 23*(1), 45. Advance online publication. DOI: 10.1186/s12879-023-07999-2 PMID: 36690945

Nimgampalle, M., Chakravarthy, H., Sharma, S., Shree, S., Bhat, A. R., Pradeepkiran, J. A., & Devanathan, V. (2023). Neurotransmitter systems in the etiology of major neurological disorders: Emerging insights and therapeutic implications. *Ageing Research Reviews, 89*, 101994. DOI: 10.1016/j.arr.2023.101994 PMID: 37385351

Niyonambaza, S., Kumar, P., Xing, P., Mathault, J., De Koninck, P., Boisselier, E., Boukadoum, M., & Miled, A. (2019). A Review of Neurotransmitters Sensing Methods for Neuro-Engineering Research. *Applied Sciences (Basel, Switzerland), 9*(21), 4719. DOI: 10.3390/app9214719

Noah, N. D. (1987). *Epidemiology of bacterial meningitis*. Bacterial Meninggitis.

Noe, C. R., Noe-Letschnig, M., Handschuh, P., Noe, C. A., & Lanzenberger, R. (2020). Dysfunction of the blood-brain barrier—A key step in neurodegeneration and dementia. *Frontiers in Aging Neuroscience, 12*, 185. DOI: 10.3389/fnagi.2020.00185 PMID: 32848697

Nonyong, P., Ekalaksananan, T., Phanthanawiboon, S., Aromseree, S., Phadungsombat, J., Nakayama, E. E., Shioda, T., Sawaswong, V., Payungporn, S., Thaewnongiew, K., Overgaard, H. J., Bangs, M. J., Alexander, N., & Pientong, C. (2021). Dengue virus in humans and mosquitoes and their molecular characteristics in northeastern Thailand 2016-2018. *PLoS One, 16*(9), e0257460. Advance online publication. DOI: 10.1371/journal.pone.0257460 PMID: 34520486

Northfield, D. W. C. (1942). The treatment of brain abscess. *Journal of Neurology, Neurosurgery, and Psychiatry, 5*(1–2), 1–9. DOI: 10.1136/jnnp.5.1-2.1 PMID: 21611397

Nowak, I., Madej, M., Secemska, J., Sarna, R., & Strzalka-Mrozik, B. (2023). Virus-Based Biological Systems as Next-Generation Carriers for the Therapy of Central Nervous System Diseases. *Pharmaceutics, 15*(7), 1931. Advance online publication. DOI: 10.3390/pharmaceutics15071931 PMID: 37514117

Nudelman, Y., & Tunkel, A. R. (2009). Bacterial meningitis: Epidemiology, pathogenesis and management update. *Drugs*, *69*(18), 2577–2596. DOI: 10.2165/11530590-000000000-00000 PMID: 19943708

Nygaard, A., Langbakk, B., & Romner, B. (1998). Neuron-specific enolase concentrations in serum and cerebrospinal fluid in patients with no previous history of neurological disorder. *Scandinavian Journal of Clinical and Laboratory Investigation*, *58*(3), 183–186. DOI: 10.1080/00365519850186403

Nygaard, Ø., Langbakk, B., & Romner, B. (1997). Age- and sex-related changes of S-100 protein concentrations in cerebrospinal fluid and serum in patients with no previous history of neurological disorder. *Clinical Chemistry*, *43*(3), 541–543. DOI: 10.1093/clinchem/43.3.541

O'Garra, A., Redford, P. S., McNab, F. W., Bloom, C. I., Wilkinson, R. J., & Berry, M. P. R. (2013). The immune response in tuberculosis. *Annual Review of Immunology*, *31*(1), 475–527. https://www.annualreviews.org/doi/10.1146/annurev-immunol-032712-095939

O'Leary, P. A. (1937). Cooperative clinical studies in the treatment of syphilis: Asymptomatic neurosyphilis. *Archives of Dermatology*, *35*(3), 387–401. DOI: 10.1001/archderm.1937.01470210013002

O'Toole, R. D., Thornton, G. F., Mukherjee, M. K., & Nath, R. L. (1969). Dexamethasone in tuberculous meningitis. *Annals of Internal Medicine*, *70*(1), 39–48. https://www.acpjournals.org/doi/abs/10.7326/0003-4819-70-1-39

Olson, J. K., Girvin, A. M., & Miller, S. D. (2001). Direct activation of innate and antigen-presenting functions of microglia following infection with Theiler's virus. *Journal of Virology*, *75*(20), 9780–9789. DOI: 10.1128/JVI.75.20.9780-9789.2001 PMID: 11559811

Organization, W. H. (1995). Meningococcal meningitis. *Weekly Epidemiological Record= Relevé Épidémiologique Hebdomadaire, 70*(15), 105–107.

Ouwens, I. M. D., Ott, A., Fiolet, A., Koehler, P. J., Vos, M., Oldhoff, J. M., & Verhoeven, W. M. A. (2019). Clinical presentation of laboratory confirmed neurosyphilis in a recent cases series. *Clinical Neuropsychiatry*, *16*(1), 17. PMID: 34908934

Ou, Y., Buchanan, A., Witt, C., & Hashemi, P. (2019). Frontiers in electrochemical sensors for neurotransmitter detection: Towards measuring neurotransmitters as chemical diagnostics for brain disorders. *Analytical Methods*, *11*(21), 2738–2755. DOI: 10.1039/C9AY00055K PMID: 32724337

Owolabi, M. O., Leonardi, M., Bassetti, C., Jaarsma, J., Hawrot, T., Makanjuola, A. I., Dhamija, R. K., Feng, W., Straub, V., Camaradou, J., Dodick, D. W., Sunna, R., Menon, B., Wright, C., Lynch, C., Chadha, A. S., Ferretti, M. T., Dé, A., Catsman-Berrevoets, C. E., & Servadei, F. (2023). Global synergistic actions to improve brain health for human development. *Nature Reviews. Neurology*, *19*(6), 371–383. DOI: 10.1038/s41582-023-00808-z PMID: 37208496

Ozturk-Engin, D., Erdem, H., Hasbun, R., Wang, S.-H., Tireli, H., Tattevin, P., Argemi, X., Ouamara-Digue, E., Gombos, A., Lakatos, B., Sırmatel, F., Cag, Y., Pekok, A. U., Senbayrak, S., Balkan, I. I., Gheno, M., Uzun, N., Kaya, S., Cicek-Senturk, G., & Vahaboglu, H. (2019). Predictors of unfavorable outcome in neurosyphilis: Multicenter ID-IRI Study. *European Journal of Clinical Microbiology & Infectious Diseases*, *38*(1), 125–134. DOI: 10.1007/s10096-018-3403-7 PMID: 30368740

Pai, M., Zwerling, A., & Menzies, D. (2008). Systematic review: T-cell–based assays for the diagnosis of latent tuberculosis infection: An update. *Annals of Internal Medicine*, *149*(3), 177–184. https://www.ncbi.nlm.nih.gov/pmc/articles/PMC2951987/

Palacios-Pedrero, M. Á., Osterhaus, A. D., Becker, T., Elbahesh, H., Rimmelzwaan, G. F., & Saletti, G. (2021). Aging and options to halt declining immunity to virus infections. *Frontiers in Immunology*, *12*, 681449. DOI: 10.3389/fimmu.2021.681449 PMID: 34054872

Paliwal, V. K., & Garg, R. K. (2021). Hydrocephalus in tuberculous meningitis - Pearls and nuances. Neurology India, 69(Suppl. 2). https://journals.lww.com/neur/fulltext/2021/69002/hydrocephalus_in_tuberculous_meningitis___pearls.12.aspx

Palmer, M. E., Andrews, L. J., Abbey, T. C., Dahlquist, A. E., & Wenzler, E. (2022). The importance of pharmacokinetics and pharmacodynamics in antimicrobial drug development and their influence on the success of agents developed to combat resistant gram negative pathogens: A review. In *Frontiers in Pharmacology* (Vol. 13). DOI: 10.3389/fphar.2022.888079

Papagni, R., Novara, R., Minardi, M. L., Frallonardo, L., Panico, G. G., Pallara, E., Cotugno, S., Ascoli Bartoli, T., Guido, G., De Vita, E., Ricciardi, A., Totaro, V., Camporeale, M., Segala, F. V., Bavaro, D. F., Patti, G., Brindicci, G., Pellegrino, C., Mariani, M. F., & Nicastri, E. (2023). Human African Trypanosomiasis (sleeping sickness): Current knowledge and future challenges. *Frontiers in Tropical Diseases*, *4*, 1087003. Advance online publication. DOI: 10.3389/fitd.2023.1087003

Parenteau, A. M., Boyer, C. J., Campos, L. J., Carranza, A. F., Deer, L. K., Hartman, D. T., & Hostinar, C. E. (2022). A review of mental health disparities during COVID-19: Evidence, mechanisms, and policy recommendations for promoting societal resilience. *Development and Psychopathology*, 1–22. PMID: 36097815

Park, I. U., Tran, A., Pereira, L., & Fakile, Y. (2020). Sensitivity and specificity of treponemal-specific tests for the diagnosis of syphilis. *Clinical Infectious Diseases*, *71*(Supplement_1), S13–S20. DOI: 10.1093/cid/ciaa349 PMID: 32578866

Pastuszczak, M., Jakiela, B., Jaworek, A. K., Wypasek, E., Zeman, J., & Wojas-Pelc, A. (2015). Association of Interleukin-10 promoter polymorphisms with neurosyphilis. *Human Immunology*, *76*(7), 469–472. DOI: 10.1016/j.humimm.2015.06.010 PMID: 26100683

Patel, V. B., Bhigjee, A. I., Paruk, H. F., Singh, R., Meldau, R., & Connolly, C. (2009). Utility of a novel lipoarabinomannan assay for the diagnosis of tuberculous meningitis in a resource-poor high-HIV prevalence setting. *Cerebrospinal Fluid Research*, *6*, 13. https://www.ncbi.nlm.nih.gov/pmc/articles/PMC2777116/

Pathakumari, B., Liang, G., & Liu, W. (2020). Immune defence to invasive fungal infections: A comprehensive review. *Biomedicine and Pharmacotherapy*, *130*, 110550. DOI: 10.1016/j.biopha.2020.110550 PMID: 32739740

Peermohamed, S., Kogilwaimath, S., & Sanche, S. (2020). Neurosyphilis. *Canadian Medical Association Journal*, *192*(29), E844–E844. DOI: 10.1503/cmaj.200189 PMID: 32690559

Pei, X., Wenjuan, Z., & Haiyang, J. (2021). Food-Origin Mycotoxin-Induced Neurotoxicity: Intend to Break the Rules of Neuroglia Cells. *Oxidative Medicine and Cellular Longevity*, *2021*(1), 1–14. DOI: 10.1155/2021/9967334 PMID: 34621467

Pellett, P. E., Mitra, S., & Holland, T. C. (2014). Basics of virology. In *Handbook of Clinical Neurology* (Vol. 123, pp. 45–66). Elsevier. DOI: 10.1016/B978-0-444-53488-0.00002-X

Peltola, H. (2000). Worldwide Haemophilus influenzae type b disease at the beginning of the 21st century: Global analysis of the disease burden 25 years after the use of the polysaccharide vaccine and a decade after the advent of conjugates. *Clinical Microbiology Reviews*, *13*(2), 302–317. DOI: 10.1128/CMR.13.2.302 PMID: 10756001

Peng, C., Trojanowski, J. Q., & Lee, V. M.-Y. (2020). Protein transmission in neurodegenerative disease. *Nature Reviews. Neurology*, *16*(4), 199–212. DOI: 10.1038/s41582-020-0313-2

Perdrup, A., Jørgensen, B. B., & Pedersen, N. S. (1981). The profile of neurosyphilis in Denmark A clinical and serological study of all patients in Denmark with neurosyphilis disclosed in the years 1971-1979 incl. by Wassermann reaction (CWRM) in the cerebrospinal fluid. *Acta Dermato-Venereologica. Supplementum*, *96*, 1–14. PMID: 6953720

Perera, A., Brock, O., Ahmed, A., Shaw, C., & Ashkan, K. (2024). Taking the knife to neurodegeneration: A review of surgical gene therapy delivery to the CNS. *Acta Neurochirurgica*, *166*(1), 136. Advance online publication. DOI: 10.1007/s00701-024-06028-8 PMID: 38483631

Pérez-Vélez, C. M., Anderson, M. S., Robinson, C. C., McFarland, E. J., Nix, W. A., Pallansch, M. A., Oberste, M. S., & Glodé, M. P. (2007). Outbreak of neurologic enterovirus type 71 disease: A diagnostic challenge. *Clinical Infectious Diseases*, *45*(8), 950–957. DOI: 10.1086/521895 PMID: 17879907

Perillo, T., Capasso, R., & Pinto, A. (2024). Neuroimaging of the Most Common Meningitis and Encephalitis of Adults: A Narrative Review. *Diagnostics, 14*(11), 1064. DOI: 10.3390/diagnostics14111064

Perrachione, T. K., & Perrachione, J. R. (2008). Brains and brands: Developing mutually informative research in neuroscience and marketing. *Journal of Consumer Behaviour*, *7*(4-5), 303–318. DOI: 10.1002/cb.257

Phar, & Bereda G. (2022). *Advances in Pharmacology and Clinical Trials Committed to Create Value for Researchers Pathophysiology and Management of Bacterial Meningitis in Pediatrics Adv in Pathophysiology and Management of Bacterial Meningitis in Pediatrics*. DOI: 10.23880/apct-16000198

Phoompoung, P., & Luong, M.-L. (2019). Treatment of Non-Aspergillus Mold Infections: A Focus on Mucormycosis and Fusariosis. *Current Treatment Options in Infectious Diseases*, *11*(4), 401–417. Advance online publication. DOI: 10.1007/s40506-019-00205-5

Pintado Maury, I., Alves, M., & Fonseca, T. (2019). Neurosyphilis prevalence at a Portuguese stroke unit care. *Aging Clinical and Experimental Research*, *31*(8), 1155–1161. DOI: 10.1007/s40520-018-1052-4 PMID: 30343380

Piperi, E., Papadopoulou, E., Georgaki, M., Dovrat, S., Bar Illan, M., Nikitakis, N. G., & Yarom, N. (2024). Management of oral herpes simplex virus infections: The problem of resistance. A narrative review. In *Oral Diseases* (Vol. 30, Issue 3, pp. 877–894). John Wiley and Sons Inc. DOI: 10.1111/odi.14635

Platt, F. M. (2018). Emptying the stores: Lysosomal diseases and therapeutic strategies. *Nature Reviews. Drug Discovery*, *17*(2), 133–150. DOI: 10.1038/nrd.2017.214 PMID: 29147032

Pokorn, M. (2004). Pathogenesis and Classification of Central Nervous System Infection. *PubMed*, *15*(3), 68–71. PMID: 29988854

Poplin, V., Boulware, D. R., & Bahr, N. C. (2020). Methods for rapid diagnosis of meningitis etiology in adults. *Biomarkers in Medicine*, *14*(6), 459–479. https://www.ncbi.nlm.nih.gov/pmc/articles/PMC7248681/

Pormohammad, A., Nasiri, M. J., McHugh, T. D., Riahi, S. M., & Bahr, N. C. (2019). A systematic review and meta-analysis of the diagnostic accuracy of nucleic acid amplification tests for tuberculous meningitis. *Journal of Clinical Microbiology*, *57*(6), e01113–e01118. https://www.ncbi.nlm.nih.gov/pmc/articles/PMC6535607/

Portela, L. V., Tort, A. B., Schaf, D. V., Ribeiro, L., Nora, D. B., Walz, R., Rotta, L. N., Silva, C. T., Busnello, J. V., Kapczinski, F., & Gonçalves, C. A. (2002). The serum S100B concentration is age dependent. *Clinical Chemistry*, *48*(6), 950–952. DOI: 10.1093/clinchem/48.6.950

Prajapati, P., Sripada, L., Singh, K., Bhatelia, K., Singh, R., & Singh, R. (2015). TNF-α regulates miRNA targeting mitochondrial complex-I and induces cell death in dopaminergic cells. *Biochimica et Biophysica Acta*, *1852*(3), 451–461. DOI: 10.1016/j.bbadis.2014.11.019 PMID: 25481834

Prasad, M. K., Kumar, A., Nalini, N., Kumar, P., Mishra, B., & Lata, D. (2023). Diagnostic accuracy of cerebrospinal fluid (CSF) adenosine deaminase (ADA) for tuberculous meningitis (TBM) in adults: A systematic review and meta-analysis. *Cureus*, *15*(6), e39896. https://www.ncbi.nlm.nih.gov/pmc/articles/PMC10316459/

Press Information Bureau, Government of India. (2024, November). https://static.pib.gov.in/WriteReadData/specificdocs/documents/2024/nov/doc2024115429801.pdf

Prevention, C. for D. C. and. (2019). Sexually transmitted disease surveillance 2018. *Atlanta: US Department of Health and Human Services, 10*.

Principi, N., Caironi, M., Venturini, F., Pani, L., & Esposito, S. (2015). Daptomycin in paediatrics: Current knowledge and the need for future research. *The Journal of Antimicrobial Chemotherapy*, *70*(3), 643–648. DOI: 10.1093/jac/dku453 PMID: 25406298

Principi, N., & Esposito, S. (2015). Enterovirus D-68: An emerging cause of infection. *Expert Review of Respiratory Medicine*, *9*(6), 711–719. DOI: 10.1586/17476348.2015.1109451 PMID: 26535922

Principi, N., & Esposito, S. (2020). Bacterial meningitis: New treatment options to reduce the risk of brain damage. *Expert Opinion on Pharmacotherapy, 21*(1), 97–105. DOI: 10.1080/14656566.2019.1685497 PMID: 31675255

Pruitt, A. A. (2018). Central Nervous System Infections in Patients Receiving Cancer Therapies. *Cancer Neurology in Clinical Practice: Neurological Complications of Cancer and its Treatment*, 377-396.

Pruitt, A. A. (2021). Central nervous system infections in immunocompromised patients. *Current Neurology and Neuroscience Reports*, *21*(7), 37. DOI: 10.1007/s11910-021-01119-w PMID: 34037866

Przybojewski, S., Andronikou, S., & Wilmshurst, J. (2006). Objective CT criteria to determine the presence of abnormal basal enhancement in children with suspected tuberculous meningitis. *Pediatric Radiology*, *36*(7), 687–696. http://link.springer.com/10.1007/s00247-006-0160-z

Qu, C., Wang, Y., Wang, X., He, R., Cao, H., Liu, B., Zhang, H., Zhang, N., Lai, Z., Dai, Z., & Cheng, Q. (2023). Global Burden and Its Association with Socio-economic Development Status of Meningitis Caused by Specific Pathogens over the Past 30 years: A Population-Based Study. *Neuroepidemiology*, *57*(5), 316–335. DOI: 10.1159/000531508 PMID: 37399794

Raabe, A., & Seifert, V. (2000). Protein S-100B as a serum marker of brain damage in severe head injury: Preliminary results. *Neurosurgical Review*, *23*(3), 136–138. DOI: 10.1007/PL00011941

Rahman, M. (2023). Magnetic resonance imaging in personalized medicine. In *Metabolomics* (pp. 199–238). Academic Press. DOI: 10.1016/B978-0-323-99924-3.00001-7

Rahman, M. H., Bajgai, J., Fadriquela, A., Sharma, S., Trinh Thi, T., Akter, R., Goh, S. H., Kim, C. S., & Lee, K. J. (2021). Redox effects of molecular hydrogen and its therapeutic efficacy in the treatment of neurodegenerative diseases. *Processes (Basel, Switzerland)*, *9*(2), 308. Advance online publication. DOI: 10.3390/pr9020308

Rahman, M. H., Bajgai, J., Fadriquela, A., Sharma, S., Trinh, T. T., Akter, R., Jeong, Y. J., Goh, S. H., Kim, C. S., & Lee, K. J. (2021). Therapeutic potential of natural products in treating neurodegenerative disorders and their future prospects and challenges. *Molecules (Basel, Switzerland)*, *26*(17), 5327. Advance online publication. DOI: 10.3390/molecules26175327

Rajasingham, R., Smith, R. M., Park, B. J., Jarvis, J. N., Govender, N. P., Chiller, T. M., Denning, D. W., Loyse, A., & Boulware, D. R. (2017). Global burden of disease of HIV-associated cryptococcal meningitis: An updated analysis. *The Lancet. Infectious Diseases*, *17*(8), 873–881. DOI: 10.1016/S1473-3099(17)30243-8 PMID: 28483415

Raksakoon, C., & Potiwat, R. (2021). Current arboviral threats and their potential vectors in Thailand. In *Pathogens* (Vol. 10, Issue 1). DOI: 10.3390/pathogens10010080

Ramachandran, P. S., & Wilson, M. R. (2021). Chronic Meningitis. In *Aminoff's Neurology and General Medicine* (pp. 839–851). Elsevier., DOI: 10.1016/B978-0-12-819306-8.00047-2

Ramakrishna, A., Giridhar, P., & Ravishankar, G. A. (2011). Phytoserotonin: A review. *Plant Signaling & Behavior*, *6*(6), 800–809. DOI: 10.4161/psb.6.6.15242 PMID: 21617371

Raman Sharma, R. (2010). Fungal infections of the nervous system: Current perspective and controversies in management. *International Journal of Surgery*, *8*(8), 591–601. DOI: 10.1016/j.ijsu.2010.07.293 PMID: 20673817

Ramchandani, M. S., Litvack, J. R., & Marra, C. M. (2020). Otosyphilis: A review of the literature. *Sexually Transmitted Diseases*, *47*(5), 296–300. DOI: 10.1097/OLQ.0000000000001155 PMID: 32149965

Ranjbarzadeh, R., Bagherian Kasgari, A., Jafarzadeh Ghoushchi, S., Anari, S., Naseri, M., & Bendechache, M. (2021). Brain tumor segmentation based on deep learning and an attention mechanism using MRI multi-modalities brain images. *Scientific Reports*, *11*(1), 10930. DOI: 10.1038/s41598-021-90428-8 PMID: 34035406

Razek, A. A. K. A., Watcharakorn, A., & Castillo, M. (2011). Parasitic Diseases of the Central Nervous System. *Neuroimaging Clinics of North America*, *21*(4), 815–841. DOI: 10.1016/j.nic.2011.07.005 PMID: 22032501

Re, D. B., Le Verche, V., Yu, C., Amoroso, M. W., Politi, K. A., Phani, S., Ikiz, B., Hoffmann, L., Koolen, M., Nagata, T., Papadimitriou, D., Willey, J., Cleveland, D. W., Henderson, C. E., & Przedborski, S. (2014). Necroptosis drives motor neuron death in models of both sporadic and familial ALS. *Neuron*, *81*(5), 1001–1008. DOI: 10.1016/j.neuron.2014.01.011

Reddy, A. B., Pinto, M., Hegde, S. P., Iqbal, A. A. M., Bejai, V., & Shenoy, M. M. (2022). A retrospective study on seroprevalence and clinical spectrum of syphilis from a tertiary care Center in South India. *APIK Journal of Internal Medicine*, *10*(3), 169–173. DOI: 10.4103/ajim.ajim_58_21

Reddy, G., Kiran, K., Padmavathi, A. R., & Nancharaiah, Y. V. (2022). Fungal infections: Pathogenesis, antifungals and alternate treatment approaches. *Current Research in Microbial Sciences*, *3*, 100137. DOI: 10.1016/j.crmicr.2022.100137 PMID: 35909631

Ricci, S., Grandgirard, D., Wenzel, M., Braccini, T., Salvatore, P., Oggioni, M. R., Leib, S. L., & Koedel, U. (2014). Inhibition of matrix metalloproteinases attenuates brain damage in experimental meningococcal meningitis. *BMC Infectious Diseases*, *14*(1), 1–10. DOI: 10.1186/s12879-014-0726-6 PMID: 25551808

Richardson, D., & Goldmeier, D. (2021). Probenecid in the treatment of neurosyphilis in men who have sex with men: A commentary. *Sexually Transmitted Infections*. PMID: 34510007

Riddell, I. V. J.IV, & Shuman, E. K. (2012). Epidemiology of central nervous system infection. *Neuroimaging Clinics of North America*, *22*(4), 543–556. DOI: 10.1016/j.nic.2012.05.003 PMID: 23122256

Rieder, H. L., Snider, D. E., & Cauthen, G. M. (1990). Extrapulmonary tuberculosis in the United States. *The American Review of Respiratory Disease*, *141*(2), 347–351. http://www.atsjournals.org/doi/abs/10.1164/ajrccm/141.2.347

Rios, P., Radhakrishnan, A., Thomas, S. M., Darvesh, N., Straus, S. E., & Tricco, A. C. (2020). Guidelines for preventing respiratory illness in older adults aged 60 years and above living in long-term care: A rapid review of clinical practice guidelines. medRxiv, 2020-03.

Rizzo, C., Napoli, C., Venturi, G., Pupella, S., Lombardini, L., Calistri, P., Monaco, F., Cagarelli, R., Angelini, P., Bellini, R., Tamba, M., Piatti, A., Russo, F., Palù, G., Chiari, M., Lavazza, A., & Bella, A. (2016). West Nile virus transmission: Results from the integrated surveillance system in Italy, 2008 to 2015. *Eurosurveillance*, *21*(37), 30340. Advance online publication. DOI: 10.2807/1560-7917.ES.2016.21.37.30340 PMID: 27684046

Rizzo, M. R., & Paolisso, G. (2021). SARS-CoV-2 emergency and long-term cognitive impairment in older people. *Aging and Disease*, *12*(2), 345. DOI: 10.14336/AD.2021.0109 PMID: 33815868

Robertson, F. C., Lepard, J. R., Mekary, R. A., Davis, M. C., Yunusa, I., Gormley, W. B., Baticulon, R. E., Mahmud, M. R., Misra, B. K., Rattani, A., Dewan, M. C., & Park, K. B. (2018). Epidemiology of central nervous system infectious diseases: A meta-analysis and systematic review with implications for neurosurgeons worldwide. *Journal of Neurosurgery*, *130*(4), 1107–1126. DOI: 10.3171/2017.10.JNS17359 PMID: 29905514

Robertson, S. J., Mitzel, D. N., Taylor, R. T., Best, S. M., & Bloom, M. E. (2009). Tick-borne flaviviruses: Dissecting host immune responses and virus countermeasures. *Immunologic Research, 43*(1–3), 172–186. DOI: 10.1007/s12026-008-8065-6 PMID: 18841330

Rock, R. B., Olin, M., Baker, C. A., Molitor, T. W., & Peterson, P. K. (2008). Central nervous system tuberculosis: Pathogenesis and clinical aspects. *Clinical Microbiology Reviews, 21*(2), 243–261. https://www.ncbi.nlm.nih.gov/pmc/articles/PMC2292571/

Rodríguez-Núñez, A., Cid, E., Eirís, J., Rodríguez-García, J., Camiña, F., Rodríguez-Segade, S., & Castro-Gago, M. (1999). Neuron-specific enolase levels in the cerebrospinal fluid of neurologically healthy children. *Brain & Development, 21*(1), 16–19. DOI: 10.1016/S0387-7604(98)00058-0

Rodríguez-Núñez, A., Cid, E., Rodríguez-García, J., Camiña, F., Rodríguez-Segade, S., & Castro-Gago, M. (2003). Neuron-specific enolase, nucleotides, nucleosides, purine bases, oxypurines and uric acid concentrations in cerebrospinal fluid of children with meningitis. *Brain & Development, 25*(2), 102–106. DOI: 10.1016/S0387-7604(02)00180-5

Rohlwink, U. K., Kilborn, T., Wieselthaler, N., Banderker, E., Zwane, E., & Figaji, A. A. (2016). Imaging features of the brain, cerebral vessels and spine in pediatric tuberculous meningitis with associated hydrocephalus. *The Pediatric Infectious Disease Journal, 35*(10), e301–e310. https://www.ncbi.nlm.nih.gov/pmc/articles/PMC5024759/

Roos, K. L., Tunkel, A. R., Van De Beek, D., & Scheld, W. M. (2014). Acute bacterial meningitis. In *Infections of the Central Nervous System: Fourth Edition* (Tenth Edit). Elsevier Inc. DOI: 10.2310/IM.1270

Rotbart, H. A. (2000). Viral meningitis. *Seminars in Neurology, 20*(3), 277–292. DOI: 10.1055/s-2000-9427 PMID: 11051293

Rubin, S., Eckhaus, M., Rennick, L. J., Bamford, C. G. G., & Duprex, W. P. (2015). Molecular biology, pathogenesis and pathology of mumps virus. *The Journal of Pathology, 235*(2), 242–252. DOI: 10.1002/path.4445 PMID: 25229387

Rychert, J. (2019). Benefits and limitations of MALDI-TOF mass spectrometry for the identification of microorganisms. Infectiology Journal, 2(4), 1–5. https://www.infectiologyjournal.com/articles/benefits-and-limitations-of-malditof-mass-spectrometry-for-the-identification-of-microorganisms.html

Sáez-Llorens, X., Ramilo, O., Mustafa, M. M., Mertsold, J., & McCracken, G. H.Jr. (1990). Molecular pathophysiology of bacterial meningitis: Current concepts and therapeutic implications. *The Journal of Pediatrics, 116*(5), 671–684. DOI: 10.1016/S0022-3476(05)82647-2 PMID: 2184210

Sahu, P. S., & Katwala, J. (2022). Pathogenesis of Fungal Infections in the Central Nervous System: Host and Pathogen Factors in Neurotropism. *Current Fungal Infection Reports, 16*(4), 221–233. DOI: 10.1007/s12281-022-00444-y

Sah, V. K., Wang, L., Min, X., Rizal, R., Feng, Z., Ke, Z., Deng, M., Li, L., & Li, H. (2015). Human schistosomiasis: A diagnostic imaging focused review of a neglected disease. *Radiology of Infectious Diseases (Beijing, China), 2*(3), 150–157. DOI: 10.1016/j.jrid.2015.11.007

Saini, A. G., Dogra, S., Kumar, R., Nada, R., & Singh, M. (2011). Primary tuberculous cerebellar abscess: Case report. *Annals of Tropical Paediatrics, 31*(4), 367–369. DOI: 10.1179/1465328111Y.0000000037

Salado-Rasmussen, K., Wessman, M., Cowan, S. A., Gerstoft, J., & Katzenstein, T. L. (2019). Syphilitic hepatitis and neurosyphilis: An observational study of Danish HIV-infected individuals during a 13-year period. *Sexually Transmitted Infections, 95*(6), 416–418. DOI: 10.1136/sextrans-2018-053921 PMID: 30923165

Salam, M. A., Al-Amin, M. Y., Salam, M. T., Pawar, J. S., Akhter, N., Rabaan, A. A., & Alqumber, M. A. (2023, July). Antimicrobial resistance: A growing serious threat for global public health. *Health Care, 11*(13), 1946. PMID: 37444780

Salazar, L., & Hasbun, R. (2017). Cranial imaging before lumbar puncture in adults with community-acquired meningitis: Clinical utility and adherence to the Infectious Diseases Society of America guidelines. *Clinical Infectious Diseases, 64*(12), 1657–1662. DOI: 10.1093/cid/cix240 PMID: 28369295

Salomon, A., Berry, I., Tuite, A. R., Drews, S., Hatchette, T., Jamieson, F., Johnson, C., Kwong, J., Lina, B., Lojo, J., Mosnier, A., Ng, V., Vanhems, P., & Fisman, D. N. (2020). Influenza increases invasive meningococcal disease risk in temperate countries. *Clinical Microbiology and Infection, 26*(9), 1257–e1. DOI: 10.1016/j.cmi.2020.01.004 PMID: 31935565

Sanchez, S. G., Bassot, E., & Cerutti, A., Hoa Mai Nguyen, Amel Aïda, Blanchard, N., & Sébastien Besteiro. (2023). The apicoplast is important for the viability and persistence of *Toxoplasma gondii* bradyzoites. *Proceedings of the National Academy of Sciences of the United States of America, 120*(34). DOI: 10.1073/pnas.2309043120

Sandler, S. J., Figaji, A. A., & Adelson, P. D. (2010). Clinical applications of biomarkers in pediatric traumatic brain injury. *Child's Nervous System, 26*(2), 205–213. DOI: 10.1007/s00381-009-0998-2

Santos, L. A., Grisolia, J. C., Malaquias, L. C. C., Paula, F. B. A., Dias, A. L. T., & Burger, E. (2020). Medication association and immunomodulation: An approach in fungal diseases and in particular in the treatment of paracoccidioidomycosis. *Acta Tropica, 206*, 105412–105412. DOI: 10.1016/j.actatropica.2020.105412 PMID: 32135141

Sarawagi, A., Soni, N. D., & Patel, A. B. (2021). Glutamate and GABA Homeostasis and Neurometabolism in Major Depressive Disorder. *Frontiers in Psychiatry, 12*, 637863. DOI: 10.3389/fpsyt.2021.637863 PMID: 33986699

Scarborough, M., & Thwaites, G. E. (2008). The diagnosis and management of acute bacterial meningitis in resource-poor settings. *Lancet Neurology, 7*(7), 637–648. DOI: 10.1016/S1474-4422(08)70139-X PMID: 18565457

Schlüter, D., & Barragan, A. (2019). Advances and Challenges in Understanding Cerebral Toxoplasmosis. *Frontiers in Immunology, 10*, 242. Advance online publication. DOI: 10.3389/fimmu.2019.00242 PMID: 30873157

Schneider, A., Sari, A. T., Alhaddad, H., & Sari, Y. (2020). Overview of therapeutic drugs and methods for the treatment of Parkinson's disease. *CNS & Neurological Disorders - Drug Targets, 19*(3), 195–206. DOI: 10.2174/1871527319666200402095644

Schuchat, A., Robinson, K., Wenger, J. D., Harrison, L. H., Farley, M., Reingold, A. L., Lefkowitz, L., & Perkins, B. A. (1997). Bacterial meningitis in the United States in 1995. *The New England Journal of Medicine, 337*(14), 970–976. DOI: 10.1056/NEJM199710023371404 PMID: 9395430

Schwartz, I. S., & Kauffman, C. A. (2020). Blastomycosis. *Seminars in Respiratory and Critical Care Medicine, 41*(1), 31–41. DOI: 10.1055/s-0039-3400281

Schwartz, S., Kontoyiannis, D. P., Harrison, T., & Ruhnke, M. (2018). Advances in the diagnosis and treatment of fungal infections of the CNS. *Lancet Neurology, 17*(4), 362–372. DOI: 10.1016/S1474-4422(18)30030-9 PMID: 29477506

Scolarici, M. J., King, C., Sterkel, A., Smith, J., Gauthier, G., & Saddler, C. (2022). The Role of Isavuconazonium Sulphate for the Treatment of Blastomycosis: A Case Series and Antifungal Susceptibility. *Open Forum Infectious Diseases, 9*(7), ofac220. Advance online publication. DOI: 10.1093/ofid/ofac220 PMID: 35821730

Seddon, J. A., Tugume, L., Solomons, R., Prasad, K., & Bahr, N. C. (2019). The current global situation for tuberculous meningitis: Epidemiology, diagnostics, treatment and outcomes. *Wellcome Open Research*, *4*, 167. https://www.ncbi.nlm.nih.gov/pmc/articles/PMC7029758/

Shahjin, F., Chand, S., & Yelamanchili, S. V. (2019). Extracellular Vesicles as Drug Delivery Vehicles to the Central Nervous System. *Journal of Neuroimmune Pharmacology, 15*(3), 443–458. DOI: 10.1007/s11481-019-09875-w

Shahzad, K., & Mati, W. (2020). Advances in magnetic resonance imaging (MRI). In *Advances in Medical and Surgical Engineering* (pp. 121-142). Academic Press.

Shaikh, M. S., Baig, M. S., Ali, S. S., Ahmad, A., Shaikh, M. M., Mahaparale, P. R., & Faiyazuddin, M. (2024). Review on cerebral malaria—Pathogenesis and role of EphA2 receptor in maintaining blood brain barrier integrity. *Health Sciences Review (Oxford, England)*, *11*, 100175. DOI: 10.1016/j.hsr.2024.100175

Shapiro, S., Miller, A., Lahat, N., Sobel, E., & Lerner, A. (2003). Expression of matrix metalloproteinases, sICAM-1 and IL-8 in CSF from children with meningitis. *Journal of the Neurological Sciences*, *206*(1), 43–48. DOI: 10.1016/S0022-510X(02)00317-9 PMID: 12480084

Sharma, S., & Sethi, G. R. (2021). *Standard Treatment Guidelines—A Manual for Medical Therapeutics, 6e*. Wolters Kluwer India Pvt. Ltd.

Shaukat, Z., Farooq, Q. U. A., Tu, S., Xiao, C., & Ali, S. (2022). A state-of-the-art technique to perform cloud-based semantic segmentation using deep learning 3D U-Net architecture. *BMC Bioinformatics*, *23*(1), 251. DOI: 10.1186/s12859-022-04794-9 PMID: 35751030

Sheikh, B. A., Bhat, B. A., & Mir, M. A. (2022). Antimicrobial resistance: New insights and therapeutic implications. *Applied Microbiology and Biotechnology*, *106*(19–20), 6427–6440. DOI: 10.1007/s00253-022-12175-8 PMID: 36121484

Shekhar, R., Rao, J. R., Devi, K. A., & Rao, R. B. (2013). CSF proteins as discriminatory markers of tubercular and pyogenic meningitis. *Journal of Clinical and Diagnostic Research : JCDR*, *7*(8), 1586–1588. https://www.ncbi.nlm.nih.gov/pmc/articles/PMC3782903/

Shelton, W. J., & Gonzalez, J. M. (2023). Outcomes of patients in Chagas disease of the central nervous system: A systematic review. *Parasitology*, 1–9. DOI: 10.1017/S0031182023001117 PMID: 37987164

Shen, Y., Dong, X., Liu, J., Lv, H., & Ge, Y. (2022). Serum interleukin-26 is a potential biomarker for the differential diagnosis of neurosyphilis and syphilis at other stages. *Infection and Drug Resistance*, *15*, 3693–3702. DOI: 10.2147/IDR.S366308 PMID: 35859909

Sheybani, F., Haddad, M., & Shirazinia, M. (2023). Epidemiology and etiology of community-acquired CNS infections in Iran: A narrative review. *Future Neurology*, *18*(4), FNL73. Advance online publication. DOI: 10.2217/fnl-2023-0017

Shields, R. K. (2024). Progress and New Challenges in Combatting the Threat of Antimicrobial Resistance: Perspective From an Infectious Diseases Pharmacist. *The Journal of Infectious Diseases*, *229*(2), 303–306. DOI: 10.1093/infdis/jiad250 PMID: 37487530

Shi, F., Qiu, X., Yu, M., & Huang, Y. (2022). Tuberculosis-specific antigen stimulated and unstimulated interferon-γ for tuberculous meningitis diagnosis: A systematic review and meta-analysis. *PLoS One*, *17*(8), e0273834. https://www.ncbi.nlm.nih.gov/pmc/articles/PMC9426936/

Shikani, H. J., Freeman, B. D., Lisanti, M. P., Weiss, L. M., Tanowitz, H. B., & Desruisseaux, M. S. (2012). Cerebral Malaria. *American Journal of Pathology*, *181*(5), 1484–1492. DOI: 10.1016/j.ajpath.2012.08.010 PMID: 23021981

Shi, M., & Mody, C. H. (2016). Fungal Infection in the Brain: What We Learned from Intravital Imaging. *Frontiers in Immunology*, *7*. Advance online publication. DOI: 10.3389/fimmu.2016.00292 PMID: 27532000

Shinjyo, N. & Kita, K. (2021). Infection and Immunometabolism in the Central Nervous System: A Possible Mechanistic Link Between Metabolic Imbalance and Dementia. *Front Cell Neurosci*. .DOI: 10.3389/fncel.2021.765217

Shrestha, G. S., Nepal, G., & Prust, M. L. (2024, March). Developing Systems of Emergency and Inpatient Neurologic Care in Resource-Limited Settings. In *Seminars in neurology*. Thieme Medical Publishers, Inc. DOI: 10.1055/s-0043-1778638

Shukla, B., Aguilera, E. A., Salazar, L., Wootton, S. H., Kaewpoowat, Q., & Hasbun, R. (2017). Aseptic meningitis in adults and children: Diagnostic and management challenges. *Journal of Clinical Virology*, *94*, 110–114. Advance online publication. DOI: 10.1016/j.jcv.2017.07.016 PMID: 28806629

Sierksma, A., Escott-Price, V., & De Strooper, B. (2020). Translating genetic risk of Alzheimer's disease into mechanistic insight and drug targets. *Science*, *370*(6512), 61–66. DOI: 10.1126/science.abb8575

Sigera, L. S. M., & Denning, D. W. (2023). Flucytosine and its clinical usage. In *Therapeutic Advances in Infectious Disease* (Vol. 10). DOI: 10.1177/20499361231161387

Sigfrid, L., Perfect, C., Rojek, A., Longuere, K. S., Lipworth, S., Harriss, E., Lee, J., Salam, A., Carson, G., Goossens, H., & Horby, P. (2019). A systematic review of clinical guidelines on the management of acute, community-acquired CNS infections. *BMC Medicine*, *17*(1), 170. Advance online publication. DOI: 10.1186/s12916-019-1387-5 PMID: 31488138

Simões, E. A. F., Bont, L., Manzoni, P., Fauroux, B., Paes, B., Figueras-Aloy, J., Checchia, P. A., & Carbonell-Estrany, X. (2018). Past, Present and Future Approaches to the Prevention and Treatment of Respiratory Syncytial Virus Infection in Children. In *Infectious Diseases and Therapy* (Vol. 7, Issue 1). DOI: 10.1007/s40121-018-0188-z

Simon, R. P. (1985). Neurosyphilis. *Archives of Neurology*, *42*(6), 606–613. DOI: 10.1001/archneur.1985.04060060112021 PMID: 3890813

Singh, A. E. (2020). Ocular and neurosyphilis: Epidemiology and approach to management. *Current Opinion in Infectious Diseases*, *33*(1), 66–72. DOI: 10.1097/QCO.0000000000000617 PMID: 31789673

Singh, G., Tucker, E. W., & Rohlwink, U. K. (2022). Infection in the developing brain: The role of unique systemic Immune Vulnerabilities. *Frontiers in Neurology*, *12*, 805643. DOI: 10.3389/fneur.2021.805643 PMID: 35140675

Singh, P., Gupta, K., Sharma, M., & Kumar, S. (2024). Molecular and Cellular Mechanism of Pathogen Invasion into the Central Nervous System: Meningitis. In *Mechanism and Genetic Susceptibility of Neurological Disorders* (pp. 317–340). Springer Nature Singapore. DOI: 10.1007/978-981-99-9404-5_14

Sivapathasundharam, B., Gururaj, N., & Ranganathan, K. (2020). Viral infections. *Shafer's Textbook of Oral Pathology E-book*, 327.

Snydman, D. R., Walker, M., Kublin, J. G., & Zunt, J. R. (2006). Parasitic Central Nervous System Infections in Immunocompromised Hosts: Malaria, Microsporidiosis, Leishmaniasis, and African Trypanosomiasis. *Clinical Infectious Diseases*, *42*(1), 115–125. DOI: 10.1086/498510 PMID: 16323101

Socha, W., Kwasnik, M., Larska, M., Rola, J., & Rozek, W. (2022). Vector-borne viral diseases as a current threat for human and animal health—One Health perspective. *Journal of Clinical Medicine*, *11*(11), 3026. DOI: 10.3390/jcm11113026 PMID: 35683413

Solaimalai, D., Gupta, A., George, L., Manesh, A., Karthik, R., Sathishkumar, D., Peter, C. V. D., Varghese, G. M., Pulimood, S. A., Kannangai, R., & Prakash, J. A. J. (2022). Upward trends of syphilis in the non-pregnant adults: A six-year report on clinical and epidemiological profile of syphilis from a tertiary care center, India. *Frontiers in Public Health, 10*, 908591. DOI: 10.3389/fpubh.2022.908591 PMID: 35958862

Song, T. J., Choi, Y. C., Lee, K. Y., & Kim, W. J. (2012). Serum and cerebrospinal fluid neuron-specific enolase for diagnosis of tuberculous meningitis. *Yonsei Medical Journal, 53*(6), 1068–1072. DOI: 10.3349/ymj.2012.53.6.1068

Songtao, X., Hongzhi, G., & Zhengde, X. (2023). [Expert consensus on the application of pathogenic diagnostic techniques for viral encephalitis and meningitis]. *National Medical Journal of China, 103 9*(9), 648–657. DOI: 10.3760/CMA.J.CN112137-20221014-02154

Sparling, P. F. (1999). *Natural history of syphilis. Sexually Transmitted Diseases* (3rd ed.). McGraw-Hill.

Spatola, M., Nziza, N., Irvine, E. B., Cizmeci, D., Jung, W., & Van, L. H. (2024). Distinctive antibody responses to Mycobacterium tuberculosis in pulmonary and brain infection. *Brain, 147*(9), 3247–3260. https://www.ncbi.nlm.nih.gov/pmc/articles/PMC11370789/

Spelber, D., & Lahijani, S. (2020). Neurosyphilis presenting as mania and psychosis after incidental treatment with cephalexin: A case report and literature review of Jarisch-Herxheimer reactions. *Psychosomatics, 61*(2), 177–180. DOI: 10.1016/j.psym.2019.06.001 PMID: 31331661

Spinella, P. C., Donoghue, A., Rajendra, A., Drott, H. R., Dominguez, T. E., & Helfaer, M. (2004). Cerebrospinal fluid levels of S-100β in children and its elevation in pediatric meningitis. *Pediatric Critical Care Medicine, 5*(1), 53–57. DOI: 10.1097/01.PCC.0000102395.31510.4E

Sridharan, S., Govindaswamy, A., Rajendran, A., & Roopesh, R. K. (2024). Challenges in management of Candida auris meningitis secondary to infected ventriculoperitoneal shunt – A case report. *Indian Journal of Medical Microbiology, 48*, 100555. Advance online publication. DOI: 10.1016/j.ijmmb.2024.100555 PMID: 38428528

Srivastava, N., Deval, H., Mittal, M., Kant, R., & Bondre, V. P. (2022). The outbreaks of acute encephalitis syndrome in Uttar Pradesh, India (1978–2020) and its effective management: A remarkable public health success story. *Frontiers in Public Health, 9*, 793268. DOI: 10.3389/fpubh.2021.793268 PMID: 35223759

Stahl, E. C., Sabo, J. K., Kang, M. H., Allen, R., Applegate, E., Kim, S. E., Kwon, Y., Seth, A., Lemus, N., Salinas-Rios, V., Soczek, K. M., Trinidad, M., Vo, L. T., Jeans, C., Wozniak, A., Morris, T., Kimberlin, A., Foti, T., Savage, D. F., & Doudna, J. A. (2023). Genome editing in the mouse brain with minimally immunogenic Cas9 RNPs. *Molecular Therapy : the Journal of the American Society of Gene Therapy*, *31*(8), 2422–2438. DOI: 10.1016/j.ymthe.2023.06.019 PMID: 37403358

Steiner, J., Bernstein, H. G., Bielau, H., Berndt, A., Brisch, R., Mawrin, C., Keilhoff, G., & Bogerts, B. (2007). Evidence for a wide extra-astrocytic distribution of S100B in human brain. *BMC Neuroscience*, *8*, 2. Advance online publication. DOI: 10.1186/1471-2202-8-2

Stelzle, D., Makasi, C., Schmidt, V., Trevisan, C., Van Damme, I., Ruether, C., Dorny, P., Magnussen, P., Zulu, G., Mwape, K. E., Bottieau, E., Prazeres da Costa, C., Prodjinotho, U. F., Carabin, H., Jackson, E., Fleury, A., Gabriël, S., Ngowi, B. J., & Winkler, A. S. (2023). Efficacy and safety of antiparasitic therapy for neurocysticercosis in rural Tanzania: A prospective cohort study. *Infection*, *51*(4), 1127–1139. DOI: 10.1007/s15010-023-02021-y PMID: 36961623

Stember, J. N., & Shalu, H. (2022). Classification of 3D MRI brain volumes using reinforcement learning and clinical reports. *Journal of Digital Imaging*, *35*(5), 1143–1152. DOI: 10.1007/s10278-022-00644-5 PMID: 35562633

Stewart, S. M. (1953). The bacteriological diagnosis of tuberculous meningitis. *Journal of Clinical Pathology*, *6*(3), 241–242. https://www.ncbi.nlm.nih.gov/pmc/articles/PMC1023629/

Stojakovic, A., Paz-Filho, G., Arcos-Burgos, M., Licinio, J., Wong, M. L., & Mastronardi, C. A. (2017). Role of the IL-1 Pathway in Dopaminergic Neurodegeneration and Decreased Voluntary Movement. *Molecular Neurobiology*, *54*(6), 4486–4495. DOI: 10.1007/s12035-016-9988-x PMID: 27356916

Straif-Bourgeois, S., Tonzel, J. L., Kretzschmar, M., & Ratard, R. (2023). Infectious disease epidemiology. In *Handbook of epidemiology* (pp. 1–79). Springer New York. DOI: 10.1007/978-1-4614-6625-3_34-1

Strein, M., Holton-Burke, J. P., Smith, L. R., & Brophy, G. M. (2019). Prevention, treatment, and monitoring of seizures in the intensive care unit. *Journal of Clinical Medicine*, *8*(8), 1177. DOI: 10.3390/jcm8081177 PMID: 31394791

Subramanian, A., Gupta, A., Saxena, S., Gupta, A., Kumar, R., Nigam, A., Kumar, R., Mandal, S. K., & Roy, R. (2005). Proton MR CSF analysis and a new software as predictors for the differentiation of meningitis in children. *NMR in Biomedicine*, *18*(4), 213–225. DOI: 10.1002/nbm.942

Sulaiman, T., Medi, S., Erdem, H., Senbayrak, S., Ozturk-Engin, D., & Inan, A. (2020). The diagnostic utility of the "Thwaites' system" and "Lancet consensus scoring system" in tuberculous vs. non-tuberculous subacute and chronic meningitis: Multicenter analysis of 395 adult patients. *BMC Infectious Diseases*, *20*, 788. https://www.ncbi.nlm.nih.gov/pmc/articles/PMC7585215/

Surianarayanan, C., Lawrence, J. J., Chelliah, P. R., Prakash, E., & Hewage, C. (2023). Convergence of Artificial Intelligence and Neuroscience towards the Diagnosis of Neurological Disorders—A Scoping Review. *Sensors (Basel)*, *23*(6), 3062. DOI: 10.3390/s23063062 PMID: 36991773

Suter, Y., Jungo, A., Rebsamen, M., Knecht, U., Herrmann, E., Wiest, R., & Reyes, M. (2019). Deep learning versus classical regression for brain tumor patient survival prediction. In A. Crimi, S. Bakas, H. Kuijf, F. Keyvan, M. Reyes, & T. van Walsum (Eds.), *Brainlesion: Glioma, multiple sclerosis, stroke and traumatic brain injuries* (pp. 429–440). Springer. DOI: 10.1007/978-3-030-11726-9_38

Suthar, R., & Sankhyan, N. (2019). Bacterial infections of the central nervous system. *Indian Journal of Pediatrics*, *86*(1), 60–69. DOI: 10.1007/s12098-017-2477-z PMID: 29297142

Sütlaş, P. N., Ünal, A., Forta, H., Şenol, S., & Kırbaş, D. (2003). Tuberculous meningitis in adults: Review of 61 cases. *Infection*, *31*(6), 387–391. DOI: 10.1007/s15010-003-3179-1

Swartz, M. N., Healy, B. P., & Musher, D. M. (1999). Late syphilis. *Sexually Transmitted Diseases*, 487–509.

Syggelou, A., Spyridis, N., Benetatou, K., Kourkouni, E., Kourlaba, G., & Tsagaraki, M. (2020). BCG vaccine protection against TB infection among children older than 5 years in close contact with an infectious adult TB case. *Journal of Clinical Medicine*, *9*(10), 3224. https://www.mdpi.com/2077-0383/9/10/3224

Taha, A. R. (2020). Central Nervous System Infection. *Highly Infectious Diseases in Critical Care: A Comprehensive Clinical Guide*, 147-174.

Tai, M. L. S., Nor, H. M., Viswanathan, S., Rose, N., Zain, M., & Pow, Z. Y. (2017). Spinal tuberculous disease is common in tuberculous meningitis. *Neurology Asia*.

Tang, X., & Li, G. (2017). The interpretation of practice guidelines for the diagnosis and management of aspergillosis: 2016 update by the Infectious Diseases Society of America. In *Chinese Journal of Infection and Chemotherapy* (Vol. 17, Issue 4). DOI: 10.16718/j.1009-7708.2017.04.021

Tan, X., Zhang, J., Li, J., Yue, X., & Gong, X. (2020). The prevalence of asymptomatic neurosyphilis among HIV-negative serofast patients in China: A meta-analysis. *PLoS One*, *15*(11), e0241572. DOI: 10.1371/journal.pone.0241572 PMID: 33147295

Tazerji, S. S., Nardini, R., Safdar, M., Shehata, A. A., & Duarte, P. M. (2022). An overview of anthropogenic actions as drivers for emerging and re-emerging zoonotic diseases. *Pathogens (Basel, Switzerland)*, *11*(11), 1376. DOI: 10.3390/pathogens11111376 PMID: 36422627

Teleanu, R., Adelina-Gabriela, N., Eugenia, R., Oana, V., Alexandru, M., Daniel, M., & Nina, K. (2022). Academic Editor Neurotransmitters—Key Factors in Neurological and Neurodegenerative Disorders of the Central Nervous System. *International Journal of Molecular Sciences*, *23*(11), 5954. DOI: 10.3390/ijms23115954 PMID: 35682631

Tenforde, M. W., Mokomane, M., Leeme, T. B., Tlhako, N., Tsholo, K., Chebani, T., Stephenson, A., Hutton, J., Mitchell, H. K., Patel, R. K. K., Hurt, W. J., Pilatwe, T., Masupe, T., Molefi, M., Guthrie, B. L., Farquhar, C., Mine, M., & Jarvis, J. N. (2019). Mortality in adult patients with culture-positive and culture-negative meningitis in the Botswana national meningitis survey: A prevalent cohort study. *The Lancet. Infectious Diseases*, *19*(7), 740–749. DOI: 10.1016/S1473-3099(19)30066-0 PMID: 31250824

Tennant, D.R. (2018). Review of Glutamate Intake from Both Food Additive and Non-Additive Sources in the European Union. *Ann. Nutr. Metab.*. DOI: 10.1159/000494778

Terreni, M., Taccani, M., & Pregnolato, M. (2021). New antibiotics for multidrug-resistant bacterial strains: Latest research developments and future perspectives. *Molecules (Basel, Switzerland)*, *26*(9), 2671. DOI: 10.3390/molecules26092671 PMID: 34063264

Testa, C. M., & Jankovic, J. (2019). Huntington disease: A quarter century of progress since the gene discovery. *Journal of the Neurological Sciences*, *396*, 52–68. DOI: 10.1016/j.jns.2018.09.022 PMID: 30419368

Teunissen, C. E., Tumani, H., Bennett, J. L., Berven, F. S., Brundin, L., Comabella, M., Franciotta, D., Frederiksen, J. L., Fleming, J. O., Furlan, R., Hintzen, R. Q., Hughes, S. G., Jiménez Jiménez, F. J., Kroksveen, A. C., Kuhle, J., Magnussen, J. S., Petzold, A., Persson, L., Villoslada, P., & Zetterberg, H. (2011). Consensus guidelines for CSF and blood biobanking for CNS biomarker studies. *Multiple Sclerosis International*, *2011*, 246412. Advance online publication. DOI: 10.1155/2011/246412

Texel, S., Camandola, S., Ladenheim, B., Rothman, S., Mughal, M., Unger, E. L., Cadet, J. L., & Mattson, M. P. (2012). Ceruloplasmin deficiency results in an anxiety phenotype involving deficits in hippocampal iron, serotonin, and BDNF. *Journal of Neurochemistry, 120*(1), 125–134. DOI: 10.1111/j.1471-4159.2011.07554.x PMID: 22035068

Thigpen, M. C., Whitney, C. G., Messonnier, N. E., Zell, E. R., Lynfield, R., Hadler, J. L., Harrison, L. H., Farley, M. M., Reingold, A., Bennett, N. M., Craig, A. S., Schaffner, W., Thomas, A., Lewis, M. M., Scallan, E., & Schuchat, A. (2011). Bacterial meningitis in the United States, 1998–2007. *The New England Journal of Medicine, 364*(21), 2016–2025. DOI: 10.1056/NEJMoa1005384 PMID: 21612470

Thomas, S. (2020). Antimicrobial Resistance: Global Challenges and Future Interventions. *Antimicrobial Resistance: Global Challenges and Future Interventions*, 1–230. DOI: 10.1007/978-981-15-3658-8/COVER

Thomas, R., Le Tulzo, Y., & Bellissant, E. (1996). Place des corticoïdes dans le traitement des méningites purulentes chez l'adulte. *Medecine et Maladies Infectieuses, 26*, 1119–1124. DOI: 10.1016/S0399-077X(96)80026-6

Thong, W. Y., Han, A., Wang, S. J., Lin, J., Isa, M. S., Koay, E. S., & Tay, S. K. (2017). Enterovirus infections in Singaporean children: An assessment of neurological manifestations and clinical outcomes. *Singapore Medical Journal, 58*(4), 189–195. DOI: 10.11622/smedj.2016099 PMID: 27245861

Thwaites, G. E., Bang, N. D., Dung, N. H., Quy, H. T., Oanh, D. T. T., Thoa, N. T. C., Hien, N. Q., Thuc, N. T., Hai, N. N., Lan, N. T. N., Lan, N. N., Duc, N. H., Tuan, V. N., Hiep, C. H., Chau, T. T. H., Mai, P. P., Dung, N. T., Stepniewska, K., White, N. J., & Farrar, J. J. (2004). Dexamethasone for the treatment of tuberculous meningitis in adolescents and adults. *The New England Journal of Medicine, 351*(17), 1741–1751. DOI: 10.1056/NEJMoa040573 PMID: 15496623

Thwaites, G. E., Caws, M., Chau, T. T. H., Dung, N. T., Campbell, J. I., & Phu, N. H. (2004). Comparison of conventional bacteriology with nucleic acid amplification (amplified Mycobacterium direct test) for diagnosis of tuberculous meningitis before and after inception of antituberculosis chemotherapy. *Journal of Clinical Microbiology, 42*(3), 996–1002. https://www.ncbi.nlm.nih.gov/pmc/articles/PMC356903/

Thwaites, G. E., Chau, T. T. H., & Farrar, J. J. (2004). Improving the bacteriological diagnosis of tuberculous meningitis. *Journal of Clinical Microbiology, 42*(1), 378–379. https://www.ncbi.nlm.nih.gov/pmc/articles/PMC321694/

Thwaites, G. E., Chau, T. T. H., Stepniewska, K., Phu, N. H., Chuong, L. V., & Sinh, D. X. (2002). Diagnosis of adult tuberculous meningitis by use of clinical and laboratory features. *Lancet, 360*(9342), 1287–1292. https://www.thelancet.com/journals/lancet/article/PIIS0140-6736(02)11318-3/fulltext

Thwaites, G. E., Macmullen-Price, J., Chau, T. T. H., Mai, P. P., Dung, N. T., & Simmons, C. P. (2007). Serial MRI to determine the effect of dexamethasone on the cerebral pathology of tuberculous meningitis: An observational study. *Lancet Neurology, 6*(3), 230–236. https://www.ncbi.nlm.nih.gov/pmc/articles/PMC4333204/

Thwaites, G., Chau, T., Mai, N., Drobniewski, F., McAdam, K., & Farrar, J. (2000). Tuberculous meningitis. *Journal of Neurology, Neurosurgery, and Psychiatry, 68*(3), 289–299. https://www.ncbi.nlm.nih.gov/pmc/articles/PMC1736815/

Tiu, S. C., Chan, W. Y., Heizmann, C. W., Schäfer, B. W., Shu, S. Y., & Yew, D. T. (2000). Differential expression of S100B and S100A6 in the human fetal and aged cerebral cortex. *Brain Research. Developmental Brain Research, 119*(2), 159–168. DOI: 10.1016/S0165-3806(99)00176-5

Towfighi, A., Berger, R. P., Corley, A. M., Glymour, M. M., Manly, J. J., & Skolarus, L. E. (2023). Recommendations on social determinants of health in neurologic disease. *Neurology, 101*(7, Supplement_1), S17–S26. DOI: 10.1212/WNL.0000000000207562 PMID: 37580147

Townend, W., & Ingebrigtsen, T. (2006). Head injury outcome prediction: A role for protein S-100B? *Injury, 37*(12), 1098–1108. DOI: 10.1016/j.injury.2006.07.014

Travassos da Rosa, J. F. S., Travassos da Rosa, A. P. A., Vasconcelos, P. F. C., Pinheiro, F. P., Rodrigues, S. G., Travassos da Rosa, E. S., & Dias, L. B. (1998). Arboviruses isolated in the Evandro Chagas Institute, including some described for the first time in the Brazilian Amazon region, their known hosts, and their pathology for man. In Travassos da Rosa, J. F. S., Travassos da Rosa, A. P. A., & Vasconcelos, P. F. C. (Eds.), *An overview of arbovirology in Brazil and neighbouring countries* (pp. 19–31). Instituto Evandro Chagas.

Tsafaras, G. P., Ntontsi, P., & Xanthou, G. (2020). Advantages and limitations of the neonatal immune system. *Frontiers in Pediatrics, 8*, 5. DOI: 10.3389/fped.2020.00005 PMID: 32047730

Tsai, H., Shi, M., Lee, S., Wann, S., Tai, M., & Chen, Y. (2011). Expression of matrix metalloproteinases and their tissue inhibitors in the serum and cerebrospinal fluid of patients with meningitis. *Clinical Microbiology and Infection, 17*(5), 780–784. DOI: 10.1111/j.1469-0691.2010.03393.x PMID: 21521415

Tsai, M., Yang, C., Lee, N., Hsieh, S., Lin, Y., Sun, H., Sheng, W., Lee, K., Yang, S., & Liu, W. (2014). Jarisch-Herxheimer reaction among HIV-positive patients with early syphilis: Azithromycin versus benzathine penicillin G therapy. *African Journal of Reproduction and Gynaecological Endoscopy*, *17*(1). PMID: 25174641

Tsukahara, H., Fujii, Y., Matsubara, K., Yamada, M., Nagaoka, Y., Saito, Y., Yashiro, M., Tsuge, M., Goto, S., Kitamura, T., & Hata, A. (2013). Prognostic value of brain injury biomarkers in acute encephalitis/encephalopathy. *Pediatrics International*, *55*(4), 461–464. DOI: 10.1111/ped.12074

Tuddenham, S., & Ghanem, K. G. (2016). Ocular syphilis: Opportunities to address important unanswered questions. *Sexually Transmitted Infections*, *92*(8), 563–565. DOI: 10.1136/sextrans-2016-052570 PMID: 27116973

Tunkel, A. R., Hartman, B. J., Kaplan, S. L., Kaufman, B. A., Roos, K. L., Scheld, W. M., & Whitley, R. J. (2004). Practice guidelines for the management of bacterial meningitis. *Clinical Infectious Diseases*, *39*(9), 1267–1284. DOI: 10.1086/425368 PMID: 15494903

Tunkel, A. R., & Scheld, W. M. (1993). Pathogenesis and pathophysiology of bacterial meningitis. *Clinical Microbiology Reviews*, *6*(2), 118–136. DOI: 10.1128/CMR.6.2.118 PMID: 8472245

Ueda, N. K., Nakamura, K., Go, H., Takehara, H., Kashiwabara, N., Arai, K., Takemura, H., Namai, Y., & Kanemitsu, K. (2018). Neonatal meningitis and recurrent bacteremia with group B Streptococcus transmitted by own mother's milk: A case report and review of previous cases. *International Journal of Infectious Diseases*, *74*, 13–15. Advance online publication. DOI: 10.1016/j.ijid.2018.06.016 PMID: 29959094

Useche, Y., Pérez, A. R., de Meis, J., Bonomo, A., & Savino, W. (2022). Central nervous system commitment in Chagas disease. *Frontiers in Immunology*, *13*, 975106. Advance online publication. DOI: 10.3389/fimmu.2022.975106 PMID: 36439149

Valluzzi, R. L., Fierro, V., Arasi, S., Mennini, M., Pecora, V., & Fiocchi, A. (2019). Allergy to food additives. *Current Opinion in Allergy and Clinical Immunology*, *19*(3), 256–262. DOI: 10.1097/ACI.0000000000000528 PMID: 30883393

Van Belle, S., de Lange, A., Tomes, H., Lucas, R., Naidoo, V., & Raimondo, J. V. (2021). Peripheral Taenia infection increases immunoglobulins in the central nervous system. *International Journal for Parasitology*, *51*(8), 685–692. DOI: 10.1016/j.ijpara.2020.12.008 PMID: 33753094

Van de Beek, D., Brouwer, M. C., Thwaites, G. E., & Tunkel, A. R. (2012). Advances in treatment of bacterial meningitis. *Lancet*, *380*(9854), 1693–1702. DOI: 10.1016/S0140-6736(12)61186-6 PMID: 23141618

Van der Linden, L., Wolthers, K. C., & van Kuppeveld, F. J. M. (2015). Replication and inhibitors of enteroviruses and parechoviruses. *Viruses*, *7*(8), 4529–4562. DOI: 10.3390/v7082832 PMID: 26266417

Van Engelen, B. G. M., Lamers, K. J. B., Gabreels, F. J. M., Wevers, R. A., Van Geel, W. J. A., & Borm, G. F. (1992). Age-related changes of neuron-specific enolase, S-100 protein, and myelin basic protein concentrations in cerebrospinal fluid. *Clinical Chemistry*, *38*(6), 813–816. DOI: 10.1093/clinchem/38.6.813

Verdon, R., Chevret, S., Laissy, J. P., & Wolff, M. (1996). Tuberculous meningitis in adults: Review of 48 cases. *Clinical Infectious Diseases*, *22*(6), 982–988. DOI: 10.1093/clinids/22.6.982

Vergnano, S., Kadambari, S., Whalley, K., Menson, E. N., Martinez-Alier, N., Cooper, M., Sanchez, E., Heath, P. T., & Lyall, H. (2015). Characteristics and outcomes of human parechovirus infection in infants (2008-2012). *European Journal of Pediatrics*, *174*(7), 919–924. DOI: 10.1007/s00431-014-2483-3 PMID: 25573462

Vijayakumar, B., Sarin, K., & Mohan, G. (2012). Tuberculous brain abscess and subdural empyema in an immunocompetent child: Significance of AFB staining in aspirated pus. *Annals of Indian Academy of Neurology*, *15*(2), 130–133. https://www.ncbi.nlm.nih.gov/pmc/articles/PMC3345591/

Villoria, M. F., Fortea, F., Moreno, S., Muñoz, L., Manero, M., & Benito, C. (1995). MR imaging and CT of central nervous system tuberculosis in the patient with AIDS. *Radiologic Clinics of North America*, *33*(4), 805–820.

Virus Prevention, Diagnosis, and Treatment. (2023). *A Guide to Virology for Engineers and Applied Scientists: Epidemiology, Emergency Management, and Optimization*, 57–74. DOI: 10.1002/9781119853169.ch4

Vives-Bauza, C., de Vries, R. L. A., Tocilescu, M., & Przedborski, S. (2010). PINK1/Parkin direct mitochondria to autophagy. *Autophagy*, *6*(2), 315–316. DOI: 10.4161/auto.6.2.11103

von Baumgarten, L., Stauss, H. J., & Lünemann, J. D. (2023). Synthetic Cell-Based Immunotherapies for Neurologic Diseases. *Neurology(R). Neuroimmunology and Neuroinflammation*, *10*(5), e200139. Advance online publication. DOI: 10.1212/NXI.0000000000200139 PMID: 37385738

Wall, E. C., Chan, J. M., Gil, E., & Heyderman, R. S. (2021). Acute bacterial meningitis. *Current Opinion in Neurology, 35*(3), 386–395. DOI: 10.1097/WCO.0000000000000934 PMID: 33767093

Wang, J. L., Han, C., Yang, F. L., Wang, M. S., & He, Y. (n.d.). Normal cerebrospinal fluid protein and associated clinical characteristics in children with tuberculous meningitis. Annals of Medicine, 53(1), 885–889. https://www.ncbi.nlm.nih.gov/pmc/articles/PMC8205029/

Wang, F., Kream, R. M., & Stefano, G. B. (2020). Long-term respiratory and neurological sequelae of COVID-19. *Medical Science Monitor, 26*, e928996–e1. DOI: 10.12659/MSM.928996 PMID: 33177481

Warsinke, A., Benkert, A., & Scheller, F. W. (2000). Electrochemical immunoassays. *Fresenius' Journal of Analytical Chemistry, 366*(6-7), 622–634. DOI: 10.1007/s002160051559

Weaver, A. K., Head, J. R., Gould, C. F., Carlton, E. J., & Remais, J. V. (2022). Environmental factors influencing COVID-19 incidence and severity. *Annual Review of Public Health, 43*(1), 271–291. DOI: 10.1146/annurev-publhealth-052120-101420 PMID: 34982587

Wehrli, W., & Staehelin, M. (1971). Actions of the rifamycins. *Bacteriological Reviews, 35*(3), 290–309. DOI: 10.1128/br.35.3.290-309.1971 PMID: 5001420

Weight, C. M., Venturini, C., Pojar, S., Jochems, S. P., Reiné, J., Nikolaou, E., Solórzano, C., Noursadeghi, M., Brown, J. S., Ferreira, D. M., & Heyderman, R. S. (2019). Microinvasion by Streptococcus pneumoniae induces epithelial innate immunity during colonisation at the human mucosal surface. *Nature Communications, 10*(1), 3060. DOI: 10.1038/s41467-019-11005-2 PMID: 31311921

Wen, S., Feng, D., Chen, D., Yang, L., & Xu, Z. (2020). Molecular epidemiology and evolution of Haemophilus influenzae. *Infection, Genetics and Evolution, 80*, 104205. DOI: 10.1016/j.meegid.2020.104205 PMID: 31981610

Whitener, D. R. (1978). Tuberculous brain abscess: Report of a case and review of the literature. *Archives of Neurology, 35*(3), 148–155. DOI: 10.1001/archneur.1978.00500270030007

Wiesmann, M., Missler, U., & Gottmann, D. (1998). Plasma S-100b protein concentration in healthy adults is age- and sex-independent. *Clinical Chemistry, 44*(5), 1056–1058. DOI: 10.1093/clinchem/44.5.1056

Wiesmann, M., Missler, U., Hagenström, H., & Gottmann, D. (1997). Plasma S-100 protein levels after aneurysmal subarachnoid haemorrhage. *Acta Neurochirurgica, 139*(12), 1155–1160. DOI: 10.1007/BF01408577

Williams, S. L., & Chiller, T. (2022). Update on the Epidemiology, Diagnosis, and Treatment of Coccidioidomycosis. *Journal of Fungi (Basel, Switzerland), 8*(7), 666. DOI: 10.3390/jof8070666 PMID: 35887423

Wilson, M. R., Sample, H. A., Zorn, K. C., Arevalo, S., Yu, G., Neuhaus, J., Federman, S., Stryke, D., Briggs, B., Langelier, C., Berger, A., Douglas, V., Josephson, S. A., Chow, F. C., Fulton, B. D., DeRisi, J. L., Gelfand, J. M., Naccache, S. N., Bender, J., & Chiu, C. Y. (2019). Clinical metagenomic sequencing for diagnosis of meningitis and encephalitis. *The New England Journal of Medicine, 380*(24), 2327–2340. DOI: 10.1056/NEJMoa1803396 PMID: 31189036

Wirantara, H., Rusli, M., Arfijanto, M. V., & Bramantono, B. (2023). Cryptococcal Meningoencephalitis in HIV/AIDS Patient Coinfected with Tuberculosis. Case Report. *Gaceta Medica de Caracas, 131*(2). Advance online publication. DOI: 10.47307/GMC.2023.131.2.15

Wongchitrat, P., Shukla, M., Sharma, R., Govitrapong, P., & Reiter, R.J. (2021). Role of Melatonin on Virus-Induced Neuropathogenesis-A Concomitant Therapeutic Strategy to Understand SARS-CoV-2 Infection. *Antioxidants*. .DOI: 10.3390/antiox10010047

Wongchitrat, P., Chanmee, T., & Govitrapong, P. (2024). Molecular Mechanisms Associated with Neurodegeneration of Neurotropic Viral Infection. *Molecular Neurobiology, 61*(5), 2881–2903. DOI: 10.1007/s12035-023-03761-6 PMID: 37946006

Woodard, J. L., & Berman, D. M. (2006). Prevention of meningococcal disease. *Fetal and Pediatric Pathology, 25*(6), 311–319. DOI: 10.1080/15513810701209538 PMID: 17696042

Woolston, S. L., Dhanireddy, S., & Marrazzo, J. (2016). Ocular syphilis: A clinical review. *Current Infectious Disease Reports, 18*(11), 1–6. DOI: 10.1007/s11908-016-0542-9 PMID: 27686678

Workowski, K. A., Bolan, G. A., & Prevention, C. for D. C. and. (2015). *Sexually transmitted diseases treatment guidelines, 2015.*

Workowski, K. A. (2021). Sexually transmitted infections treatment guidelines, 2021. *MMWR. Recommendations and Reports*, 70. PMID: 34292926

World Health Organization. (2007). Global tuberculosis control: Surveillance, planning, financing (WHO/HTM/TB/2007.376). https://iris.who.int/bitstream/handle/10665/43629/9789241563141_eng.pdf?sequence=1

World Health Organization. (2011). Automated real-time nucleic acid amplification technology for rapid and simultaneous detection of tuberculosis and rifampicin resistance: Xpert MTB/RIF system (WHO/HTM/TB/2011.4).

World Health Organization. (2016). The use of molecular line probe assay for the detection of resistance to isoniazid and rifampicin: Policy update. Author. https://iris.who.int/handle/10665/250586

World Health Organization. (2021). *Consolidated guidelines on HIV prevention, testing, treatment, service delivery and monitoring: recommendations for a public health approach*. World Health Organization.

World Health Organization. (2022). *Line probe assays for detection of drug-resistant tuberculosis: Interpretation and reporting manual for laboratory staff and clinicians*. Author.

World Health Organization. (2022). *WHO consolidated guidelines on tuberculosis. Module 5: Management of tuberculosis in children and adolescents*. Author.

World Health Organization. (2024a). *Global Tuberculosis Report 2024*.

World Health Organization. (2024b). *WHO consolidated guidelines on tuberculosis: Module 3. Diagnosis—Rapid diagnostics for tuberculosis detection* (3rd ed.). Author.

World Health Organization. 2. (2020). *Guidance on COVID-19 for the care of older people and people living in long-term care facilities, other non-acute care facilities and home care* (No. WPR/DSE/2020/015). WHO Regional Office for the Western Pacific.

Wu, F., Hu, W., Xu, B., & Wang, Q. (2018). Effects of Treponema pallidum on the expression of chemokine ligand 6, 8, 10 in human brain microvascular endothelial cells. *Zhonghua Pifuke Zazhi*, 358–362.

Wu, K.-X., Wang, X.-T., Hu, X.-L., Jiang, X.-Y., Zhuang, J.-C., Xu, Y.-Z., Lin, L.-R., Tong, M.-L., Yang, T.-C., & Liu, L.-L. (2021). LncRNA-ENST00000421645 upregulates kank1 to inhibit IFN-γ expression and promote T cell apoptosis in neurosyphilis. *Frontiers in Microbiology*, *12*, 749171. DOI: 10.3389/fmicb.2021.749171 PMID: 34917045

Wunrow, H. Y., Bender, R. G., Vongpradith, A., Sirota, S. B., Swetschinski, L. R., Novotney, A., Gray, A. P., Ikuta, K. S., Sharara, F., Wool, E. E., Aali, A., Abd-Elsalam, S., Abdollahi, A., Abdul Aziz, J. M., Abidi, H., Aboagye, R. G., Abolhassani, H., Abu-Gharbieh, E., Adamu, L. H., & Kyu, H. H. (2023). Global, regional, and national burden of meningitis and its aetiologies, 1990–2019: A systematic analysis for the Global Burden of Disease Study 2019. *Lancet Neurology*, *22*(8), 685–711. DOI: 10.1016/S1474-4422(23)00195-3 PMID: 37479374

Wu, S. C., Cao, Z. S., Chang, K. M., & Juang, J. L. (2017). Intestinal microbial dysbiosis aggravates the progression of Alzheimer's disease in Drosophila. *Nature Communications*, *8*, 24. Advance online publication. DOI: 10.1038/s41467-017-00040-9

Wu, S., Ye, F., Wang, Y., & Li, D. (2024). Neurosyphilis: Insights into its pathogenesis, susceptibility, diagnosis, treatment, and prevention. *Frontiers in Neurology*, *14*, 1340321. DOI: 10.3389/fneur.2023.1340321 PMID: 38274871

Xiang, L., Zhang, T., Zhang, B., Zhang, C., Hou, S., & Yue, W. (2021). The associations of increased cerebral small vessel disease with cognitive impairment in neurosyphilis presenting with ischemic stroke. *Brain and Behavior*, *11*(6), e02187. DOI: 10.1002/brb3.2187 PMID: 33998172

Xu, W., Wong, G., Hwang, Y. Y., & Larbi, A. (2020, October). The untwining of immunosenescence and aging. *Seminars in Immunopathology*, *42*(5), 559–572. DOI: 10.1007/s00281-020-00824-x PMID: 33165716

Yadav, N., & Upadhyay, R. K. (2023). Global effect of climate change on seasonal cycles, vector population and rising challenges of communicable diseases: A review. *Journal of Atmospheric Science Research*, *6*(1), 21–59. DOI: 10.30564/jasr.v6i1.5165

Yamaguchi, R., Matsuo, K., Yamazaki, A., Abe, C., Nagai, S., & Terasaka, K. (1989). Cloning and characterization of the gene for immunogenic protein MPB64 of Mycobacterium bovis BCG. *Infection and Immunity*, *57*(1), 283–288. https://www.ncbi.nlm.nih.gov/pmc/articles/PMC313089/

Yi, M., Li, H., Wu, Z., Yan, J., Liu, Q., Ou, C., & Chen, M. (2018). A promising therapeutic target for metabolic diseases: Neuropeptide Y receptors in humans. *Cellular Physiology and Biochemistry*, *45*(1), 88–107. DOI: 10.1159/000486225 PMID: 29310113

Yimtae, K., Srirompotong, S., & Lertsukprasert, K. (2007). Otosyphilis: A review of 85 cases. *Otolaryngology - Head and Neck Surgery*, *136*(1), 67–71. DOI: 10.1016/j.otohns.2006.08.026 PMID: 17210336

Yushchenko, M., Weber, F., Mäder, M., Schöll, U., Maliszewska, M., Tumani, H., Felgenhauer, K., & Beuche, W. (2000). Matrix metalloproteinase-9 (MMP-9) in human cerebrospinal fluid (CSF): Elevated levels are primarily related to CSF cell count. *Journal of Neuroimmunology, 110*(1–2), 244–251. DOI: 10.1016/S0165-5728(00)00339-8 PMID: 11024556

ZainEldin, H., Gamel, S. A., El-Kenawy, E.-S. M., Alharbi, A. H., Khafaga, D. S., Ibrahim, A., & Talaat, F. M.ZainEldin. (2022). Brain tumor detection and classification using deep learning and sine-cosine fitness grey wolf optimization. *Bioengineering (Basel, Switzerland), 10*(1), 18. DOI: 10.3390/bioengineering10010018 PMID: 36671591

Zammarchi, L., Bonati, M., Strohmeyer, M., Albonico, M., Requena-Méndez, A., Bisoffi, Z., Nicoletti, A., García, H. H., & Bartoloni, A. (2017). Screening, diagnosis and management of human cysticercosis and*Taenia solium*taeniasis: Technical recommendations by the COHEMI project study group. *Tropical Medicine & International Health, 22*(7), 881–894. DOI: 10.1111/tmi.12887 PMID: 28449318

Zender, H. O., Olivier, P., & Genné, D. (2009). Méningites bactériennes communautaires aiguës chez l'adulte. *Revue Medicale Suisse, 5*(220), 1968–1974. DOI: 10.53738/REVMED.2009.5.220.1968 PMID: 19908635

Zhang, X. M., Huang, J., Ni, X. Y., Zhu, H. R., Huang, Z. X., Ding, S., Yang, X. Y., Tan, Y. Di, Chen, J. F., & Cai, J. H. (2024). Current progression in application of extracellular vesicles in central nervous system diseases. *European Journal of Medical Research, 29*(1), 1–14. DOI: 10.1186/s40001-023-01606-5

Zhang, A., Sun, H., Wang, P., Han, Y., & Wang, X. (2012). Recent and potential developments of biofluid analyses in metabolomics. *Journal of Proteomics, 75*(4), 1079–1088. DOI: 10.1016/j.jprot.2011.10.027

Zhang, C., Qiu, M., & Fu, H. (2024). Oligodendrocytes in central nervous system diseases: The effect of cytokine regulation. *Neural Regeneration Research, 19*(10), 2132–2143. DOI: 10.4103/1673-5374.392854 PMID: 38488548

Zhang, R.-L., Zhang, J.-P., & Wang, Q.-Q. (2014). Recombinant Treponema pallidum protein Tp0965 activates endothelial cells and increases the permeability of endothelial cell monolayer. *PLoS One, 9*(12), e115134. DOI: 10.1371/journal.pone.0115134 PMID: 25514584

Zhou, J., Zhang, H., Tang, K., Liu, R., & Li, J. (2022). An Updated Review of Recent Advances in Neurosyphilis. *Frontiers in Medicine, 9*(September), 1–10. DOI: 10.3389/fmed.2022.800383 PMID: 36203756

Zhou, X.-J., Yang, Q., Tan, Q.-H., Zhang, L.-Y., Shi, L.-B., & Zou, J.-X. (2021). Paragonimus and its hosts in China: An update. *Acta Tropica*, *223*, 106094–106094. DOI: 10.1016/j.actatropica.2021.106094 PMID: 34389330

Zhu, L., Gu, X., Peng, R.-R., Wang, C., Gao, Z., Zhou, P., Gao, Y., Shi, M., Guan, Z., & Seña, A. C. (2014). Comparison of the cerebrospinal fluid (CSF) toluidine red unheated serum test and the CSF rapid plasma reagin test with the CSF venereal disease research laboratory test for diagnosis of neurosyphilis among HIV-negative syphilis patients in China. *Journal of Clinical Microbiology*, *52*(3), 736–740. DOI: 10.1128/JCM.02522-13 PMID: 24335955

Zinserling, V. (2022). *Infectious Lesions of the Central Nervous System*. Springer Nature. DOI: 10.1007/978-3-030-96260-9

About the Contributors

Tabish Qidwai is working as Professor and Director of Institute of Biosciences and Technology, SRM University, India. He has done M.Tech and PhD in Biotechnology Engineering from Dr APJ Kalam Technical University, Lucknow. He has worked as a faculty member at BB Ambedkar Central University, Lucknow and Raja Balwant Singh College, Agra. He received various prestigious awards including the Rashtriya Gaurav Award for remarkable contributions to Science and Technology, Certificate of Excellence in Science and Technology, University Gold Medal, Research Excellence Award, Teaching and Learning Innovation Award and several certificate of appreciation for significant contribution to academics. He has 13 years of teaching and research experience in genomics and immunology and infectious diseases. He has published nearly 60 book chapters, research articles, review articles in peer-reviewed international journals and authored/edited 5 books as a single author/editor. He has I10 index 25 and h index 20 and more than 1000 citations. Currently, He is supervising 5 PhD students and 3 PhDs are awarded under his supervision. He is a member of many national and international scientific societies and organizations. His research interests are focused on the functional genomics, immunology, and infectious disease research including malaria and COVID-19.

* * *

Senthil Kumar A. V. is working as a Professor and Principal, Nehru Institute of Information Technology and Management, Coimbatore, India. He has worked as Professor and Director, PG and Research Department of Computer Applications, Hindusthan College of Arts & Science, Coimbatore, Tamilnadu for 15 years and as Senior Grade Lecturer in CMS College of Science and Commerce for 14 years. To his credit he has industrial experience for five years and teaching experience of 29 years. He has also received his Doctor of Science (D.Sc in Computer Science).

He has to his credit 86 Book Chapters, 234 papers in International and National Journals, 85 papers in International Conferences in International and National Conferences, and edited 17 books and 3 Text books. He is as Associate Editor of IEEE Access. He is an Editor-in-Chief for many journals and Key Member for India, Machine Intelligence Research Lab (MIR Labs). He is an Editorial Board Member and Reviewer for various International Journals. He is also a Committee member for various International Conferences. He has guided 16 Ph.D scholars and guiding 3 Ph. D scholars now.

Abraham Olufemi Asuku is a neurophysiologist with special interest in neurotoxicity, neurodegenerative diseases, neurodevelopmental disorders and neuroinformatics. He has published in many high impact factors journals and also contributed to many book chapters. He is a member of Neuroscience Society of Nigeria and the Physiological Society, UK. Dr Asuku is an editor of the book titled "Non-pharmacological interventions for dementia" published by CRC Press Taylor and Francis.

Hanane El Fatimi is a PhD student in neuroscience, Laboratory of Neuroscience and Cellular Physiology, Mohammed VI University of Health Sciences, Morocco.

Bilal El-Mansoury, PhD, is a Professor in the Department of Biology at the Faculty of Sciences, Chouaib Doukkali University. He previously served as a Postdoctoral Researcher in Neuroscience at the Royal College of Surgeons in Ireland (RCSI), University of Medicine and Health Sciences. His research focuses on elucidating the role of glial cells dysfunction in the pathophysiology of hepatic encephalopathy and a range of neurodegenerative disorders. Dr. El-Mansoury has also investigated the regulatory role of microRNAs (miRNAs) in CDKL5 deficiency disorder, aiming to identify novel therapeutic targets for this rare and severe epileptic encephalopathy. In addition to his research activities, he is the editor of some scholarly books, including "Physiology and Function of Glial Cells in Health and Disease".

Grace Ayobami Fajemidagba is a certified physiologist and biomedical researcher with utmost interest in neuroscience. She currently works as a lecturer in the Department of Human Physiology, Redeemers University, Ede, Osun State, Nigeria. Her research interests are in brain and mental health, neuroinflammatory diseases, cognition, phytomedicine and drug discovery.

Jagadamba G. is working as Asst. Professor in the Department of Information Science and Engineering, Siddaganga Institute of Technology, Tumakuru, Karnataka. She obtained her BE, M.Tech, and Ph.D. degree from VTU, Belagavi.

She is having 22 years of teaching and 17 years of research experience. Her research interests include analysis of diseases through electronic health records/images, security issues in the ubiquitous computing environment, adaptive and biometric authentication systems, trust and context-based security systems, and applications for e-commerce, e-learning, m-banking, and healthcare. She has published many book chapters in CRC press and IGI publications. She has also authored many research articles in reputed international journals, and national/international conferences. Apart from teaching, she has completed many industry projects and conducted many certification courses. She also delivered many seminars, webinars, and faculty development workshops. She has secured the "Best Project Award" in national level competition, "Best Paper Award" in conferences, "Best teacher Award 2021" from the Institute of Scholars, "Best Scholar Award 2022" from the International Research Awards on Science, Health and Engineering, 2021, and "Instructor of the Year 2021 " from CISCO, Bangalore. Apart from academic activities, she has been very keen on serving society and the environment. With a group of like-minded friends, she has planted more than 5000 seedlings in dry lands around Tumakuru by keeping a motto of going green.

Vanishree G. has rich experience, 28 years in Academics & administration. Having worked as HOD, Principal, and vice principal in Vignan Institutions, Institute of Aeronautical Engineering, Badruka, St. Patricks, St. Joseph College, Kristu Jayanti College, etc. She also worked as Director for Kempe Gowda institute of management studies and research Bangalore. Presently she is working as a professor at IBS-B Bangalore. Prof has been a credit participator in several National seminars & conferences and published journal articles. She has won the best teacher, parent, and Adarsh yuvathi awards. She makes herself suited to the position placed. She is responsible and inspiring, good attitude and believes in ethical norms. Having a good record of good results, she believes in statement, "Learning is a continuous process."

Vaishali Mishra is a senior product manager specializing in data and AI and has expertise in data quality, data governance, analytics, and artificial intelligence (AI). She has significant experience in the travel tech, healthcare, and biomedical industries and has worked on several high-impact projects.

Ayyoub Skaou holds a PhD in Biology (2025) from Cadi Ayyad University, a Master's degree in Physiopathology (2020), and a Bachelor's degree in Cellular and Molecular Biology (2018). He is trained in the biological sciences, with a broad background in the study of living systems.

Index

A

B

C

D

www.ingramcontent.com/pod-product-compliance
Lightning Source LLC
LaVergne TN
LVHW082346011026
849160LV00024B/1183